M.D. ANDERSON SOLID TUMOR ONCOLOGY SERIES

Series Editor
Raphael E. Pollock, M.D., Ph.D.

Springer Science+Business Media, LLC

FORTHCOMING IN THE
M.D. ANDERSON SOLID TUMOR ONCOLOGY SERIES

Breast Cancer
Edited by S. Eva Singletary, M.D.

Melanoma
Edited by Jeffrey E. Lee, M.D.

Gastric Cancer
Edited by Paul F. Mansfield, M.D.

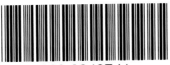

369 0246741

This book is due for return on or before the last date shown below.

Steven A. Curley, M.D.
Department of Surgical Oncology
Division of Surgery
The University of Texas M.D. Anderson Cancer Center
Editor

Liver Cancer

With 58 Illustrations

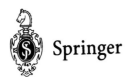

Springer

Steven A. Curley, M.D.
Professor of Surgery
Chief, Gastrointestinal Tumor Surgery, Department of Surgical Oncology
Division of Surgery
The University of Texas M.D. Anderson Cancer Center
1515 Holcombe Boulevard
Houston, TX, 77030, USA

Series Editor
Raphael E. Pollock, M.D., PH.D.
Head, Division of Surgery
Professor and Chairman, Department of Surgical Oncology
The University of Texas M.D. Anderson Cancer Center
1515 Holcombe Boulevard
Houston, TX 77030, USA

Library of Congress Cataloging-in-Publication Data
Curley, Steven A.
    Liver cancer/Steven A. Curley.
        p. cm. — (M.D. Anderson solid tumor oncology series)
        Includes bibliographical references and index.
    ISBN 978-1-4612-7236-6   ISBN 978-1-4612-1666-7 (eBook)
    DOI 10.1007/978-1-4612-1666-7
    1. Liver—Cancer.   I. Title.   II. Series.
    [DNLM: 1. Liver Neoplasms—diagnosis. 2. Liver Neoplasms-
    -therapy. WI 735   C975L 1998]
    RC280.L5C86 1998
    616.99´436—dc21   97-41042

Printed on acid-free paper.

Production managed by Timothy Taylor; manufacturing supervised by Jeffrey Taub.
Typeset by KP Company, Brooklyn, NY.

9 8 7 6 5 3 2 1

This book is dedicated to Beverlee, Niel, and Emily, who remind me daily of the wonders in life; and to the patients we serve.

"Not everything that is faced can be changed, but nothing can be changed until it is faced."

JAMES BALDWIN

"The Greeks bequeathed us one of the most beautiful words in our language, the word enthusiam—en theos—the god within. The grandeur of human actions is measured by the inspiration from which they spring. Happy is the person who bears a god within, and who obeys it. The ideas of art, of science, are lighted by reflection from the infinite."

PAUL TILLICH

Series Preface

The field of solid tumor oncology is changing at an astonishing rate. To learn about new developments, generate fresh research perspectives, and then integrate these advancements into clinical practice is a daunting challenge confronting all who work in the oncology arena. The onset and rapid deployment of internet capacities worldwide has created a mileau of global and instantaneous information access. The task of staying current is becoming even more challenging, and in some ways, more difficult to accomplish.

Against this information pressure backdrop, how can yet more didactic material for the already overburdened oncology physician be justified? Based on the premise that we all must remain in a learning mode if we are to remain relevant, The University of Texas M.D. Anderson Annual of Solid Tumor Oncology is designed to focus on a single disease site in each volume. It is our belief that there is an information "gray zone" that lies between the peer reviewed (and increasingly electronically available) individual research report and the large comprehensive multiauthored textbook. Between these two loci there exists an information gap that will be best served by a succinct disease site-focused volume that provides an indepth analysis of current multimodality care for a specific solid tumor system, as well as the areas of basic, translational, and clinical research that will emerge for future clinical application. Each volume in this series is authored by an academic surgical oncologist of national repute in practice at the Department of Surgical Oncology at the University of Texas M.D. Anderson Cancer Center. Under the leadership of these individuals, outstanding experts throughout the world have been tapped to contribute to this effort.

The target audience is physicians who are focusing on solid tumor oncology. However, it is our hope that medical students and physicians-in-training who aspire to a career in solid tumor oncology will also find these volumes to be of value. In this new era, we are now beginning to understand the molecular determinants driving solid tumor carcinogenesis, proliferation, and dissemination. These molecularly-based insights are moving rapidly into the clinical armamentarium. This poses a tremendous challenge to those of us who are not yet fully conversant, yet these developments also give confidence that we are about to enter what will certainly be the most exciting era yet in solid tumor oncology. The tumors afflicting our patients compel us to be our best, as does our own dedication to fighting this disease cluster that will surpass cardiovascular illness as a cause of mortality worldwide early in the next millennium. On behalf of my faculty colleague authors at the University of Texas M.D. Anderson Cancer Center and our many contributing experts, I would like to thank you for your willingness to participate with us in this exciting new project.

RAPHAEL E. POLLOCK
Houston, Texas

Contents

Contributors

CHUSLIP CHARNSANGAVEJ, M.D.
Professor of Radiology
Department of Diagnostic Radiology
The University of Texas M.D. Anderson Cancer Center
1515 Holcombe Blvd.
Houston, TX 77030, USA

JUDY CHASE, PHARM. D.
Department of Pharmacy
The University of Texas M.D. Anderson Cancer Center
1515 Holcombe Blvd.
Houston, TX 77030, USA

CHUL HO CHO M.D., PH.D.
Department of Cell Biology
The University of Texas M.D. Anderson Cancer Center
1515 Holcombe Blvd.
Houston, TX 77030, USA

STEVEN A. CURLEY, M.D.
Professor of Surgery
Chief, Gastrointestinal Tumor Surgery
Department of Surgical Oncology
The University of Texas M.D. Anderson Cancer Center
Houston, TX 77030, USA

LEE M. ELLIS, M.D.
Assistant Professor of Surgery
Departments of Surgical Oncology and and Cell Biology
The University of Texas M.D. Anderson Cancer Center
1515 Holcombe Blvd.
Houston, TX 77030, USA

FRANCESCO FIORE, M.D.
Associate Professor of Radiology
National Cancer Institute of Naples
Via M. Semmola 1
80131 Naples, Italy

DANIEL J. GAGNÉ, M.D.
Division of Surgical Oncology
Department of Surgery
Allegheny General Hospital
320 East North Avenue
Pittsburgh, PA 15212, USA

REVATHY IYER, M.D.
Assistant Professor of Radiology
Department of Diagnostic Radiology
The University of Texas M.D. Anderson Cancer Center
1515 Holcombe Blvd.
Houston, TX 77030, USA

FRANCESCO IZZO, M.D.
Associate Professor of Surgery
Department of Surgical Oncology "C"
National Cancer Institute of Naples
Via M. Semmola 1
80131 Naples, Italy

DENNIE V. JONES, Jr., M.D.
Clinical Scientist
Genentech, Inc.
Section of BioOncology
Department of Medical Affairs
One DNA Way
S. San Francisco, CA 94080-4990, USA

KELLY M. MCMASTERS, M.D., PH.D.
Assistant Professor of Surgical Oncology
Department of Surgery
James Graham Brown Cancer Center
University of Louisville
529 S. Jackson St.
Louisville, KY 40292, USA

YEHUDA Z. PATT, M.D.
Associate Professor of Medicine
Department of Gastrointestinal Medical Oncology and Digestive Diseases
The University of Texas M.D. Anderson Cancer Center
1515 Holcombe Blvd.
Houston, TX 77030, USA

ROBERT RADINSKY, PH.D.
Assistant Professor
Department of Cell Biology
The University of Texas M.D. Anderson Cancer Center
1515 Holcombe Blvd.
Houston, TX 77030, USA

TYVIN RICH, M.D.
Chairman and Professor, Department of Radiation Therapy
University of Virginia Health Sciences Center
Hospital Drive, Box 383
Charlottesville, VA 22908, USA

MARK S. ROH, M.D.
Director, Division of Surgical Oncology
Allegheny General Hospital
320 East North Avenue
Pittsburgh, PA 15212, USA

CHARLES R. SHUMATE, M.D.
Clinical Associate Professor of Surgery
Surgical Oncology and General Surgery
2018 Brookwood Medical Center Drive
Suite G2
Birmingham, AL 77030, USA

TODD M. TUTTLE, M.D.
Department of Surgery
Park Nicollet Clinic
3900 Park Nicollet Blvd.
Minneapolis, MN 55416, USA

CARLO deWERRA, M.D.
Associate Professor of Surgery
University of Naples
Via Panzini 5
80131 Naples, Italy

1

Imaging Studies for Hepatobiliary Tumors

REVATHY IYER AND CHUSILP CHARNSANGAVEJ

Surgical techniques with curative intent are becoming more common-place for both primary and metastatic tumors of the liver. The development of aggressive surgical techniques has allowed the surgeon to view a patient with a primary hepatic tumor or certain types of metastatic disease as a possible candidate for curative resection rather than as a patient with end stage disease. It is therefore important to detect and characterize hepatic lesions to determine if a patient is a surgical candidate and, if so, to plan operative strategies. It is the goal of hepatic imaging to identify and stage lesions for hepatic surgeons. The issues imaging must address include (1) whether hepatic lesions are present and, if so, how many; (2) the character of any such lesions; and (3) whether malignant tumors are resectable.[1,2] These queries are now being answered more easily with advances in imaging.

Hepatic imaging has improved significantly as a result of advances in the technology of such modalities as nuclear medicine, ultrasonography (US), and computed tomography (CT) as well as the advent of new cross-sectional imaging modalities such as magnetic resonance imaging (MRI). Single photon emission computed tomography (SPECT) has improved the resolution of nuclear scans, and Doppler ultrasonography has proved useful for assessing hepatic lesions. Helical CT scanners allow rapid imaging of the liver during various phases of contrast enhancement. MRI uses no ionizing radiation, allows multiplanar imaging, and provides excellent contrast between tissues. This chapter discusses each of the above-mentioned modalities and then turns to a discussion of the imaging appearances of common liver tumors.

Nuclear Medicine

Radionuclide scanning has been unique in its ability to provide physiologic information to define disease processes more clearly. Liver spleen scans using technetium-99m (^{99m}Tc)–sulfur colloid were at one time widely used to evaluate liver masses. Advances in US, CT, and MRI have now superseded liver spleen scans for the detection of liver lesions. Nuclear medicine scans are generally used for lesion characterization rather than detection. The scan most widely utilized in this capacity is the red blood cell (RBC)-labeled blood pool scan, which employs the radionuclide ^{99m}Tc for characterizing hemangiomas. Scans employing ^{99m}Tc-sulfur colloid or iminodiacetic acid derivatives are used to characterize focal nodular hyperplasia. Furthermore, scintigraphic techniques employing gallium-67 (^{67}Ga) citrate are used to characterize primary hepatocellular neoplasms such as adenomas and hepatomas.[3]

Hepatic arterial perfusion scintigraphy (HAPS) is a technique that localizes the distribution of chemotherapeutic agents via surgically implanted hepatic artery catheters. This technique is now being used to detect early metastatic disease. Both planar and SPECT images are obtained after injecting ^{99m}Tc-macroaggregated albumin into the common hepatic artery just distal to the origin of the gastroduodenal artery. Most primary and metastatic liver malignancies derive their blood supply from the hepatic artery, so these lesions appear as areas of increased radiotracer uptake. It should be noted that this technique is invasive, requiring catheterization of the hepatic artery.[3]

Ultrasonography

Ultrasonography is widely available in most practice settings and is often used to evaluate the liver initially. Sonographers scan the liver using a combination of subcostal and intercostal approaches with transducers that vary between 3 and 5 megahertz (MHz) depending on patient body habitus. US is well suited to imaging because it is relatively inexpensive, produces no ionizing radiation, is noninvasive, and is both fast and portable. Advances in US include the advent of real-time scanning, which produces fewer artifacts than static scanning. Furthermore, duplex or color flow Doppler US for definition of vascular structures is now available on most units.

Although US has all of the aforementioned advantages, routine transabdominal sonographic evaluation of the liver for purposes of presurgical staging of liver tumors is of limited value. The sensitivity and specificity are low, with an overall false negative rate estimated at more than 50%.[1] Lesions at the dome of the liver adjacent to the lung base may be difficult to image. Patient body habitus comes into play in that large patients with more subcutaneous fat are more difficult to image. Fatty infiltration of the liver, which is a relatively common condition in oncology patients, does not allow adequate imaging of the liver owing to poor sound beam transmission. Furthermore, the examination is operator-dependent, and results may be difficult to reproduce for purposes of comparison. Determining whether a lesion is of benign or malignant etiology is rarely possible.

Intraoperative US, on the other hand, is often considered the gold standard for lesion detection.[4] Using transducers on the order of 5–8 MHz it has the ability to image, with excellent resolution, subcentimeter nodules that may not even be palpable surgically. Intraoperative US is not used as a screening tool because it is highly invasive, and by definition it is not a preoperative screening procedure. The skill of the sonographer also comes into play as does cooperation between the surgeon and the sonographer.

Contrast agents for US are under study to determine their clinical utility. These agents, composed of stabilized microbubbles, are injected intravenously and pass safely through the microcirculation of the lungs and enter the systemic arterial system. These microbubbles, of which only small volumes are injected, undergo resonant oscillation which produces enhancement of Doppler US signals. Increased Doppler signals may therefore be detected around hepatic tumors that incite neovascularity.[5]

Computed Tomography

The latest generation of CT scanner is the spiral, or helical, scanner. These scanners are similar to conventional CT scanners in that they acquire images using x-rays, but they are unique in their ability to obtain a volume of data in which the data set corresponds to a series of projections arranged as a helix. Such a helical data set is obtained by moving the table on which the patient lies at constant speed while the x-ray tube continuously rotates, providing a sustained exposure. This process of helical data acquisition is made possible by improvements in the gantry system, which allow continuous rotation, improved detector efficiency, and greater tube cooling capabilities.[6]

The primary advantage of helical CT scanners over conventional CT scanners is the increased speed with which data may be acquired. Scans of the liver may be obtained in less than 45 seconds with helical CT, compared to 90–120 seconds with a conventional CT scanner. Rapid data acquisition allows repetitive scanning of the abdomen, which in turn provides images of the liver during the various phases of contrast enhancement. It should be noted that helical CT scanners still rely on the use of intravenous iodinated contrast agents to detect and characterize hepatic lesions. The ability of CT to detect abnormalities in the liver relies largely on the difference between the density of the normal parenchyma and that of the lesion. To improve lesion conspicuity, intravenous contrast enhancement is used to increase the density difference between the normal parenchyma and the lesion.

Following delivery of a bolus of contrast material, three phases of enhancement in the liver have been observed: an early vascular or arterial phase, a portal venous phase, and a delayed phase. During the early arterial phase only the hepatic artery and aorta enhance, and the hepatic parenchyma remains minimally enhanced. As contrast material passes through the splanchnic circulation and returns to the liver via the portal vein, there is a rapid increase in the density of the hepatic parenchyma, which receives its blood supply largely from the portal venous system with minimal contribution from the hepatic artery. Subsequently, there is gradual washout of contrast during the delayed phase. The arterial and portal venous phases of contrast enhancement occur 20 seconds to 2 minutes after the start of the injection, depending on the rate of injection. The ability to obtain images during the early arterial phase is important because such early images aid in the detection of hypervascular lesions, such as hepatocellular carcinoma, focal nodular hyperplasia, or metastatic neuroendocrine tumors, which may become isodense to the normal surrounding liver tissue and thus invisible on delayed scans (Fig. 1.1).[7] The portal dominant phase is important to detect hypovascular tumors, such as metastatic adenocarcinoma or cholangiocarcinoma, because during this phase the difference in tissue density between the hepatic parenchyma and the tumor is maximum, thereby, allowing the lesion to be seen better.

Another advantage of helical CT is its ability to display images in three-dimensional and multiplanar formats. The volume acquisition of data accomplished with helical CT allows data processing to display images in three-dimensional and multiplanar formats. Multiplanar reformatting is also possible with conventional CT, but misregistration artifacts degrade the quality of the images.

Computed tomography during arterial portography (CTAP) is an even more sensitive means of hepatic imaging by CT. This invasive procedure requires catheterization of the superior mesenteric artery, usually via a femoral arterial approach, and intraarterial injection of iodinated contrast immediately before CT scanning. High concentrations of iodine are thus delivered to the liver via the portal venous system, resulting in intense enhancement of the normal liver, which receives both portal venous blood supply and some hepatic arterial supply. Tumors, which have primarily hepatic arterial supply, are seen as filling defects in the intensely staining background of normal liver.[1, 8-10] CTAP showed more than twice as many metastatic deposits in the liver as conventional CT in two separate studies.[9,10] Although extremely sensitive, CTAP has less than perfect specificity. Perfusion defects produce high false positive rates.[1,11,12] Furthermore, small benign lesions such as cysts may be indistinguishable from malignancy. CTAP is useful for delineating vascular anatomy. Such delineation of anatomy is of importance to the surgeon preoperatively.

Magnetic Resonance Imaging

Magnetic resonance imaging is the latest in our array of imaging tools. The major advantage of MRI over other imaging modalities is its ability to display inherent tissue contrast. MRI relies on the differing hydrogen content and T1 and T2 relaxation times of various tissues to provide contrast between these tissues. The hydrogen content of most soft tissue varies by about 20%, and the variation of T1 and T2 relaxation times is considerably greater.[13] Different imaging problems require different imaging techniques. Radiolo-

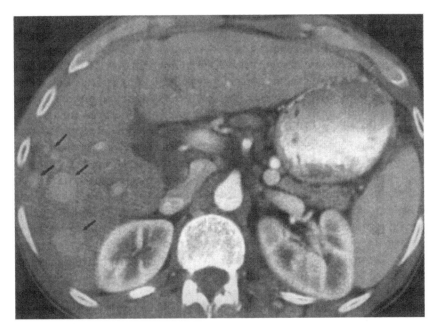

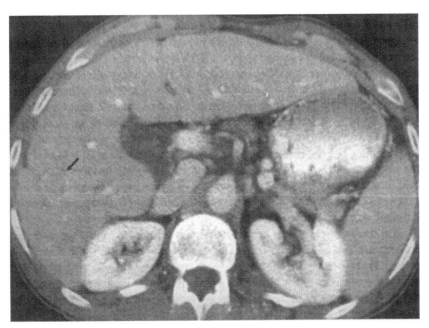

FIGURE 1.1. Multifocal hepatocellular carcinoma. (A) CT image during early vascular or arterial phase shows multiple enhancing nodules within the right lobe of the liver (arrows). (B) CT image obtained at the same axial level 45 seconds later shows only one barely perceptible nodule (arrow).

gists select imaging techniques to combine these three components variably and thereby alter image contrast to answer a specific clinical question.

Magnetic resonance imaging has a distinct advantage over CT in that it does not rely on the use of contrast agents for detecting lesions. Patients with iodine allergy or renal insufficiency are therefore not excluded and may be imaged without complications related to the administration of iodinated contrast. Although MRI does not rely on contrast agents for detection of disease, MR contrast agents may be used to gain additional information about the character of any lesions that may be present. For example, the use of a contrast agent is important for specific characterization of lesions such as hemangiomas.[14–17] Gadolinium, a rare earth metal that is injected intravenously as an ionic or nonionic chelate, remains the agent most widely used for this purpose. Other MR contrast agents, such as manganese and super paramagnetic iron oxide particles, are being studied to determine their clinical value. These agents are used to increase specificity of lesions. For example, manganese (II) N,N'-dipyridoxylethylenediamine-N,NPPP-di acetate-5,5'-bis(phosphate) (MnDPDP), a manganese chelate of a vitamin B_6 derivative, is taken up and metabolized by hepatocytes but not by metastatic lesions. As a result, tumors of hepatocellular origin enhance whereas metastatic lesions do not.[18] In the case of super paramagnetic iron oxide, the normal reticuloendothelial (RE) cells of the liver phagocytize the iron oxide particles, which results in a sharp contrast between normal liver with Kupffer cells and liver tumors that have no RE function.[19,20]

Apart from its ability to display inherent tissue contrast and to detect lesions without using contrast agents, MRI has two other distinct advantages. First, it permits direct multiplanar imaging. By allowing direct coronal and sagittal imaging, it improves localization of lesions, thereby further facilitating surgical planning for resectable disease. Second, the MR image quality is less likely to be affected by the presence of objects such as surgical clips. Surgical clips in patients who have undergone prior biliary or hepatic surgery may produce streak artifacts on CT scans, which limit the ability to evaluate the surrounding liver. Although ferrogmagnetic surgical clips may also affect MR image quality by producing signal voids, the nickel content of many surgical clips is sufficiently high to render them nonferromagnetic, thereby eliminating the problem of image quality when using MRI.[13]

Despite its many advantages, MRI is not without its drawbacks. Some patients are excluded from MR imaging, such as those with pacemakers or certain types of metallic implants which are in danger of being deflected within the confines of the strong magnetic fields. Claustrophobia is a potential problem in many individuals, although the anxiety patients feel may be alleviated by anxiolytics. Some, however, require general anesthesia before imaging is accomplished. Although improved scan techniques have shortened MR examinations, the scan times remain relatively long especially compared to helical CT. Motion artifacts are a greater problem for MRI than CT because of these longer scan times.

Overall, MRI is more sensitive for hepatic lesion detection than other noninvasive modalities, including intravenous enhanced CT.[9,10] CTAP does display more sensitivity than MRI for detecting focal lesions, but the inherent drawbacks of this technique are its invasive nature and lack of specificity. For most patients who require imaging evaluation of the liver for contemplated resection, correlative imaging is performed. A combination of MRI and CTAP is advocated as a means of detecting the largest number of lesions and characterizing these lesions preoperatively.[10] Detection of extrahepatic disease such as adenopathy or extrahepatic extension is also important when determining if a patient is a surgical candidate; and, again, correlative imaging is valuable preoperativley.

Focal Liver Lesions

Cysts

Hepatic cysts are commonly encountered during abdominal imaging. They may be congenital, postinflammatory, posttraumatic, or parasitic in origin. It is estimated that the overall incidence of benign congenital hepatic cysts is approximately 2.5%.[21,22] US is the most efficient and reliable means for defining simple hepatic cysts. These benign lesions are typically anechoic with smooth margins and no perceptible wall. The fluid content of cysts show a relative lack of absorption and reflection of sound compared to normal hepatic parenchyma, resulting in distal acoustic enhancement.[21] US may demonstrate thin septations. When this typical sonographic appearance is not present, the differential considerations include an abscess, hematoma, necrotic metastasis, or echinococcal cyst.[23] Small subcentimeter lesions and lesions near the dome of the liver may be difficult to visualize and thus to characterize adequately using US.

The CT and MRI appearances of hepatic cysts are characteristic. In the case of CT, the definitive diagnosis is based on finding a nonenhancing lesion with fluid density and a thin wall. In cysts measuring less than 1 cm, the CT attenuation values obtained may not be accurate because of partial volume effects.[24] The MRI appearance of a hepatic cyst is that of a well circumscribed lesion that is markedly hypointense on T1-weighted images and markedly hyperintense on T2-weighted images because of the fluid content.[25,26] The differential considerations may include hemangiomas or necrotic metastases. Gadolinium administration improves specificity because cysts do not enhance, whereas hemangiomas and metastases do.

The subcentimeter cyst remains a diagnostic dilemma in many cases. Because of the improved resolution of CT, CTAP, and MRI, radiologists now more frequently detect such lesions. However, because of their small size these lesions remain difficult to characterize by any modality. The only solution currently available is follow-up imaging. These lesions should be followed on subsequent scans to determine stability and thereby exclude malignant disease.[1]

Cavernous Hemangioma

Cavernous hemangioma, the most common benign liver tumor, is found in 0.4–20.0% of the population with a 5:1 female to male predominance. Although they are usually solitary, 10–30% of patients have multiple lesions.[21,27,28]

On US, the typical cavernous hemangioma is a well circumscribed, homogeneous, hyperechoic mass. This typical appearance is found in 70–80% of lesions. Distal acoustic enhancement appears in some cases but is not specific. A hypoechoic central area may be seen that represents fibrosis or necrosis.[21,27,28] Atypical sonographic appearances of hemangioma are not uncommon, constituting about 15–20% of all lesions. Such lesions may be hypoechoic or isoechoic to surrounding liver especially in patients with fatty infiltration of the liver because the hepatic substrate demonstrates increased echogenicity owing to the increased lipid content.[21,29] The sonographic appearance of a typical hyperechoic lesion is not entirely specific and metastatic disease should be included in the differential diagnosis. Correlative imaging is necessary for further evaluation.

On noncontrast CT scans cavernous hemangiomas appear as low attenuation well circumscribed masses, an appearance that is not helpful for characterization. The most useful sign on CT is the enhancement pattern demonstrated on dynamic contrast-enhanced CT.[30] Hemangiomas characteristically demonstrate intense, nodular, mural enhancement with a gradual increase in the size of the enhancing nodules, which eventually coalesce and completely fill the lesion during the delayed equilibrium phase (Fig. 1.2). This nodular or globular enhancement pattern has a reported sensitivity of 88% and a specificity of 84–100%, particularly when the enhancement is similar to that of the aorta.[31] Nevertheless, small lesions measuring less than 1 cm may show homogeneous hyperdense enhancement during the dynamic phase, making it difficult to distinguish them from hypervascular metastases.[32] Thrombosis within hemangiomas also confounds this typical nodular or globular enhancement pattern.

Magnetic resonance imaging displays greater sensitivity and specificity than contrast-enhanced CT when differentiating hemangiomas from other

---

FIGURE 1.2. Cavernous hemangioma. (A) CT image during early vascular phase shows a hypodense mass in the left lobe of the liver with several globular or nodular foci of enhancement (arrows). (B) CT image obtained at the same axial level several minutes later shows complete filling in of the lesion. (C) Axial T2-weighted MR image of the same patient shows a hyperintense lesion (arrow). (D) Axial SPECT image of the same patient after administration of technetium 99-radiolabeled red blood cells shows the lesion (arrow). Uptake is also seen within the normal spleen (arrowhead).

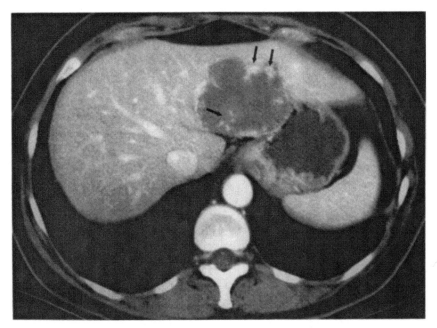

FIGURE 1.2-A.

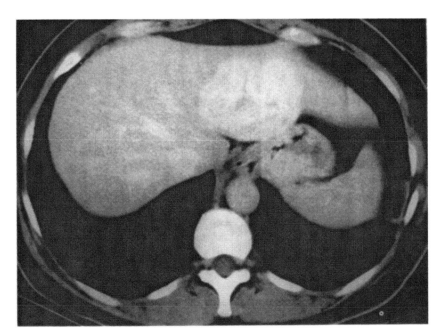

FIGURE 1.2-B.

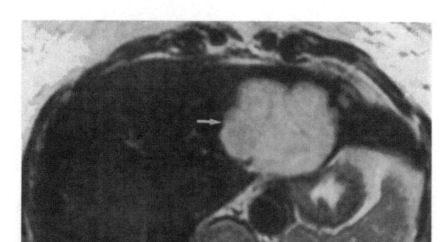

FIGURE 1.2-C.

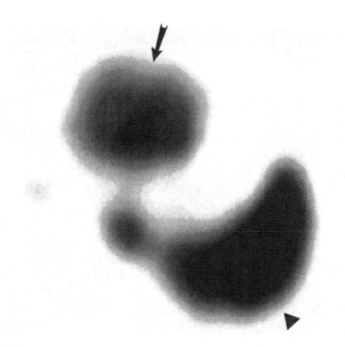

FIGURE 1.2-D.

lesions, having an accuracy reported at about 90%.[33-35] MRI relies on morphologic features, signal characteristics, and enhancement patterns. On T1-weighted scans hemangiomas are hypointense to surrounding liver and appear similar to other liver tumors. T2-weighted images increase the specificity and sensitivity of MRI. Hemangiomas are characteristically hyperintense on T2-weighted images, and this hyperintensity increases as scans are more heavily T2-weighted.[36] This hyperintense signal is likely a result of the slowly flowing or stagnant blood in the cavernous spaces. Hemangiomas are most commonly homogeneous in T2 signal intensity. Most malignant lesions, on the other hand, show an inhomogeneous appearance on T2-weighted images.[37] Some overlap in appearance still exists, however, because thrombosis, fibrosis, or hemorrhage within a hemangioma may cause an atypical appearance.[38] The contrast agent gadolinium proves useful for further improving specificity. After intravenous administration of gadolinium dynamic MRI displays a nodular enhancement pattern similar to that seen on contrast-enhanced CT. Delayed scans obtained several minutes after contrast administration show complete filling in of the lesion, which becomes hyperintense to surrounding liver.[39,40]

Technetium-99m-radiolabeled red blood cells (RBCs) comprise another means to characterize hemangiomas. RBCs are radiolabeled with the isotope ^{99m}Tc and reinjected. Dynamic imaging shows blood flow with slow, uniform radiotracer accumulation on delayed images that peaks about 30–50 minutes after injection. Routine planar imaging detects lesions larger than 3 cm, and SPECT has improved the detection rate of small lesions on the order of 1–2 cm with a reported sensitivity as high as 93%.[3] Hepatocellular carcinoma may rarely show the same scintigraphic pattern as a hemangioma on RBC labeled scans. A rare liver tumor, angiosarcoma has an appearance identical to that of a hemangioma.[3,41]

The foregoing indicates that multiple modalities are available to image hemangiomas. When incidental liver lesions are identified by CT or US and are suspected of being hemangiomas, a particularly valuable approach for characterization that we use at our institution and that has been advocated by others is as follows: When the lesion is larger than 2.5 cm, a ^{99m}Tc-RBC-tagged study is used for confirmation. If the lesion is smaller than 2.5 cm, MRI is useful for further evaluation.[28] Subcentimeter lesions are difficult to characterize by any modality and should be followed.

Focal Nodular Hyperplasia

Focal nodular hyperplasia (FNH) is a rare benign hepatic tumor. It consists of hepatocytes, bile ducts, and Kupffer cells often surrounding a central scar.[42] The sonographic appearance of FNH is variable. Lesions are well marginated and have variable echogenicity. The central scar may not be evident. Both CT and MRI rely on the vascular nature of these tumors for characterization. FNH may be difficult to detect on noncontrast CT because the CT attenuation of these lesions is similar to that of surrounding liver. The hypodense central scar, when present, aids in detection. During the early arterial phase of a dynamic contrast-enhanced CT scan, this focal lesion demonstrates marked enhancement—much greater than that of surrounding liver. Rapid washout of contrast occurs, and the FNH becomes isoattenuating to the liver during the portal venous and delayed phases (Fig. 1.3). The early arterial phase of imaging is therefore most important for characterization of FNH.[24,43] The central scar usually remains hypodense but is seen in fewer than 50% of lesions. When the scar is not present, FNH has a CT appearance similar to that of hepatic adenomas.[43] Fibrolamellar hepatocellular carcinoma, a small, well differentiated hepatocellular carcinoma, or a hypervascular metastasis, particularly when small, may show a similar pattern of enhancement on CT.

The MR signal characteristics of FNH are similar to those of surrounding liver, resulting in low lesion-to-liver contrast. T1- and T2-weighted scans usually show a lesion isointense to surrounding liver,[44,45] although FNH may appear hypointense on T1-weighted images and hyperintense on T2-weighted images.[46] The central scar, when present, is low signal on T1-weighted images and hyperintense on T2-weighted images.[47] As with CT, dynamic gadolinium-enhanced MRI displays the extreme vascular nature of these tumors. Early arterial images show dense homogeneous enhancement; and during the portal venous and delayed phases FNH becomes isointense to normal liver. The central scar may show late enhancement.[48,49]

The liver spleen scan, which uses ^{99m}Tc-sulfur colloid, sometimes helps distinguish FNH from other tumors such as hepatic adenomas. FNH contains Kupffer cells that phagocytize the labeled sulfur colloid. Because most FNH has a high enough concentration of Kupffer cells, roughly 70% of these lesions exhibit radiotracer uptake. In contrast, tumors such as hepatocellular adenoma and hepatocellular carcinoma rarely take up the agent and thus appear as focal defects.[43]

Hepatocellular Adenoma

Hepatic adenomas, which are less common than FNH, are hepatic tumors composed of benign hepatocytes. Bile duct epithelium is not present, and only rare Kupffer cells are seen.[50] These adenomas occur primarily in women of childbearing age. There is a well known association between the tumors and the use of oral contraceptives. Hepatic adenomas, unlike FNH, may require surgical intervention because adenomas may hemorrhage, rupture, or in rare instances transform into malignant tumors.[21,24]

The US appearance of hepatic adenomas is variable depending on the presence of complications such as hemorrhage or necrosis. Lesions are well demarcated and may show foci of increased echogenicity likely corresponding to areas of necrosis or hemorrhage. Areas of sonolucency may represent evolving hemorrhage. It is not possible to distinguish these tumors from FNH sonographically.[21]

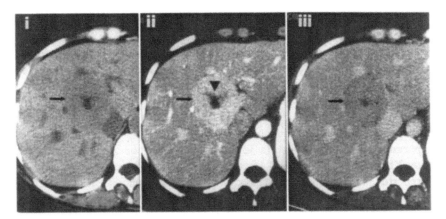

FIGURE 1.3-A.

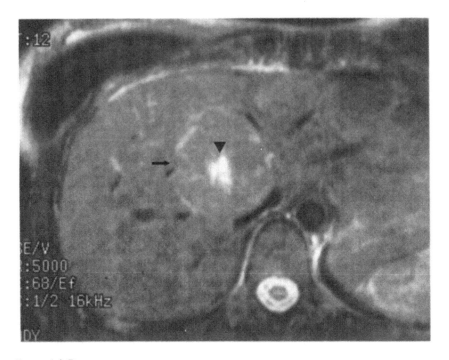

FIGURE 1.3-B.

FIGURE 1.3. Focal nodular hyperplasia. (A) Serial CT images obtained without contrast (i), during the early vascular phase (ii), after contrast administration and several minutes later (iii) demonstrate a homogeneously enhancing mass that rapidly becomes isodense to surrounding liver (arrows). Note the hypodense central scar (arrowhead). (B) Axial T2-weighted MR image in the same patient shows the lesion isointense to surrounding liver parenchyma (arrow). The central scar is hyperintense (arrowhead).

Hepatic adenomas are typically hypodense or isodense to the liver on noncontrast CT. Administration of contrast and dynamic scanning shows early arterial enhancement of the mass which becomes isoattenuating on delayed scans. A fibrous capsule is seen occasionally. A central scar is not present. Adenomas may appear inhomogeneous because of complications such as hemorrhage.[24]

On MR images hepatic adenomas commonly display a peripheral rim, heterogeneity, and T1 hyperintensity.[51] The peripheral rim corresponds to a pseudocapsule seen by histologic analysis. This peripheral rim is hypointense on T1-weighted images and of variable signal on T2-weighted images; it is reported in up to one-third of cases. Most hepatic adenomas have a heterogeneous appearance on all pulse sequences relating to hemorrhage and necrosis. The tumors are usually hyperintense on T1- and T2-weighted images. T1 hyperintensity corresponds to the presence of fat and blood products which is a relatively specific finding in liver masses found in young women.[25] Contrast uptake is similar to that of FNH in that these tumors enhance early, but adenomas show heterogeneous enhancement compared to the dense, homogeneous enhancement of FNH.[51]

Fatty Infiltration of the Liver

Lipid commonly deposits within hepatocytes and may be secondary to a variety of conditions ranging from diabetes to malignancy. Numerous drugs also contribute to fatty change in the liver. Patients with an underlying malignancy who may have been treated with chemotherapy are prone to fatty change in the liver. The fat deposition may be focal or diffuse. Focal fatty deposits may be particularly difficult to distinguish from more threatening lesions such as metastasis. Similarly, focal areas of sparing may occur in a diffusely fatty liver, causing a diagnostic dilemma. Typically, a focal fatty deposit or focal sparing is located near the surface of the liver, where it is close to the attachment of hepatic ligaments such as in segment IV along the falciform ligament (Fig. 1.4).

Hepatic sonography may be difficult to perform in a patient with a diffusely fatty liver because the larger quantity of lipid causes increased echogenicity of the liver parenchyma and attenuation and scattering of the sound beam.[52] In contrast, focal fatty infiltration of the liver causes focal pseudolesions. These focal fatty deposits demonstrate no mass effect and show a normal distribution of vessels in and around the pseudolesion (Fig. 1.5). Characterization of nonuniform fat deposition remains difficult with US.[53]

Focal fatty deposits appear as low attenuation lesions on CT scans of the liver. Lack of a mass effect and the presence of normal vessels in and around the lesion is used, as with US, to characterize focal fat.[52] These findings may not be present in all cases, and benign fatty infiltration may be confused with metastatic disease, resulting in diagnostic dilemmas.[54]

With its superior ability to characterize fat, MRI is most helpful for distin-

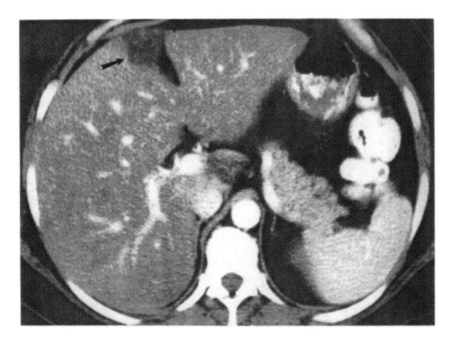

FIGURE 1.4. Focal fatty deposit (arrow) involving segment IV, adjacent to the falciform ligament as shown by CT.

guishing cases of benign fatty infiltration from other liver lesions (Fig. 1.6). Chemical shift MRI is the technique used to diagnose focal fatty infiltration. This subtraction technique relies on the fact that fat and water protons resonate in and out of phase with each other. Signal dropout occurs in areas primarily containing fat when fat resonates out of phase with water, allowing a specific diagnosis of focal fatty deposits.[55] It should be noted that conventional spin echo imaging and routine fat saturation sequences are usually not helpful for diagnosing focal fatty infiltration.

Metastatic Disease

Metastatic disease is the most common hepatic malignancy in the United States. Multiple focal lesions are more common than solitary lesions, and diffusely infiltrative disease may occur.

Hepatic metastases have varying appearance on US; they may be hypoechoic, hyperechoic, isoechoic, or mixed. Although it is not possible to classify a lesion histologically based on its sonographic appearance, some generalizations may be made. For example, hepatic metastatic disease from the colon is frequently hyperechoic, whereas melanoma, which tends to enlarge and necrose, is usually hypoechoic. Calcification in metastatic-mucin

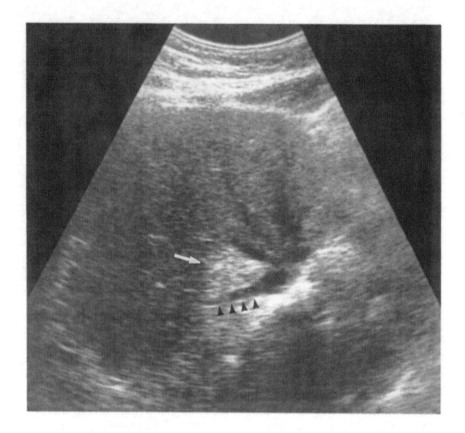

FIGURE 1.5-A.

FIGURE 1.5. Focal fatty infiltration. (A) Hepatic sonogram obtained in the axial plane at the level of the hepatic vein confluence shows a hyperechoic lesion (white arrow) with a normal right hepatic vein (arrowheads) passing through the lesion. (B) CT scan obtained on the same patient at the same level shows a markedly low attenuation lesion (arrow) in keeping with focal fat.

producing tumors appears as a dense, echogenic focus with distal acoustic shadowing. Because portal vein occlusion occurs in up to 8% of cases of metastatic disease, Doppler evaluation of the hepatic vessels may help exclude invasion and thrombosis of the portal vein.[21]

The CT appearance of metastatic disease varies with the primary tumor type. Tumors of the colon, breast, and lung account for the largest numbers of hepatic metastases because of the prevalence of these tumors. On contrast-enhanced CT, most metastatic tumors appear as hypodense foci relative to surrounding liver. This hypoattenuation is the result of hypovascularity or

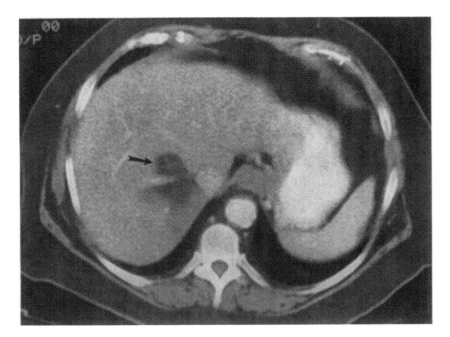

necrosis. Some hypodense metastases show rim enhancement of the periphery. This enhancing rim corresponds to vascularized viable tumor at the periphery of the lesion with necrosis at the center. Viable tumors receive this vascular supply from the hepatic artery, and rim enhancement has been noted more frequently after hepatic artery administration of contrast material.[56] If the viable periphery of the tumor does not enhance to a greater extent than the surrounding liver, the true size of lesions may be underestimated. This problem can be made less severe by using a bolus enhanced dynamic technique, whereby early images generally show some enhancement of the rim compared to later images, where this enhancing rim may become isointense to surrounding liver.

Some malignancies demonstrate hypervascular metastases. Examples of hypervascular tumors include neuroendocrine, renal, and thyroid malignancies. Metastases from breast carcinoma are also occasionally hypervascular. Nonenhanced CT and early arterial images are most important for detecting these lesions, which enhance early and quickly become isointense to surrounding liver.[32] At our institution we routinely perform both non-contrast- and contrast enhanced images for this group of tumors. Similarly, the initial work-up of any new patient should include nonenhanced and enhanced images to detect unsuspected hypervascular lesions.

Magnetic resonance imaging displays hepatic metastases as low intensity lesions on T1-weighted images and hyperintense lesions on T2-weighted

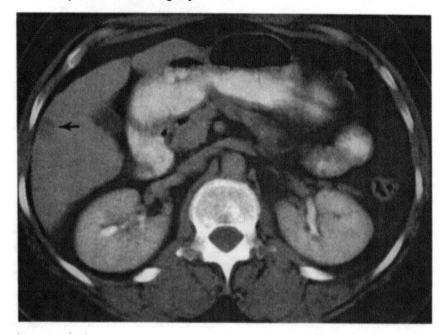

FIGURE 1.6-A

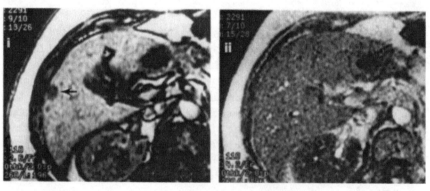

FIGURE 1.6-B.

FIGURE 1.6. Focal fatty deposit. (A) CT scan shows a low attenuation focus in the right lobe of the liver (arrow) in a patient with breast cancer. The differential diagnosis includes metastatic disease. (B) Axial out-of-phase MR image (i) in the same patient shows the lesion (arrow). The in-phase image (ii) does not show the lesion, which therefore represents benign fat.

images. Hemorrhagic hepatic metastases and those of malignant melanoma are characteristically hyperintense on non-contrast-enhanced T1-weighted images. MR signs of hepatic metastases as seen on T2-weighted images include an amorphous or inhomogeneous mass with irregular, poorly defined borders. A target appearance may be seen, with a hyperintense central area that corresponds to central necrosis. A peripheral halo, if present, likely corresponds to peritumoral edema.[37]

There is disagreement regarding the optimal pulse sequence for lesion detection.[25] We use multiple pulse sequences employing T1 and T2 weighting to optimize lesion detection. Contrast agents such as ferrumoxides, which are super paramagnetic iron oxides, may also be of value in detecting lesions.[57] Gadolinium is administered to help characterize lesions that may have been detected on non-contrast-enhanced images (Fig. 1.7).

Hepatocellular Carcinoma

Although relatively uncommon in the United States, primary hepatocellular carcinoma (HCC) ranks high in incidence in other parts of the world. HCC is commonly associated with liver cirrhosis secondary to viral hepatitis. Various patterns of tumor occur in the liver, such as solitary masses, multifocal masses, or diffuse disease. Invasion of the portal and hepatic venous systems is common. Imaging plays a role in the detection of tumors because of the relative insensitivity of clinical signs and laboratory studies.[21]

Ultrasonography is more widely available and less expensive than either CT or MRI and may therefore be used as a screening tool along with the serum α-fetoprotein, level, which is elevated in up to 75% of patients with HCC.[21,58] The US appearance of these tumors varies with their varying morphology. Diffusely infiltrating tumors are the most difficult to detect. When tumor nodules are present they are usually hypoechoic, although echogenicity is variable. Hyperechoic foci may represent fatty elements.[59] Doppler evaluation may be useful for evaluating venous invasion and thrombosis. Intraoperative US may be helpful for defining the extent of tumor and its relation to vessels when resection is attempted.[21]

The CT appearance of HCC also varies with the morphologic presentation. In the case of mass lesions, non-contrast-enhanced CT shows hypodense masses. A nodular type of HCC may be recognized as an enhancing lesion, particularly during the early bolus (arterial) phase of intravenous contrast enhancement. A hypodense capsule can frequently be identified during the bolus phase that becomes hyperdense during the delayed phase. Large lesions frequently show a mosaic pattern demonstrating multinodularity within the lesion (Fig. 1.8). Areas of tumor hemorrhage and necrosis can also be defined, which are features not seen with FNH. Early visualization of the portal venous system may occur because of arteriovenous shunting. Advanced tumors may grow outside the capsule and invade the hepatic or portal veins Tumor thrombus within the hepatic or portal veins appears as an enhancing, expansile, intraluminal mass. Daughter, or satellite, nodules and tumor growth beyond the capsule is also seen with advanced disease. In our experience, it may be difficult to distinguish a small (< 2 cm) HCC that enhances uniformly

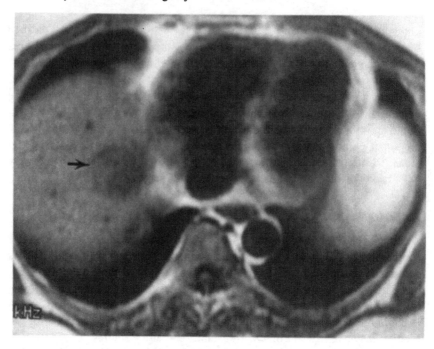

FIGURE 1.7-A.

FIGURE 1.7. Metastatic colon carcinoma. (A) Axial T1-weighted MR image shows a hypointense lesion at the dome of the lever (arrow). (B) Sagittal gradient image in the same patient obtained after gadolinium administration shows peripheral ring-like enhancement (arrows) of the lesion, which is in contrast to the globular enhancement typical of hemangiomas.

from a small hypervascular hepatic metastasis or FNH unless there are stigmata of hepatic cirrhosis, which point to HCC as the diagnosis.

As in the case of US and CT, the MRI appearance of HCC is variable. T1-weighted images show hypointense masses that may have areas of hyperintensity related to hemorrhage or lipid content. T2-weighted scans show hyperintense lesions. This appearance contrasts with the MRI appearance of regenerating nodules, which are frequently found in a background of cirrhosis and may be mistaken for HCC by US or CT. Regenerating nodules are usually hyperintense on T1-weighted images and hypointense on T2-weighted images.

Dynamic scans obtained after administering gadolinium show heterogeneous enhancement of HCC that gradually becomes more homogeneous and eventually fades.[60] Administration of the tissue-specific agent MnDPDP, which is taken up by hepatocytes and lesions of hepatocellular origin, causes enhancement of these primary tumors.[18]

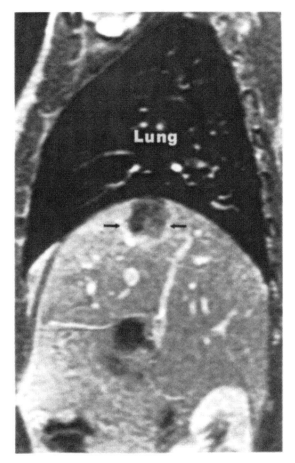

FIGURE 1.7-B.

Gallium-67 (^{67}Ga) scans may also be used to characterize HCC. More than 90% of these tumors accumulate ^{67}Ga. Among these gallium-avid tumors, more than 50% show uptake greater than that of the surrounding liver, which also takes up this agent. Regenerating nodules, on the other hand, rarely accumulate ^{67}Ga.[3]

Fibrolamellar HCC is an uncommon type that occurs in young patients and has a slightly better prognosis. Imaging of fibrolamellar HCC usually shows a central scar similar to that of FNH. Enhancement patterns of these tumors are similar to those of FNH. The presence of central calcification in fibrolamellar HCC has been used to help distinguish this malignant neoplasm from benign FNH, although this finding is not always specific.[61]

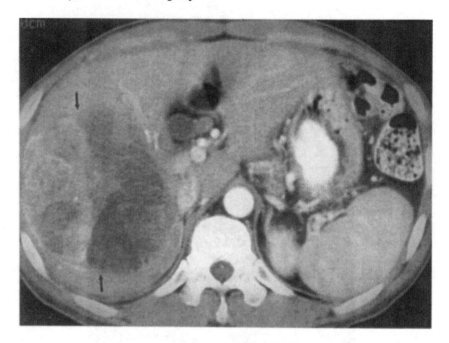

FIGURE 1.8. Hepatocellular carcinoma. Axial CT image obtained after contrast administration shows a large, inhomogeneous mass (arrows) within the right lobe of the liver. Multiple hypervascular nodules with areas of necrosis and hemorrhage are seen within the mass, which is typical of the nodular type of hepatocellular carcinoma.

Cholangiocarcinoma

Cholangiocarcinoma, an uncommon malignancy, may arise from a major bile duct (the usual case) or from small bile ductules within the hepatic parenchyma. Lesions arising from a major bile duct are frequently smaller at diagnosis because they may cause obstructive jaundice, prompting the patient to seek medical attention early. Intrahepatic cholangiocarcinomas are frequently larger at diagnosis, as they can form masses in the hepatic parenchyma without causing symptoms. As they grow larger, intrahepatic cholangiocarcinomas can also cause obstruction of major bile ducts.

When cholangiocarcinoma occurs in the extrahepatic biliary tree, it may be difficult to visualize the tumor mass by imaging. US and CT show dilated biliary radicals with abrupt termination of dilated ducts at the site of the tumor. Hilar cholangiocarcinoma often infiltrates the surrounding periductal fat and involves adjacent vessels. Lymphatic spread is common as well. Although calculi causing obstruction can usually be excluded, benign strictures may appear similar, with an abrupt transition from dilated to normal caliber ducts.[62,63] Intrahepatic cholangiocarcinoma which is less common has an entirely nonspecific CT appearance; its scan is similar to that of metastatic adenocarcinoma of various primaries including carcinoma of the colon, pancreas, and breast. Intrahepatic cholangiocarcinoma frequently contains areas of fibrosis, necrosis, and mucin. The vascularity of these tumors is variable depending on the degree of solid tumor present. The lesions therefore tend to enhance irregularly at the periphery during the bolus phase, with the degree of enhancement vary (Fig. 1.9). Areas of fibrosis are generally hypodense during the bolus phase but may slowly enhance later, whereas areas of necrosis and pools of mucin usually remain hypodense during the various phases. The presence of segmental or lobar bile duct dilatation and associated atrophy of hepatic parenchyma may favor the diagnosis of cholangiocarcinoma (Fig. 1.10).

Conclusions

The goals of hepatic imaging are constantly changing as greater clinical demands are placed on diagnostic radiology by the introduction of new surgical and medical procedures. The evolution of imaging technology has been rapid over the past decades, providing answers to questions that previously could not be addressed. The limits of resolution of liver imaging continue to

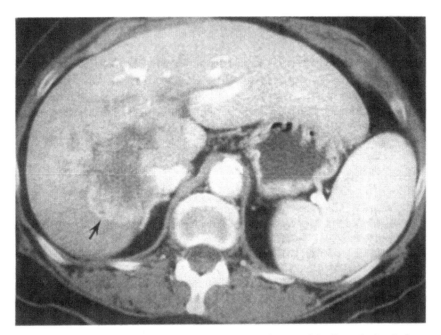

FIGURE 1.9. Intrahepatic cholangiocarcinoma. Axial CT image of the liver obtained after contrast administration shows a mass in the right lobe with irregular peripheral enhancement (arrow) and low-attenuation fibrosis in the center.

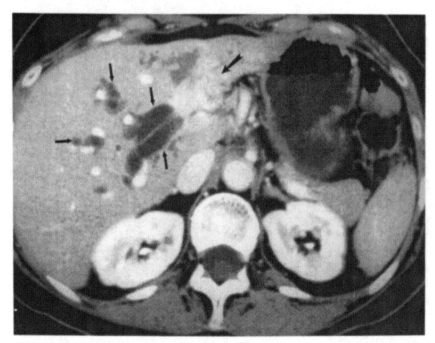

FIGURE 1.10. Cholangiocarcinoma. CT scan obtained after contrast administration shows an enhancing mass (large arrow) with resulting biliary dilatation (small arrows). There is atrophy of the left lobe of the liver.

improve, allowing detection of smaller and smaller lesions. Tissue specific characterization, however, remains difficult in many cases. The development of more tissue-specific contrast agents and faster imaging techniques may ultimately allow evaluation of organ and tumor perfusion kinetics, which would further our understanding of hepatic pathology.

References

1. Ferruci JT. Liver tumor imaging: current concepts. AJR 155:473, 1990
2. Sugarbaker PH. Surgical decision making for large bowel cancer metastatic to the liver. Radiology 174:621, 1990
3. Davis LP, McCarroll K. Correlative imaging of the liver and hepatobiliary system. Semin Nucl Med 24:208, 1994
4. Rifkin ND, Rosato FE, Brauk M, et al. Intra-operative ultrasound of the liver: an important adjunctive tool for decision making in the operating room. Ann Surg 205:466, 1987
5. Burns PN. Ultrasound contrast agents in radiological diagnosis. Radiologia Medica 87:71, 1994
6. Zemen RK, Fox SH, Silverman PM, et al. Helical (spiral) CT of the abdomen. AJR 160:719, 1993

7. Foley WD. Dynamic hepatic CT. Radiology 170:617, 1989
8. Matsui O, Takashima T, Kadaya M, et al. Liver metastases from colorectal cancers: detection with CT during arterial portography. Radiology 165:65, 1987
9. Heiken JP, Weyman PJ, Lee JKT, et al. Detection of focal hepatic masses: prospective evaluation with CT, delayed CT, CT during arterial portography, and MR imaging. Radiology 171:47, 1989
10. Nelson RC, Chezmar JL, Sugarbaker PH, Bernardino ME. Hepatic tumors: comparison of CT during arterial portography, delayed CT, and MR imaging for preoperative evaluation. Radiology 172:27, 1989
11. Freeny PC, Marks WM. Hepatic perfusion abnormalities during CT angiography. Radiology 159:685, 1986
12. Van Beers B, Pringot J, Gigot JF, Dauterbande J, Mathurin P. Non-tumorous attenuation differences on computed tomographic portography. Gastrointest Radiol 15:107, 1990
13. Moss AA, Goldberg HI, Stark DB, et al. Hepatic tumors: magnetic resonance and CT appearance. Radiology 150:141, 1984
14. Ohtomo K, Itai Y, Yoshikawa K et al. Hepatic tumors: dynamic MR imaging. Radiology 163:27, 1987
15. Hamm B, Wolf KJ, Felix R. Conventional and rapid MR imaging of the liver with Gd-DTPA. Radiology 164:313, 1987
16. Van Beers, Demeure R, Pringot J, et al. Dynamic spin echo imaging with Gd-DTPA: value in the differentiation of hepatic tumors. AJR 154:515, 1990
17. Edelman RR, Siegal JB, Singer A, Dupuis K, Longmaid HE. Dynamic MR imaging of the liver with Gd-DTPA: initial clinical results. AJR 153:1213, 1989
18. Hamm B, Vogel TJ, Branding G, et al. Focal liver lesion: MR imaging with Mn-DPDP-initial clinical results in 40 patients. Radiology 182:167, 1992
19. Vogl TJ, Hammerstingl R, Schwarz W, et al. Superparamagnetic iron-oxide-enhanced MR imaging for differential diagnosis of focal liver lesions. Radiology 198:881, 1996
20. Stark DD, Weissleder R, Elizondo G, et al. Superparamagnetic iron oxide: clinical application as a contrast agent for MR imaging of the liver. Radiology 168:297, 1988
21. Marn CS, Bree RL, Silver TM. Ultrasonography of the liver: technique and focal and diffuse disease. Radiol Clin North Am 29:1151, 1991
22. Gaines PA, Sampson MA. The prevalence and characterization of simple hepatic cysts by ultrasound examination. Br J Radiol 62:335, 1989
23. Spiegel RM, King DL, Green WM. Ultrasonography of primary cysts of the liver. AJR 131:235, 1978
24. Foley WD, Jochen RJ. Computed tomography: focal and diffuse liver disease. Radiol Clin North Am 29:1213, 1991
25. Kanzer GK, Weinreb JC. Magnetic resonance imaging of diseases of the liver and biliary system. Radiol Clin North Am 29:1259, 1991
26. Haaga JR. Magnetic resonance imaging of the liver. Radiol Clin North Am 22:879, 1984
27. Bree RL, Schwab RE, Glazer GM, et al. The varied appearances of hepatic cavernous hemangiomas with sonography, computed tomography, magnetic resonance imaging and scintigraphy. Radiographics 7:1153, 1987
28. Nelson RC, Chezmar JL. Diagnostic approaches to hepatic hemangiomas. Radiology 176:11, 1990

29. Marsh JI, Gibney RG, Li DKB. Hepatic hemangioma in the presence of fatty infiltration: an atypical sonographic appearance. Gastrointest Radiol 14:262, 1989
30. Quinn SF, Benjamin GG. Hepatic cavernous hemangioma: simple diagnostic sign with dynamic bolus CT. Radiology 182:545, 1992
31. Leslie DF, Johnson CD, MacCarthy RL, et al. Single-pass CT of hepatic tumors: value of globular enhancement in distinguishing hemangiomas from hypervascular metastases. AJR 165:1403, 1995
32. Bressler EL, Alpern MB, Glazer GM, et al. Hypervascular hepatic metastases:CT evaluation. Radiology 162:49, 1987
33. Stark DD, Felder RC, Wittenberg J, et al. Magnetic resonance imaging of cavernous hemangioma of the liver: tissue-specific characterization. AJR 145:213, 1985
34. Ohtomo K, Itai Y, Furui S, et al. Hepatic tumor differentiation by transverse relaxation time (T2) of magnetic resonance imaging. Radiology 155:421, 1985
35. Egglin TK, Rummeny E, Stark DD, et al. Hepatic tumors: quantitative tissue characterization with MR imaging. Radiology 176:107, 1990
36. McFarland EG, Mayo-Smith WW, Saini S, et al. Hepatic hemangiomas and malignant tumors: improved differentiation with heavily T2-weighted conventional spin-echo MR imaging. Radiology 193: 43, 1994
37. Wittenberg J, Stark DD, Forman BH, et al. Differentiation of hepatic metastases from hepatic hemangiomas and cysts by using MR imaging. AJR 151:79, 1988
38. Ros PR, Lubbers PR, Olmsted WW, et al. Hemangioma of the liver: heterogeneous appearance on T2 weighted images. AJR 149:1167, 1987
39. Hamm B, Fischer E, Taupitz M. Differentiation of hepatic hemangiomas from metastases by dynamic contrast-enhanced MR imaging. J Comput Assist Tomogr 14:205, 1990
40. Whitney WS, Herfkens RJ, Jeffrey RB, et al. Dynamic breath-hold multiplanar spoiled gradient-recalled MR imaging with gadolinium enhancement for differentiating hepatic hemangiomas from malignancies at 1.5 T. Radiology 189:863, 1993
41. Drane WE. Nuclear medicine techniques for the liver and biliary system: update for the 1990Æs. Radiol Clin North Am 29:1129, 1991
42. Wanless IR, Mawdsely C, Adams R. Pathogenesis of focal nodular hyperplasia. Hepatology 5:1194, 1985
43. Welch TJ, Sheedy PF II, Johnson CM, et al. Focal nodular hyperplasia and hepatic adenoma: comparison of angiography, CT, ultrasound, and scintigraphy. Radiology 156:593, 1985
44. Rummeny E, Weissleder R, Stark DD, et al. Primary liver tumors: diagnosis by MR imaging. AJR 152:63, 1989
45. Lee MJ, Saini S, Hamm B, et al. Focal nodular hyperplasia of the liver: MR findings in 35 proved cases. AJR 156:317, 1991
46. Mattison GR, Glazer GM, Quint LE, et al. MR imaging of focal nodular hyperplasia: characterization and distinction from primary malignant hepatic tumors. AJR 148:711, 1987
47. Rummeny E, Weissleder R, Stark DD, Sironi S, et al. Central scars in primary liver tumors: MR features, specificity, and pathologic correlation. Radiology 171:323, 1989
48. Mathieu D, Rahmouni A, Anglade MC, et al. Focal nodular hyperplasia of the liver: assessment with contrast enhanced turbo-FLASH MR imaging. Radiology 180:25, 1991

49. Mahfouz AE, Hamm B, Taupitz M, et al. Hypervascular liver lesions: differentiation of focal nodular hyperplasia from malignant tumors with dynamic gadolinium-enhanced MR imaging. Radiology 186:133, 1993

50. Lubbers PR, Ros PR, Goodman ZD, et al. Accumulation of technetium-99m sulfur colloid by hepatocellular adenoma: scintigraphic-pathologic correlation. AJR 148:1105, 1987

51. Arrive L, Flejou JF, Vilgrain V, et al. Hepatic adenoma: MR findings in 51 pathologically proved lesions. Radiology 193:507, 1994

52. Scartarige JC, Scott WW, Donovan PJ, et al. Fatty infiltration of the liver: ultrasonographic and computed tomographic correlation. J Ultrasound Med 3:9, 1984

53. Wang SS, Chiang JH, Bai YT, et al. Focal hepatic fatty infiltration as a cause of pseudotumors: ultrasonographic patterns and clinical differentiation. J Clin Ultrasound 18:401, 1990

54. Yates CH, Streight FA. Focal fatty infiltration of the liver simulating metastatic disease. Radiology 159:83, 1986

55. Mitchell DG. Focal manifestations of diffuse liver disease at MR imaging. Radiology 185:1, 1992

56. Moss AA, Dean BP, Axel L, et al. Dynamic CT of hepatic masses with intravenous and intra-arterial contrast material. AJR 138:847, 1982

57. Seneterre E, Taourel P, Bouvier Y, et al. Detection of hepatic metastases: ferrumoxides-enhanced MR imaging versus unenhanced MR imaging and CT during arterial portography. Radiology 200:785, 1996

58. Curati WL, Halevy A, Gibson RN, et al. Ultrasound, CT, and MRI comparison in primary and secondary tumors of the liver. Gastrointest Radiol 13:123, 1988

59. Tanaka S, Kitamura T, Imaoka Y, et al. Hepatocellular carcinoma: Sonographic and histologic correlation. AJR 140:701, 1983

60. Larson RE, Semelks RC, Bagley AS, et al. Hypervascular malignant liver lesions: comparison of various MR imaging pulse sequences and dynamic CT. Radiology 192:393, 1994

61. Caseiro-Alves F, Zins M, Mahfouz AE et al. Calcification in focal nodular hyperplasia: a new problem for differentiation from fibrolamellar hepatocellular carcinoma. Radiology 198:889, 1996

62. Cohen SM, Kurtz AB. Biliary sonography. Radiol Clin North Am 29:1171, 1991

63. Baron RL. Computed tomography of the biliary tree. Radiol Clin North Am 29:1235, 1991

2

Surgical Management of Hepatocellular Carcinoma

STEVEN A. CURLEY

Hepatocellular carcinoma (HCC) is one of the 10 most common cancers in the world. Although relatively uncommon in Western Countries, HCC is probably the most common solid cancer in the world.[1,2] Worldwide annual incidence of HCC is estimated to be at least one million new patients.[3-5] HCC is also one of the most lethal human malignancies, with a mortality index of 0.94.[6]

In general, the incidence of HCC increases with age, occurring most often between the third and fifth decades of life.[7] There is a pronounced geographic variation in the incidence of HCC. High incidence regions include sub-Saharan Africa, the southeastern coastline of China, Southeast Asia, Taiwan, Singapore, and Hong Kong. In areas of high incidence with high risk populations, defined as more than 30 new cases per 100,000 population each year, HCC occurs in younger age groups.[8] Men are affected by HCC at a much higher rate than women in all high and intermediate risk populations studied. In Ethiopia HCC is the second most common cancer in men (9.8% incidence), but only the fifteenth most common cancer in women (1.3% incidence).[9] In high incidence regions of the world, HCC is frequently a predominant cause of mortality in men in the population. For example, in Taiwan, HCC is the leading cause of death for men over 40 years of age.[10]

Intermediate incidence rates are found in central and southern Europe, northern Africa, Japan, and Swaziland and in Inuits, Native Americans, and Alaskan Aleuts.[11] Low incidence rates for HCC are reported in northern Europe, northern America, Australia, and the United Kingdom. In the United States the overall incidence of HCC is 2.8 per 100,000.[11]

Risk Factors Associated with Hepatocellular Cancer

The marked disparity in the incidence of HCC based on geographic region suggests a role for environment-related causative factors. Additionally, individuals with a variety of hereditary biochemical abnormalities affecting the liver are known to have an increased risk of developing HCC. The environmental and hereditary factors related to HCC are listed in Table 2.1.

TABLE 2.1. Factors associated with increased risk to develop hepatocellular carcinoma

Hepatitis B virus infection
Hepatitis C virus infection
Aflatoxin B_1 ingestion
Cirrhosis
Chronic ethanol ingestion
Primary biliary cirrhosis
Hemochromatosis
α_1-Antitrypsin deficiency
Glycogen storage diseases
Hypercitrullinemia
Porphyrias
Hereditary tyrosinemia
Wilson's disease
Hepatotoxin exposure (Thoratrast, polyvinyl chloride, carbon tetrachloride)

There is a striking correspondence between areas where HCC is common and hepatitis B virus (HBV) is endemic. In geographic regions with a high incidence of HCC, the chance of developing this cancer is more than 160 times greater in HBV carriers than in HBV-free individuals.[10] The most compelling evidence causally linking HBV infection and HCC has come from prospective studies. In 1975 a prospective study was initiated in Taiwan of 22,707 male Chinese government employees to evaluate the incidence and relative risk of HCC in relation to HBV infection.[12] HBV infection is hyperendemic in Taiwan, and only 5.6% of the men tested were negative for all HBV markers. HBV carriers [hepatitis B surface antigen (HBsAg)-positive] represented 15.2% (3454) of the men; 68.6% were positive for antibody to the HBsAg (anti-HBsAg), and 9.9% had antibody to the core antigen of HBV (anti-HBc). HCC caused the death of 152 men in this study; 143 deaths occurred among the 3454 men who were HBV carriers and the remaining 9 in the group of men who expressed antibody to HBV. Thus the relative risk of HCC among HBsAg carriers was 98.4%, indicating a more than 200-fold increased risk of HCC in HBV carriers.

Hepatitis C virus (HCV) infection is a serious, common complication of blood transfusion, occurring in 7–10% of all patients who receive a transfusion.[13] HCV is a single-stranded RNA virus, whereas HBV is a double-stranded DNA virus. Although HCV is molecularly unrelated to HBV, chronic HCV or HBV infection increases the risk of developing HCC. Unlike HBV infection, most patients who develop HCV infection develop chronic infection and a carrier state. A study based on liver biopsy samples stored over a 10-year period indicated that patients with anti-HCV antibodies had a significantly higher risk of developing HCC than did those who were anti-HCV-negative.[14] Interestingly, this biopsy study provided histologic proof that anti-HCV-positive patients had chronic hepatitis or cirrhosis in more than 75% of cases. The cumulative risk of HCV carriers to develop HCC is significant and sobering. An epidemiologic study of 62,280 Japanese suggests that 28% of male and 6% of female HCV carriers develop HCC.[15] It may be possible to predict the chronic HCV patients at greatest risk to develop HCC, as a report revealed that HCV patients with high rates of DNA synthesis in hepatocytes have a fivefold higher incidence of HCC than patients with low rates of hepatocyte DNA synthesis.[16]

The aflatoxins are the group of compounds with the strongest epidemiologic evidence for involvement in human HCC. They are produced by the molds *Aspergillus flavus* and *Aspergillus parasiticus*. Aflatoxin B_1 (AFB$_1$) occurs in foods and grains stored under humid conditions and has the highest potency among the aflatoxins as a toxin and a carcinogen.[17] In hepatocytes AFB$_1$ is metabolized into its active form, AFB$_1$-8,9-epoxide, which forms bulky adducts with nuclear DNA.[18,19] On a molar basis, activated AFB$_1$ is one of the most potent mutagens identified, a property that correlates well with carcinogenicity. Orally administered AFB$_1$ has been found to be hepatocarcinogenic in multiple laboratory animals. AFB$_1$ also induces activating mutations in proto-oncogenes and inactivating mutations in the tumor suppressor gene *p53*.[18–20]

Alcohol-related cirrhosis probably is the most important cause of HCC is the Western world.[21] In France, a country with intermediate HCC incidence, liver cirrhosis was present in 70.9% of patients with HCC reported from 1976 to 1983.[22] Cirrhosis was associated with excessive alcohol consumption in 92% of the HCC cases. The male/female ratio of HCC was 8.1:1.0 in the cirrhotic group and 1.5:1.0 in the noncirrhotic group. Of the 247 cases of HCC, markers for HBV were found in 30.6% of the cirrhotic group and 18.7% of the noncirrhotic group.

In low-incidence countries, HCC develops almost exclusively in individuals with underlying cirrhosis. For example, 93% of patients with HCC in Germany were found to have cirrhosis, but only 9.3% were HBsAg-positive.[23] Other western European countries have similar figures associating cirrhosis with HCC: Italy 96.4%, Spain 94%, and Austria 79%. Studies in the United States have demonstrated that populations shown to be at excess risk for cirrhosis-related mortality are also at increased risk to develop HCC.[24] A feature of many hereditary disorders that affect the liver (e.g., hemochromatosis, α_1-antitrypsin deficiency, type I glycogen storage disease, hypercitrullinemia, porphyria, tyrosinemia, Wilson's disease) is the development of cirrhosis. Some of these disorders are more common than others, but an increased risk for HCC has been associated with each.[17,25–27]

Diagnosis

Since the discovery during the 1960s of an association between elevated serum α-fetoprotein (AFP) levels and HCC, measurement of serum AFP levels has been the most useful laboratory test to suggest a diagnosis of HCC in a patient with a liver tumor. More recently, des-γ-carboxy prothrombin (DCP) has been shown to be tumor-specific in human HCC.[28] This marker seems less sensitive than AFP and is totally independent of AFP. Thus AFP-negative patients may have increased DCP.[29,30] In addition to being less sensitive than serum AFP levels, DCP disappears from the plasma if the patient is given vitamin K. Other laboratory studies, including measurement of serum levels of fucosylated AFP or hepatocyte growth factor, tumor cell levels of P-glycoprotein, and hepatocyte γ-glutamyltranspeptidase MRNA species, may have a role in improving early diagnosis and establishing a prognosis; these findings must be confirmed in larger trials.[31–34]

Serum AFP concentrations are normally less than 20 ng/ml in healthy adults. Transient increases in serum AFP levels may occur in benign chronic liver disease, especially during exacerbations of hepatitis.[35] Fewer than 10% of patients with chronic hepatitis have AFP levels over 100 ng/ml, and only 1–3% have levels higher than 400 ng/ml. For HCCs less than 5 cm in diameter, fewer than 15% of patients have AFP levels higher than 1000 ng/ml.[36] Furthermore, in patients with these small HCCs, up to 40% of patients have serum AFP levels that are less than 20 ng/ml, and 30–50% have AFP levels less than 200 ng/ml (Table 2.2).

When considering all patients with a diagnosis of HCC, approximately two-thirds have elevated serum AFP levels.[37] Serum AFP levels do not correlate with the size of the primary HCC, extent of intrahepatic disease, or presence of metastases. When evaluated histologically, well differentiated HCC or anaplastic HCC tends to be associated with minimal or no elevation of serum AFP levels.[38] Fewer than 50% of fibrolamellar HCCs are associated with elevated serum AFP levels, and in patients with elevated levels the value rarely exceeds 250 ng/ml.[39]

TABLE 2.2. Serum α-fetoprotein levels at the time of diagnosis in 606 patients with hepatocellular carcinomas of varying size

Tumor size	No.	α-Fetoprotein level (ng/ml)					
		0–20	20–200	200–1000	1000–5000	5000–10,000	>10,000
≤ 2 cm	47	19 (40.4%)	15 (31.9%)	10 (21.3%)	3 (6.4%)	0	0
2–3cm	54	13 (24.1%)	27 (50.0%)	10 (18.5%)	3 (5.6%)	1 (1.9%)	0
3–5cm	98	27 (27.6%)	34 (34.7%)	20 (20.4%)	8 (8.2%)	5 (5.1%)	4 (4.1%)
5–50%[a]	207	45 (21.7%)	49 (23.7%)	38 (18.4%)	42 (20.3%)	10 (4.8%)	23 (11.1%)
>50%[a]	200	21 (10.5%)	34 (17.0%)	19 (9.5%)	40 (20.0%)	37 (18.5)	49 (24.5%)

Adapted from Nomura et al.,[36] with permission.

[a]5–50% = percent of liver involved by tumor; >50% = more than 50% of liver involved by tumor.

Serum AFP levels are not elevated in a significant proportion of patients with early, potentially resectable HCC; and no more reliable serum marker for early disease has been identified. However, from our laboratory Izzo et al. reported that serum levels of soluble interleukin-2 receptor (sIL-2R) increase with increasing severity of liver damage in patients with chronic HCV infection.[40] Serum sIL-2R levels were highest in patients who developed HCC, and several patients with normal serum sIL-2R levels and no evidence of HCC at initial screening developed increased sIL-2R levels when they were later diagnosed with a small, early-stage HCC. Screening high risk populations has demonstrated that a small number of HCCs can be detected using only serum AFP as a screening tool in individuals who have no other clinical evidence of HCC.[41] In four studies performed in China, a total of 3,618,988 individuals in high HCC incidence regions (23–60 HCC cases per 100,000 population per year) were screened for serum AFP.[42] Altogether 301 individuals with asymptomatic HCC were diagnosed, representing 41.5% of the HCC cases diagnosed by an elevated serum AFP level. In this small subset of aysmptomatic patients, it is estimated that detection of small tumors by this method increased the number of surgically resectable lesions and improved the survival rate from 15% to 80% after 1 year and from 5% to 62% after 3 years.

Studies from moderate to high risk regions of the world have shown that serum AFP determination combined with real-time ultrasonography is the most accurate and cost-effective method to screen for HCC.[43–46] The frequency of AFP and ultrasound tests varies in these studies between 3 and 12 months, but all have demonstrated that ultrasonography is more accurate than AFP determination for detecting tumors less than 3 cm in diameter. These studies that screen high risk patients with serum AFP determination and ultrasonography have consistently demonstrated that almost 60% of patients in whom tumors develop have AFP levels that are either normal or fluctuate between normal and abnormal.[44–46] Screening high risk populations with ultrasonography and serum AFP levels produces a diagnosis in one-third to one-half of the patients with HCC at a stage where the tumor is resectable.[47,48] It is not yet clear whether these patients have an improved survival benefit because of the small number of resectable cases, the lack of long-term follow-up, and the reported high incidence of hepatic and distant metastases in the undergoing resection. Diagnostic accuracy in detecting early-stage HCC is improved using high-resolution computed tomography (CT), CT angioportography, and magnetic resonance imaging (MRI) in high risk patients with borderline ultrasound findings of AFP elevations.[49]

My pretreatment and diagnostic evaluation is based on the patterns of HCC spread (Table 2.3). In order of decreasing frequency, the five most common sites of HCC metastasis are regional lymph nodes, lungs, adrenal glands, bone, and peritoneal surfaces. Clinically detectable metastases, based on physical findings and radiographic studies, are present in 20–50% of HCC patients. The serum prothrombin time and liver function tests assess the se-

TABLE 2.3. Diagnostic and pretreatment evaluation of hepatocellular carcinoma patients

Physical examination
Serum laboratory tests
   Complete blood count, platelets
   PT and PTT
   Liver function tests[a]
   Hepatitis B and C screen (if not already known)
   α-Fetoprotein
   Carcinoembryonic antigen
Chest radiograph (CT chest only if plain radiography suggests metastases, but not definitively)
CT portography, CT abdomen
CT or ultrasound-guided fine-needle aspiration of hepatic tumor
Bone scan performed only in patients with symptomatic evidence of bone metastases

PT = prothrombin time; PTT = partial thromboplastin time; CT = computed tomography.
[a]Total bilirubin, alkaline phosphatase, aspartate aminotransferase, alanine aminotransferase, γ-glutamyltranspeptidase, albumin.

verity of hepatic dysfunction secondary to cirrhosis or extensive hepatic tumor. Baseline AFP levels are used to follow the response to treatment or to screen for recurrent disease following hepatic resection. A good two-view plain chest radiograph generally is sufficient to screen for pulmonary metastases. High-resolution CT portography that includes sections through the entire abdomen is used to evaluate the size of the primary liver tumor, the presence of intrahepatic spread of tumor, and the presence of portal or hepatic venous invasion by tumor; it is also used to detect evidence of nodal, organ, or peritoneal metastases.[50] Histologic confirmation of diagnosis is obtained using CT- or ultrasound-guided fine-needle aspiration of the liver tumor. Because bone metastases occur in 20% or fewer HCC patients, a bone scan is included for pretreatment evaluation only in patients with bone pain or radiographic evidence of bone destruction (chest radiography, CT of the abdomen).

Surgical Options

Assessment of Functional Hepatic Reserve

If the pretreatment evaluation reveals HCC confined to a potentially resectable area of the liver, determination of the functional hepatic reserve should be considered, particularly in cirrhotic patients. Unfortunately, many HCC patients with liver-only disease are not candidates for resection because of the tumor size or location with involvement of major vascular structures or because of limited hepatic reserve secondary to cirrhosis (Fig. 2.1). Postoperative liver failure and death are the consequence of an ill-planned hepatic

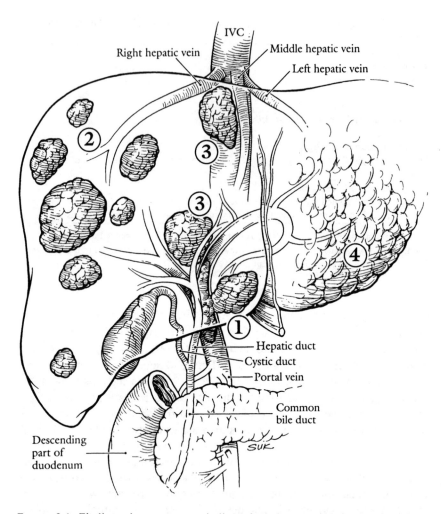

FIGURE 2.1. Findings that may contraindicate hepatic resection for hepatocellular cancer. (1) Direct tumor invasion into segmental or main portal or hepatic vein branches. (2) Multicentric tumor or satellite nodules. (3) Tumor proximity to major vascular structures precluding margin-negative resection. (4) Severe liver cirrhosis with insufficient functional hepatic reserve, which would result in hepatic failure and death following a partial liver resection.

resection, so assessing functional hepatic reserve is crucial before subjecting a cirrhotic HCC patient to surgery. The size and location of an HCC mandate the type of surgery that must be performed to achieve a margin-negative liver resection. A significant amount of hepatic parenchyma is lost with major liver resections; the average amount of liver parenchyma resected during a right trisegmentectomy is 85%, a right lobectomy 65%, and a left lobectomy 35%.[51]

Segmental or wedge resections of the liver entail loss of less functional hepatic tissue, ranging from 3% to 15%.

An HCC patient with a shrunken liver, intractable ascites, hepatic encephalopathy, prothrombin time less than 60% of control, serum albumin less than 3.0 g/dl, and serum aminotransferase levels higher than 150 IU/L does not tolerate a liver resection and should be considered only for nonsurgical treatment. In series of liver resections for HCC where the only preoperative assessment of liver function was based on clinical grounds using the Child-Turcotte classification (Table 2.4) or a modification thereof, the postresection liver failure and mortality rates for class A and B patients ranged from 8% to 25%.[52–55] In Child-Turcotte class A or B patients being considered for resection of HCC, addition of quantitative or functional hepatic studies can improve patient selection, determine the extent of hepatic parenchymal resection that can be tolerated, and reduce the postoperative mortality rate from liver failure to between 0% and 5%.[56–58]

Functional studies of the liver employ compounds that normally are rapidly acquired and metabolized or cleared by hepatocytes. Metabolism and clearance are decreased in cirrhotic livers. Some of the compounds used in functional studies have a clearance rate that is determined principally by the route of delivery rather than metabolism. Hence these compounds reflect changes in hepatic microcirculation and reductions in blood flow associated with cirrhosis. Other compounds are less affected by delivery, and their metabolism is a more accurate indicator of functional hepatocyte mass. Indocyanine green (ICG), an anionic dye bound by plasma lipoproteins, is cleared rapidly by the liver and excreted unconjugated in bile.[59,60] Hepatic clearance is limited by both the hepatic blood flow rate and uptake by hepatocytes. Following an intravenous bolus of ICG, the kinetics of its disappearance from plasma due to hepatic clearance can be used to estimate the functional hepatic reserve in cirrhotic patients, even in the presence of hyperbilirubinemia.

Intrinsic hepatic clearance of ICG appears to be superior to the Child-Turcotte classification system for assessing liver reserve in cirrhotic patients.[61] There are three ICG kinetic values commonly employed to assess functional hepatic reserve and the risk of liver failure following hepatic resection: ICG-R_{15}, the percent ICG still present in the plasma 15 minutes after bolus ad-

TABLE 2.4. Child-Turcotte classification of hepatic dysfunction in cirrhotic patients

Parameter	Criteria, by class		
	A	B	C
Nutritional status	Excellent	Good	Poor
Ascites	None	Minimal, controlled	Moderate to severe
Encephalopathy	None	Minimal, controlled	Moderate to severe
Serum bilirubin	<2	2–3	>3
Serum albumin (g/dl)	>3.5	2.8–3.5	<2.8
Prothrombin time (% of control)	>70	40–70	<40

ministration; ICG-Rmax, the maximal rate of ICG removal; and ICG-Rmax[residual], the maximal rate of ICG removal coupled with the estimated volume of the liver that would remain following hepatic resection. The ICG-R_{15} can be used to predict the extent of resection that will be tolerated without postoperative liver failure in cirrhotic patients: A value of 15–20% indicates that a lobectomy or two-segment resection will be tolerated, 21–30% indicates a single segment or wedge resection will be tolerated, and a value greater than 40% indicates that liver failure will probably occur even with a minimal hepatic resection.[62–65] In a normal, noncirrhotic liver, the average ICG-Rmax is 3.5 mg/kg/min.[66] In cirrhotic patients with HCC, an ICG-Rmax value greater than 1.0 mg/kg/min was associated with no postoperative liver resection mortality when lobectomy was performed.[66] In contrast, an ICG-Rmax less than 0.4 mg/kg/min was associated with 100% postoperative mortality from liver failure if any type of liver resection, including wedge resection, was performed. For values between 0.4 and 1.0 mg/kg/min, hepatic lobectomy produced high postoperative mortality rates due to liver failure ($\geq$ 50%), and segmental or wedge resections were associated with a postresection liver failure rate of slightly more than 10%. The ICG-Rmax[residual] also can predict the risk of liver failure following hepatic resection in cirrhotic HCC patients; the fatal liver failure risk with a value greater than 0.8 mg/kg/min is 0%, 0.40–0.79 mg/kg/min 10%, and 0.20–0.39 mg/kg/min 50%; less than 0.2 mg/kg/min is commensurate with a 100% risk of postresection liver failure.[57,66] The accuracy of the ICG-R_{15} can be combined with measurement of the amount of liver to be resected based on CT volumetric studies to improve the predictive accuracy for postresection hepatic failure.[67]

The advantages of ICG clearance determinations are that is a widely used and readily available test, and the values obtained can be used to predict risk for liver failure and mortality following hepatic resection. The two principal disadvantages of ICG clearance are (1) this test is not a true measure of hepatocellular function, as it is limited in part by cirrhosis-related altered blood flow to the liver; and (2) for patients whose values fall in the middle of the risk assessment range, the test cannot predict accurately a given individual's postoperative risk for liver failure and death. Further assessment is required for the latter individuals.

For patients with an ICG-Rmax[residual] value between 0.2 and 0.8 mg/kg/min, a large tumor or tumor location that would require resection of a lobe would be associated with excessive risk for liver failure and death. Therefore these patients should be considered for nonsurgical therapy. If it is possible to resect a smaller, more peripheral HCC with a wedge, segmental, or bisegmental resection, further studies can be performed in an attempt to define the operative risk more accurately.

The aminopyrine breath test measures the rate of aminopyrine N-demethylation by liver microsomal enzymes. Aminopyrine clearance is a true measure of hepatocyte uptake.[68,69] The aminopyrine breath test is reasonably simple to perform: The patient ingests a trace dose (approximately

1.5 µCi) of [^{14}C] aminopyrine and 2 hours later breathes into an apparatus that collects expired CO_2. The amount of exhaled $^{14}CO_2$ is then used to calculate the percentage of the [^{14}C] aminopyrine dose undergoing hepatic demethylation in 2 hours. The aminopyrine breath test has been used widely as a prognostic test for liver failure in patients with alcoholic liver disease or chronic active hepatitis or undergoing liver transplantation.[70,71] It also can predict accurately the risk of liver failure and death following abdominal surgery. In a study of 38 known cirrhotic patients undergoing surgery, there were no postoperative deaths among the patients who had an aminopyrine breath test value of more than 2.3%, whereas all six patients who died of postoperative liver failure had values less than 2.3%.[72] Unfortunately, this study included various types of abdominal operations, and the aminopyrine breath test has not been studied extensively in patients undergoing only liver resection.

Another promising method for assessing functional hepatic reserve is the clearance rate of the lidocaine metabolite monoethylgylinexylidide (MEGX). This test is less expensive, is simpler, and provides an answer more rapidly than other clearance studies.[73,74] However, it has not yet been widely applied, and larger studies of MEGX clearance rates before liver resection must be performed in cirrhotic patients.

There are two types of invasive study that can be performed to define operative risk better in cirrhotic HCC patients. The first is cannulation of the hepatic vein or veins draining the liver that remains after the proposed resection.[65] The hepatic vein catheter can be used to calculate blood flow in the vein and determine ICG removal in the segments of liver drained by the cannulated vein. In one study a blood flow rate of less than 600 ml/min and a quantity of ICG removed of less than 0.1 mg/min indicated 100% probability of liver failure and death following hepatic resection.[65] The second invasive study is transcatheter hepatic arterial embolization.[75,76] The changes in serum liver function tests and ICG clearance following this procedure may indicate if a hepatic resection will be tolerated. If selective embolization of the arterial branches supplying the tumor-bearing region of the liver is not associated with significant changes in liver function tests and ICG clearance, and particularly if compensatory hypertropy of the nonembolized regions of the liver occurs, it is probable that the patient will tolerate resection of the malignant portion of the liver.

Another method to assess surgical risk in cirrhotic HCC patients is the application of survival prediction equations.[64,77] Two multiple regression equations were developed to predict the risk of posthepatectomy liver failure.

Score 1 = −84.6 + 0.933(A) + 1.12 (B) + 0.999(C)
Score 2 = −110 + 0.942(A) + 1.36(B) + 1.17(C) + 5.94(D)

Where A is the CT volume of resected normal liver minus the CT volume of the tumor divided by the CT volume of the entire liver minus the CT volume of the tumor, then multiplied times 100; B is the ICG-R$_{15}$; C is the patient's age in years; and D is the ICG-Rmax. Using these equations, it was noted that all patients who did not survive a liver resection had scores of more than 50 points, and all survivors had scores of 50 points or less.

Resection

The optimal treatment for HCC is curative surgical excision. Unfortunately, in high-incidence regions of the world, only 10–15% of newly diagnosed HCC patients are candidates for resection, whereas in lower-incidence Western countries 15–30% of patients present with potentially resectable tumors.[65,78–81] The number of patients who undergo a truly curative resection probably is less than these numbers; 45–65% of patients referred to surgical departments with clinically apparent liver-only disease are found to have unresectable lesions because of multifocal hepatic disease, extrahepatic metastases, or inadequate functional hepatic reserve.[65,81,82]

The reported long-term survival rates following curative resection of HCC are widely variable. In Western countries where HCC is less frequently associated with HBV infection or cirrhosis, 2- and 3-year survival rates range from 23.5% to 51.0%,[82,83] and studies with longer follow-up periods report 5-year survivals ranging from 27% to 49%.[80,81,84] Studies from the Pacific rim of Asia, where most patients have a history of HBV infection and cirrhosis, report 5-year survival rates between 10.7% and 39%.[65,78,79,85–87] Two other series reported 10-year survival rates of approximately 19% for 709 patients undergoing resection for HCC.[88,89]

The variation in survival rates following resection of HCC is explained by reviewing patient selection criteria and prognostic factors. When limited hepatic resections for small tumors (< 5 cm in diameter) are performed in Child-Turcotte class A cirrhotic patients, the long-term survival is 40% or more.[81,83] Conversely, studies with lower long-term survival rates usually include populations of patients with hepatic dysfunction because of cirrhosis (Child-Turcotte class B or C) or tumors larger than 8 cm in diameter requiring resection of a significant proportion of the hepatic parenchyma. As a result of these two factors, the patients have higher operative mortality rates and poor tumor-related prognostic variables, which reduces the long-term survival rates.[86]

Several prognostic variables are useful for establishing the probability of long-term survival following resection of HCC. The tumor-free resection margin is important; in a series of 225 patients undergoing hepatic resection for HCC, the 3-year survival was 76.8% if the tumor-free margin was more than 1.0 cm compared to a 21% three-year survival for patients with a margin less than 1.0 cm.[90] The presence of cirrhosis is also a negative prognostic indicator; the 4-year survival rate in patients without cirrhosis was 81.2% compared to 34.8% in cirrhotic individuals.[80] This difference in survival may be explained in part by the higher frequency of multicentric HCC in cirrhotic patients (69%) than in those without cirrhosis (46%).[80] Vascular invasion by HCC is one of the most important prognostic variables. Preoperative imaging studies and intraoperative ultrasonography are useful for determining if adequate tumor-free margins can be attained and if there is gross portal or hepatic venous invasion by tumor. In one study, gross or microscopic tumor invasion of branches of the portal or hepatic veins was associated with rapid postresection tumor recurrence and no 3-year survivors.[64] The patients who had no evidence of vascular invasion had a 32% five-year survival rate. This finding has been corroborated by a large group of patients from Japan, where it was noted that tumor invasion of secondary or tertiary portal or hepatic venous branches was associated with markedly reduced 2- and 3-year survival rates, and involvement of the main trunks of the portal or hepatic veins was associated with postresection survival of less than 12 months.[78] These poor survival figures were explained by a meticulous pathologic study of resected HCC specimens, which revealed that the presence of tumor microsatellites or venous invasion is usually associated with residual disease in the remaining liver, even when the gross resection margins are more than 1 cm.[91] Other indicators of a poor prognosis following resection of HCC include absence of a tumor capsule, preresection serum AFP level higher than 10,000 ng/ml, tumor invasion of the capsule, poor performance status, and advanced tumor grade (Edmondson-Steiner grade III or IV).[92] In carefully selected patients who had no vascular invasion by tumor, solitary lesions without intrahepatic metastasis, tumor diameter of 5 cm or less, and a negative surgical margin of more than 1 cm, the 5-year survival rate following resection was as high as 78%.[64]

Improvements in intraoperative decision-making, surgical techniques, and instrumentation have combined to improve the selection of patients likely to benefit from resection of HCC and to reduce intraoperative blood loss and postoperative mortality. Intraoperative ultrasonography of the liver can determine the size of the primary tumor, detect portal or hepatic venous invasion and tumor thrombi, detect intrahepatic tumor metastases, assess the proximity of the tumor to major intrahepatic vascular structures, and be used to guide segmental or nonanatomic resections.[93-96] Segmental or nonanatomic liver resection is important in cirrhotic patients to maintain the largest possible volume of functional hepatic parenchyma (Fig. 2.2). I use intraoperative ultrasonography routinely in patients undergoing laparotomy for possible resection of HCC.

As noted in the preceding section on evaluation of functional hepatic reserve, operative mortality related to postresection liver failure is a major problem in HCC patients. The 30-day operative mortality in modern series has ranged from 3.6% to 19.0% (average 10.0%).[65,78-88] Fewer than 10% of the deaths are due to uncontrolled hemorrhage at the time of the liver resection; most of the deaths are caused by postoperative liver failure. The presence of cirrhosis is the most important predictor of postresection liver failure and death; the 30-day postoperative mortality for cirrhotics ranges from 14.3%

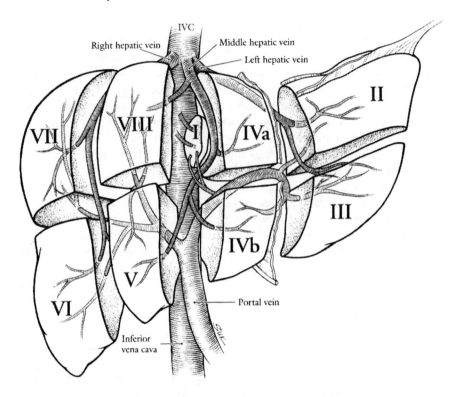

FIGURE 2.2. Segmental anatomy of the liver with the eight segments as designated by Couinaud. Segment I is the caudate lobe; segments II and III comprise the lateral segments of the left lobe; segment IV is the medial segment of the left lobe, and segments I–VIII comprise the right lobe.

to 23.8%, compared to 0.8% to 7.3% for noncirrhotics.[65,84,97] In cirrhotic HCC patients, two additional factors are important in the development of postoperative liver failure. Intraoperative blood loss of more than 1500 ml during liver resection or postoperative infection of any type significantly increases the risk for developing liver failure in these patients.[80,98] An important surgical advance was the recognition that vascular inflow occlusion of the portal vein and hepatic artery or total vascular exclusion of the liver (inflow occlusion combined with supra- and infrahepatic isolation of the vena cava) markedly reduces intraoperative blood loss and is well tolerated in cirrhotic patients if inflow occlusion does not exceed 60 minutes.[99,100] The morbidity and mortality associated with liver resection is reduced by judicious use of intraoperative vascular inflow occlusion. The livers of patients with cirrhosis tolerate liver ischemia for 30–60 minutes much better than they tolerate excessive blood loss and multiple transfusions.

In current series of liver resections for HCC, the operative mortality rate is less than 10% because of better preoperative evaluation of functional hepatic reserve, increased experience of the surgeons, and improved operative techniques. However, the postoperative morbidity rate following liver resection in HCC patients remains high, with a reported incidence between 40% and60%.[78–88,97] Reported nonfatal complications occurring after HCC resection are listed in Table 2.5. Similar to the postoperative mortality, the incidence of postoperative complications is three- to fivefold higher in cirrhotics than in noncirrhotics. Many of the complications, such as hemorrhage from gastroesophageal varices, liver insufficiency, ascites, and coagulopathy, occur almost exclusively in cirrhotic patients. Portal vein thrombosis is a particularly difficult, frequently fatal complication following hepatic resection. Portal vein thrombosis should be excluded using duplex Doppler ultrasonography in patients who develop liver dysfunction following hepatic resection. Prevention of any type of infection is important in cirrhotic patients undergoing liver resection to reduce the risk of postoperative liver insufficiency. Early diagnosis and aggressive treatment of postoperative infection is required to prevent liver failure and death.

The long-term survival figures following curative resection of HCC indicate that tumor recurrence is a major problem in these patients. The remaining liver is the most common site of recurrence in patients undergoing liver resection for HCC. Liver recurrence is the site of first failure in 45–70% of patients following resection.[83,86] Eighty-five percent of these hepatic recurrences develop within 2 years of the primary tumor resection. In 10–20% of cases the hepatic recurrence is itself resectable, but long-term survival following a second liver resection is limited by a high rate of liver and extrahepatic tumor recurrence, although long-term disease-free survival does occur rarely.[84,101–104] The prospects for long-term survival in patients undergoing hepatic resection for recurrent HCC are poor if the recurrence develops within 12 months of the primary HCC resection or if there are multiple tumors rather than a single recurrent nodule.[105] The high incidence of hepatic recur-

TABLE 2.5. Nonfatal complications after hepatic resection of hepatocellular carcinoma

Hemorrhage from gastroesophageal varices
Hemorrhage from gastritis or gastroduodenal ulceration
Hemorrhage from the cut surface of the liver
Liver insufficiency
Renal insufficiency
Subphrenic abscess
Biliary fistula
Wound infection
Pneumonia
Pleural effusion
Ascites
Small bowel obstruction
Portal vein thrombosis
Mesenteric artery thrombosis
Coagulopathy (disseminated intravascular coagulopathy)
Adult respiratory distress syndrome

rence of HCC is related in most cases to pathologic evidence of portal venous invasion by the primary tumor. Thus although complete surgical excision of HCC remains the best chance for long-term survival and cure, the group of patients with favorable prognostic factors who benefit from surgical excision as their sole treatment comprises fewer than 2% of all patients with HCC.

Cryosurgery

There is a rapidly developing experience in the use of hepatic cryosurgery to treat multiple or bilobar unresectable primary and metastatic liver tumors. Hepatic cryosurgery is based on the principle that the rapid freezing of tumor tissue using an intratumoral circulating liquid nitrogen probe causes tumor cell death by a combination of mechanisms, including osmotic dehydration, protein denaturation, perforation of cell membranes by ice crystals, destruction of tumor microvasculature, and nonspecific effects of "cold shock."[106-108] Experimental studies have demonstrated that the most important variable to achieve cytodestruction is the coldest temperature reached in the tissue; to ensure killing of tumor cells, at least 3 minutes at -35ºC is necessary.[107-108] Other important variables are the cooling rate, duration of freezing, and thawing rate, with the most effective tumor cell killing occurring by fast freezing (30ºC drop per minute), slow thawing (5ºC warming per minute) to increase intracellular ice crystal formation, and 3–5 minutes at a temperature of at least -35°C.

There are several key points related to the physics of tissue cooling by the cryoprobe. The greater the distance from the probe, the slower is the cooling of tissue. The size of the probe determines the maximum zone that can achieve a tissue temperature of at least −35ºC. For example, an 8 mm probe creates a 3 cm diameter zone of cell killing, a 10 mm probe creates a 3.6–4.0 cm diameter zone, and a 12 mm probe creates a 4.5–5.0 cm diameter zone of cytodestruction. Thermal gradients are 8°–10°C/ml, so at the freeze front the temperature is 0°C to −10°C, which is insufficient for cell killing. This factor is the reason it is important to use intraoperative ultrasonography to monitor the tissue solidification interface, also known as the leading edge of the iceball.[109-110] The leading edge of the iceball, which is hyperechoic on ultrasonography, should be 0.5–1.0 cm larger than the diameter of the tumor to ensure that the entire tumor is at least−35°C.

Cryosurgery usually requires a celiotomy, although a laparoscopic probe has been used in selected patients. Because each freeze-thaw cycle requires approximately 20 minutes, it is difficult to treat more than three or four tumors. Postoperatively, most patients develop an asymptomatic right pleural effusion. Mild leukocytosis and elevation of liver function tests (alkaline phosphatase, lactic dehydrogenase, alanine aminotransferase, and aspartate aminotransferase) are common but transient, generally returning to normal values by 5 days after treatment.[110,111] Temperature elevations to as high as

39°C are noted in most patients for the first 3–5 days following treatment because of acute tumor necrosis. The more serious complications that occur following hepatic tumor cryosurgery include major intraoperative hemorrhage from the cryoprobe tract, bile duct fistula, hepatic abscess, subphrenic abscess, and renal insufficiency related to myoglobinuria. Thus, it is necessary to evaluate baseline renal function prior to performing cryosurgery and to maintain optimal hydration and renal function during the immediate postoperative period.

Most reports of hepatic cryosurgery have involved the treatment of various tumor histologies, although there is a reported series of 60 HCC patients treated with cryosurgery.[111] Approximately one-half of the patients in this study had biopsy-proved cirrhosis, and slightly more than one-half were HBV-positive. The intraoperative treatments were not identical for the 60 patients; 27 (45%) underwent cryosurgical tumor ablation alone, 18 (30%) had cryosurgery and intraoperative hepatic arterial infusion chemotherapy or hepatic arterial ligation, and 15 (25%) were treated with cryosurgery and resection of the liver tumors. The survival of the 60 HCC patients treated with cryosurgery in this series is presented in Table 2.6. The pattern of failure in patients treated with cryosurgery is not mentioned in this study, although intrahepatic recurrence of tumor is frequently the cause of failure following cryoablation. It was noted that 49 of the 60 patients had elevated serum AFP levels prior to treatment; serum AFP decreased significantly in 38 of the 49 patients (77.6%) after cryosurgery.

The same authors updated their experience with cryoablation of HCC in 1993.[112] They treated 107 HCC patients by cryosurgery with no operative deaths. The 5- and 10-year survival rates for these 107 HCC patients were 22.0% and 8.2%, respectively. For a subset of 32 patients with small (< 5 cm diameter) solitary HCCs treated with cryosurgery, the 5- and 10-year survival rates were 48.8% and 17.1%, respectively.

Liver Transplantation

The HCC patients with liver-only disease who are not candidates for curative partial hepatectomy because of tumor size, location, multicentricity, or

TABLE 2.6. Survival of 60 patients with hepatocellular carcinoma treated with hepatic cryosurgery

Patient group	Survival (%)				
	1 Year	2 Years	3 Years	4 Years	5 Years
All (60 patients)	51.7	33.9	20.8	15.6	11.4
Tumor <5 cm (m = 21)	76.2	61.9	52.4	41.2	37.5
Cryosurgery only (m = 27)	33.3	23.1	12.5	8.7	4.3
Cryosurgery + hepatic artery chemotherapy or ligation (m = 18)	52.9	23.5	17.6	15.4	7.7

inadequate functional hepatic reserve have been treated with total hepatectomy and orthotopic liver transplantation (OLT).[84,113,114] The risk factors that
predict cancer recurrence following OLT are similar to those that predict a
high risk for recurrence after partial hepatectomy. Gross vascular invasion
by the primary tumor is a poor prognostic factor; patients with this finding
had an incidence of recurrence 42 times higher than that of patients with no
gross vascular invasion.[115] Other factors associated with a higher risk for
disease recurrence are tumor size more than 5 cm, multiple hepatic tumors,
microscopic vascular invasion, absence of a pseudocapsule, lymph node
metastases, and TNM stage III or IV disease. The presence of any of these
negative prognostic factors predicts a higher risk for tumor recurrence in
patients with either nonfibrolamellar or fibrolamellar HCC. Reports of OLT
in HCC patients describe 5-year survival rates of less than 10% to as high as
38%.[84,113–115] The higher survival rates come from studies that include patients with fibrolamellar variant and patients with small tumors (many of
which were found incidentally and not diagnosed prior to OLT). These survival rates are still poor compared to those for patients undergoing OLT for
nonmalignant liver disease where 5-year survival rates are at least 67%.

Based on the limited availability of organs and the high risk for recurrent
cancer, the use of OLT for nonfibrolamellar HCC or large fibrolamellar HCC
is highly controversial. OLT as the sole treatment for unresectable
nonfibrolamellar HCC is of questionable value. However, neoadjuvant chemotherapy, postoperative chemotherapy, and preoperative chemoembolization
have been used in attempts to decrease the rate of cancer recurrence following OLT.[116–118] A pilot study of 20 patients who underwent preoperative, intraoperative, and post-OLT systemic doxorubicin infusion resulted in an
overall survival of 59% and a disease-free survival of 54% at 3 years.[116] The
cumulative dose of doxorubicin administered was low (200 mg/m^2), and the
outcome results may be improved by delivering full-dose or combination
chemotherapy. Currently, OLT for nonfibrolamellar HCC should be considered only as part of a multimodality protocol-based regimen to treat HCC
confined to the liver.

Multimodality Therapy

Single-modality treatments such as surgical excision, systemic or regional chemotherapy, and radition therapy fail to provide long-term survival benefit for
most HCC patients. As previously noted, approximately 90% of HCC patients
present with unresectable tumors; and even among patients undergoing curative
resection most subsequently develop hepatic or systemic recurrence of disease.
Clearly, application of multimodality treatment combinations must be studied
in attempts to impove the outcome of HCC patients.

A study of 482 patients from China determined to have unresectable HCC during exploratory laparotomy describes the results of a variety of multimodality treament.[119] Patients who received no further treatment after exploratory laparotomy had a 1-year survival of 19%, with no 5-year survivors. A combination of hepatic arterial infusion chemotherapy, hepatic arterial ligation, and radioimmunotherapy produced significant cytoreduction in most of the patients treated; 30.6% of these patients were downstaged sufficiently to allow a curative surgical resection. Overall, 6.8% of the patients in this series underwent resection of their residual hepatic tumors following multimodality theraphy. The 1- and 5-year survival rates in these resected patients were 85.6% and 63.2%, respectively.

The probability of long-term survival is better for patients with resectable HCC than for those with unresectable tumors, even when the latter are treated with multimodality therapy. It appears that the use of multimodality therapy to convert unresectable to resectable HCC is associated with survival rates equivalent to those of patients who present with resectable tumors. In a study of 35 American patients, 21 presented with resectable lesions.[120,121] These 21 patients underwent resection with curative intent, with no postoperative deaths and a 5-year survival rate of 45%. The 14 patients initially presenting with unresectable liver-only disease were treated with external beam radiation therapy (2100 cGy in 300-cGy fractions) with concomitant systemic chemotherapy consisting of doxorubicin and 5-fluorouracil. Of the 14 patients, 10 also received.[131]I-antiferritin. The 14 initially unresectable tumors had at least 50% reduction in size, and all were resected successfully with no postoperative mortality or increased morbidity. The 5-year survival rate for these patients was 48%, which is similar to the 45% five-year survival rate of the 21 patients presenting with resectable HCC.

Preoperative hepatic arterial chemoembolization has been applied as part of a multimodality treatment program in patients undergoing resection of HCC.[122–125] The intent of the hepatic arterial chemoembolization treatments is to achieve cytoreduction of the tumor and reduce the incidence of postresection hepatic recurrences. Patients who receive preoperative hepatic arterial chemoembolization may have a higher incidence of intraoperative complications.[122] The studies also report that significant necrosis is present in many of the treated tumors, but there is no improvement in long-term survival rates for patients treated with preoperative hepatic arterial chemoembolization compared to patients treated with resection alone.[125] Portal vein embolization may improve resectability rates and enhance compensatory hypertrophy but has not been studied carefully in a large cohort of HCC patients.[126,127] Despite the small number of patients treated with multimodality regimens and the limited success achieved in improving the resectability rate and long-term survival, multimodality treatment programs for HCC patients must be developed and studied to improve the quality of life and outcome of HCC patients.

References

1. Beasley R. Hepatitis B virus: the major etiology of hepatocellular carcinoma. Cancer 61:1942, 1988
2. Di Bisceglie A. Hepatocellular carcinoma: molecular biology of its growth and relationship to hepatitis B virus infection. Med Clin North Am 73:985, 1989
3. Arya S, Ashraf S, Parande C, et al. Hepatitis B and delta markers in primary hepatocellular carcinoma patients in the Gizan area of Saudi Arabia. APMIS Suppl 3:30, 1988
4. Bridbord K. Pathogenesis and prevention of hepatocellular carcinoma. Cancer Detect Prev 14:191, 1989
5. Di Bisceglie A, Rustgi V, Hoofnagle J, et al. NIH conference on hepatocellular carcinoma. Ann Intern Med 108:390, 1988
6. Rustgi V. Epidemiology of hepatocellular cancer. Ann Intern Med 108:390, 1988
7. Anonymous. Hepatocellular cancer: differences between high and low incidence regions. Lancet 2:1183, 1987
8. Zuckerman A. Prevention of primary liver cancer by immunization. Cancer Detect Prev 14:309, 1989
9. Lindtjorn B. Cancer in southern Ethiopia. J Trop Med Hyg 90:181, 1987
10. Beasley RP, Hwang LY. Epidemiology of hepatocellular carcinoma. In: Vyas GN, Dienstag JL, Hoofnagle JH (eds) Viral Hepatitis and Liver Disease. Orlando, Grune & Stratton, 1984, p. 209
11. Falk H. Liver. In: Schottenfeld D, Fraumeni J (eds) Cancer Epidemiology and Prevention. Philadelphia, Saunders, 1982, p. 668
12. Beasley RP, Hwang LY, Lin CC, Chien CS. Hepatocellular carcinoma and hepatitis B virus: a prospective study of 22 707 men in Taiwan. Lancet 2:1129, 1981
13. Esteban J, Gonzalez A, Hernandez J, et al. Evaluation of antibodies to hepatitis C virus in a study of transfusion-associated hepatitis. N Engl J Med 323:1107, 1990
14. Verbaan H, Widell A, Lindgren S, et al. Hepatitis C in chronic liver disease: an epidemiological study based on 566 consecutive patients undergoing liver biopsy during a 10-year period. J Intern Med 232:33, 1992
15. Tanaka H, Hiyama T, Tsukuma H, et al. Cumulative risk of hepatocellular carcinoma in hepatitis C virus carriers: statistical estimations from cross-sectional data. Jpn J Cancer Res 85:485, 1994
16. Tarao K, Ohkawa S, Shimizu A, et al. Significance of hepatocellular proliferation in the development of hepatocellular carcinoma from anti-hepatitis C virus-positive cirrhotic patients. Cancer 73:1149, 1994
17. Lisker-Melman M, Martin P, Hoofnagle J. Conditions associated with hepatocellular carcinoma. Med Clin North Am 73:999, 1989
18. Sinha S, Webber C, Marshall CJ, et al. Activation of *ras* oncogene in aflatoxin-induced rat liver carcinogenesis. Proc Natl Acad Sci USA 85:3673, 1988
19. McMahon G, Davis EF, Huber LJ, et al. Characterization of c-Ki-*ras* and N-*ras* oncogenes in aflatoxin B_1-induced rat liver tumors. Proc Natl Acad Sci USA 87:1104, 1990

20. Aguilar F, Hussain SP, Cerutti P: Aflatoxin B$_1$ induces the transversion of GÙT in codon 249 of the p53 tumor suppressor gene in human hepatocytes. Proc Natl Acad Sci USA 90:8586, 1993

21. Hardell L, Bengtsson NO, Jonsson U, et al. Aetiological aspects on primary liver cancer with special regard to alcohol, organic solvent and acute intermittent porphyria: an epidemiological investigation. Br J Cancer 50:389, 1984

22. Boutron M, Faivre J, Milan C, et al. Primary liver cancer in Cote D-Or (France). Int J Epidemiol 17:21, 1988

23. Rockelein G, Hecken-Emmel M. Risk factors of hepatocellular carcinoma in Germany: hepatitis B or liver cirrhosis? Hepatogastroenterology 35:151, 1988

24. Fleisher JM. Occupational and non-occupational risk factors in relation to an excess of primary liver cancer observed among residents of Brooklyn, New York. Cancer 65:180, 1990

25. Hollands M, Huang J, Adams W, Little J. Hepatocellular carcinoma in western Sydney. Ann Acad Med Singapore 17:89, 1988

26. Tabor E. Hepatocellular carcinoma: possible etiologies in patients without serologic evidence of hepatitis B virus infection. J Med Virol 27:1 1989

27. Polio J, Enriquez RE, Chow A, et al. Hepatocellular carcinoma as a complication of Wilson's disease: case report and review of the literature. J Clin Gastroenterol 11:220, 1989

28. Okuda H, Obata H, Nakanishi T, et al. Production of abnormal prothrombin (des-QQQ-carboxy prothrombin) by hepatocellular carcinoma: a clinical and experimental study. J Hepatol 4:357, 1987

29. Suehiro T, Sugimachi K, Matsumata T, et al. Protein induced by vitamin K absence or antagonist II as a prognostic marker in hepatocellular carcinoma. Cancer 73:2464, 1994

30. Kasahara A, Hayashi N, Fusamoto H, et al. Clinical evaluation of plasma descarboxy prothrombin as a marker protein of hepatocellular carcinoma in patients with tumors of various sizes. Dig Dis Sci 38:2170, 1993

31. Yamashita F, Tanaka M, Satomura S, Tanikawa K. Prognostic significance of Lens culinaris agglutinin A-reactive α-fetoprotein in small hepatocellular carcinoma. Gastroenterology 111:996, 1996

32. Yamazaki H, Oi H, Matsumoto K, et al. Biphasic changes in serum hepatocyte growth factor after transarterial chemoembolization therapy for hepatocellular carcinoma. Cytokine 8:178, 1996

33. Soini Y, Virkajärvi N, Raunio H. Pääkkö P. Expression of P-glycoprotein in hepatocellular carcinoma: a potential marker of prognosis. J Clin Pathol 49:470, 1996

34. Tsutsumi M, Sakamuro D, Takada A, et al. Detection of a unique QQQ-glutamyl transpeptidase messenger RNA species closely related to the development of hepatocellular carcinoma in humans: a new candidate for early diagnosis of hepatocellular carcinoma. Hepatology 23:1093, 1996

35. Liaw YF, Tai DI, Chem TJ, et al. Alpha-fetoprotein changes in the course of chronic hepatitis: relation to bridging hepatic fibrosis and hepatocellular carcinoma. Liver 6:133, 1986

36. Nomura F, Ohnishi K, Tanabe Y. Clinical features and prognosis of hepatocellular carcinoma with reference to serum alpha-fetoprotein levels: analysis of 606 patients. Cancer 64:1700, 1989

37. Golondi L, Benzi G, Santi V, et al. Relationship between α-fetoprotein serum levels, tumour volume and growth rate of hepatocellular carcinoma in a western population. Ital J Gastroenterol 22:190, 1990
38. Thung SN, Gerber MA, Sarno E, Popper H. Distribution of five antigens in hepatocellular carcinoma. Lab Invest 41:101, 1979
39. Rolfes DB. Fibrolamellar carcinoma of the liver. In: Okuda K, Ishak KG (eds) Neoplasms of the Liver. Tokyo, Springer, 1987 p. 137
40. Izzo F, Curley SA, Maio P, et al. Soluble interleukin-2 receptor levels correlate with severity of hepatitis C virus liver injury and risk to develop hepatocellular cancer. Surgery 120:100, 1996
41. Kobayashi K, Sugimoto T, Makino H, et al. Screening methods for early detection of hepatocellular carcinoma. Hepatology 5:1100, 1985
42. Sell S. Detection of cancer by tumor markers in the blood: a view to the future. Crit Rev Oncog 4:419, 1993
43. Cottone M, Turri M, Caltagirone M, et al. Early detection of hepatocellular carcinoma associated with cirrhosis by ultrasound and alpha fetoprotein: a prospective study. Hepatogastroenterology 35:101, 1989
44. Liaw YF, Tai DI Chu CM, et al. Early detection of hepatocellular carcinoma in patients with chronic type B hepatitis: a prospective study. Gastroenterology 90:263, 1989
45. Maringhini A, Cottone M, Sciarrino E, et al. Ultrasonography and alpha-fetoprotein in diagnosis of hepatocellular carcinoma in cirrhosis. Dig Dis Sci 33:47, 1988
46. Colombo M, de Franchis R, del Nino E, et al. Hepatocellular carcinoma in Italian patients with cirrhosis. N Engl J Med 325:675, 1991
47. Curley SA, Izzo F, DeBellis M, Cremona F, Parisi V. Identification and screening of 416 patients with chronic hepatitis at high risk to develop hepatocellular cancer. Ann Surg 222:375, 1995
48. Izzo F, Cremona F, Ruffolo F, et al. Outcome of 67 hepatocellular cancer patients detected during screening of 1,125 chronic hepatitis patients. Ann Surg (in press)
49. Unoura M, Kaneko S, Matsushita E, et al. High-risk groups and screening strategies for early detection of hepatocellular carcinoma in patients with chronic liver disease. Hepatogastroenterology 40:305, 1993
50. Baron RL. Detection of liver neoplasms: techniques and outcomes. Abdom Imaging 19:320, 1994
51. Stone HH, Long WD, Smith RB, et al. Physiologic considerations in major hepatic resection. Am J Surg 117:78, 1969
52. Chlebowski RT, Tong M, Weissman J, et al. Hepatocellular carcinoma: diagnostic and prognostic features in North American patients. Cancer 53:2701, 1984
53. Lim RC Jr, Bongard FS. Hepatocellular carcinoma: changing concepts in diagnosis and management. Arch Surg 119:637, 1984
54. Lung G, Florence L, Hohgnasen K. Hepatocellular carcinoma: a 5-year institutional experience. Am J Surg 149:591, 1985
55. Ottow RT, August DA, Sugarbaker PH. Surgical therapy of liver cancer. In: Bottino JC, Opfell RW, Muggia FM (eds) Liver Cancer. Boston, Martinus Nijhoff, 1985, p. 99
56. Lee CS, Chi-Ching C, Lin TY. Partial hepatectomy on cirrhotic liver with a right lateral tumor. Surgery 98:942, 1985

57. Noguchi T, Imai T, Mizumoto R. Preoperative estimation of surgical risk of hepatectomy in cirrhotic patients. Hepatogastroenterology 37:165, 1990
58. Gholson CF, Provenza JM, Bacon BR. Hepatologic considerations in patients with parenchymal liver disease undergoing surgery. Am J Gastroenterol 85:487, 1990
59. Paumgartner G, Probst P, Kraines R, Leevy CM. Kinetics of indocyanine green removal from the blood. Ann NY Acad Sci 170:134, 1970
60. Moody FG, Rikkers LF, Aldrete JS. Estimation of the functional reserve of human liver. Ann Surg 180:592, 1974
61. Barbara JC, Poupon RE, Jaillon R, et al. Intrinsic hepatic clearance and Child-Turcotte classification for assessment of liver function in cirrhosis. J Hepatol 1:253, 1985
62. Matsumata T, Kanematsu T, Yoshida Y, et al. The indocyanine green test enables prediction of postoperative complications after hepatic resection. World J Surg 11:678, 1987
63. Kanematsu T, Takenaka K, Matsumata T, et al. Limited hepatic resection effective for selected cirrhotic patients with primary liver cancer. Ann Surg 199:51, 1984
64. Yamanaka N, Okamoto E, Toyosaka A, et al. Prognostic factors after hepatectomy for hepatocellular carcinomas: a univariate and multivariate analysis. Cancer 65:1104, 1990
65. Tsuzuki T, Sugioka A, Ueda M. Hepatic resection for hepatocellular carcinoma. Surgery 107:511, 1990
66. Mizumoto R, Kawarada Y, Noguchi T. Preoperative estimation of operative risk in liver surgery, with special reference to functional reserve of the remant liver following major hepatic resection. Jpn J Surg 9:343, 1979
67. Okamoto E, Kyo A, Yamanaka N, et al. Prediction of the safe limits of hepatectomy by combined volumetric and functional measurements in patients with impaired hepatic function. Surgery 95:586, 1984
68. Reichen J, Arts B, Schafroth U, et al. Aminopyrine N-demethylation by rats with liver cirrhosis; evidence for the intact cell hypothesis: a morphometric-functional study. Gastroenterology 93:719, 1987
69. Reichen J, Egger B, Ohara N, et al. Determinants of hepatic function in liver cirrhosis in the rate: multvariate analysis. J Clin Invest 82:2069, 1988
70. Henry DA, Kitchingman G, Langman MJ. ^{14}C-Aminopyrine breath analysis and conventional biochemical tests as predictors of survival in cirrhosis. Dig Dis Sci 30:813, 1985
71. Lashner BA, Jonas RB, Tang HS, et al. Chronic hepatitis: disease factors at diagnosis predictive of mortality. Am J Med 85:609, 1988
72. Gill RA, Goodman MW, Golfus GR, et al. Aminopyrine breath test predicts surgical risk for patients with liver disease. Ann Surg 198:701, 1983
73. Scudamore CH, Hemming A, Chow Y. Resection of hepatocellular carcinoma in the cirrhotic patient. In: Tabor E, Di Bisceglie AM, Purcell RH (eds) Etiology, Pathology, and Treatment of Hepatocellular Carcinoma in North America. The Woodlands, Portfolio Publishing, 1991, p. 293
74. Oellerich M, Burdelski M, Lautz HU, et al. Lidocaine metabolite formation as a measure of liver function in patients with cirrhosis. Ther Drug Monit 12:219, 1990
75. Miyoshi S, Minami Y, Kawata S, et al. Changes in hepatic functional reserve after transcatheter embolization of hepatocellular carcinoma. J Hepatol 6:332, 1988

76. Fujio N, Saiki K, Kinoshita H, et al. Results of treatment of patients with hepato-cellular carcinoma with severe cirrhosis of the liver. World J Surg 13:211, 1989

77. Yamanaka N, Okamoto E, Kuwata K, Tanaka N. A multiple regression equation for prediction of posthepatectomy liver failure. Ann Surg 200:658, 1984

78. Liver Cancer Study Group of Japan. Primary liver cancer in Japan: clinico-pathologic features and results of surgical treatment. Ann Surg 211:277, 1990

79. Choi TK, Lai Edward CS, Fan ST, et al. Results of surgical resection for hepatocellular carcinoma. Hepatogastroenterology 37:172, 1990

80. Nagorney DM, van Heerden JA, Ilstrup DM, Adson MA. Primary hepatic malig-nancy: surgical management and determinants of survival. Surgery 106:740, 1989

81. Paquet K-J, Koussouris P, Mercado MA, et al. Limited hepatic resection for selected cirrhotic patients with hepatocellular or cholangiocellular carcinoma: a prospective study. Br J Surg 78:459, 1991

82. Franco D, Capussotti L, Smadja C, et al. Resection of hepatocellular carcinoma: results in 72 European patients with cirrhosis. Gastroenterology 98:733, 1990

83. Cottone M, Virdone R, Fusco G, et al. Asymptomatic hepatocellular carcinoma in Child's A cirrhosis: a comparison of natural history and surgical treatment. Gas-troenterology 96:1566, 1989

84. Ringe B, Pichlmayr R, Wittekind C, Tusch G. Surgical treatment of hepato-cellular carcinoma: experience with liver resection and transplantation in 198 patients. World J Surg 15:270, 1991

85. Tsuzuki T, Ogata Y, Iida S, Shimazu M. Hepatic resection in 125 patients. Arch Surg 119:1025, 1984

86. Nagao A, Inoue U, Goto S, et al. Hepatic resection for hepatocellular carci-noma: clinical features and long-term prognosis. Ann Surg 205:33, 1987

87. Kim ST, Kim KP. Hepatic resections for primary liver cancer. Cancer Chemother Pharmacol 33:S18, 1994

88. Kosuge T, Makuuchi M, Takayama T, et al. Long-term results after resection of hepatocellular carcinoma: experience of 480 cases. Hepatogastroenterology 40:328, 1993

89. Nagasue N, Kohno H, Chang Y-C, et al. Liver resection for hepatocellular carcinoma: results of 229 consecutive patients during 11 years. Ann Surg 217:375, 1993

90. Ozawa K, Takayasu T, Kumada K, et al. Experience with 225 hepatic resections for hepatocellular carcinoma over a 4-year period. Am J Surg 161:677, 1991

91. Lai ECS, You K-T, Ng IOL, Shek TWH. The pathological basis of resection margin for hepatocellular carcinoma. World J Surg 17:786, 1993

92. Sugioka A, Tsuzuki T, Kanai T. Postresection prognosis of patients with hepa-tocellular carcinoma. Surgery 113:612, 1993

93. Parker GA, Lawrence W Jr, Horsley S III et al. Intraoperative ultrasound of the liver affects operative decision making. Ann Surg 209:569, 1989

94. Makuuchi M, Hasegawa H, Kamazaki S, et al. The use of operative ultra-sound as an aid to liver resection in patients with hepatocellular carcinoma. World J Surg 11:615, 1987

95. Clarke MP, Kane RA, Steele G, et al. Prospective comparison of preoperative imaging and intraoperative ultrasonography in the detection of liver tumors. Br J Surg 76:1323, 1989

96. Sheu JC, Lee CS, Sung IL, et al. Intraoperative hepatic ultrasonography—an indispensable procedure in resection of small hepatocellular carcinomas. Surgery 97:97, 1985

97. Bozzetti F, Gennari L, Regalia E, et al. Morbidity and mortality after surgical resection of liver tumors: analysis of 229 cases. Hepatogastroenterology 39:237, 1992

98. Takenaka K, Kanematsu T, Fukuzawa K, Sugimachi K. Can hepatic failure after surgery for hepatocellular carcinoma in cirrhotic patients be prevented? World J Surg 14:123, 1990

99. Bismuth H, Castaing D, Garden OJ. Major hepatic resection under total vascular exclusion. Ann Surg 210:13, 1989

100. Delva E, Camus Y, Nordlinger B, et al. Vascular occlusions for liver resections. Ann Surg 209:297, 1989

101. Kanematsu T, Matsumata T, Takenaka K, et al. Clinical management of recurrent hepatocellular carcinoma after primary resection. Br J Surg 75:203, 1988

102. Nagao T, Inoue S, Yoshimi F, et al. Postoperative recurrence of hepatocellular carcinoma. Ann Surg 211:28, 1990

103. Huguet C, Bona S, Nordlinger B, et al. Repeat hepatic resection for primary and metastatic carcinoma of the liver. Surg Gynecol Obstet 171:398, 1990

104. Hu R-H, Lee P-H, Yu S-C, et al. Surgical resection for recurrent hepatocellular carcinoma: prognosis and analysis of risk factors. Surgery 120:23, 1996

105. Shimada M, Takenaka K, Gion T, et al. Prognosis of recurrent hepatocellular carcinoma: a 10-year surgical experience in Japan. Gastroenterology 111:720, 1996

106. Jacob G, Li AKC, Hobbs KEF. A comparison of cryodestruction with excision or infarction of an implanted tumor in rate liver. Cryobiology 21:148, 1984

107. Gage AA, Guest K, Montes M, et al. Effect of varying freezing and thawing rates in experimental cryosurgery. Cryobiology 22:175, 1985

108. Shier WT. Studies on the mechanisms of mammalian cell killing by a freeze-thaw cycle: conditions that prevent cell killing using nucleated freezing. Cryobiology 22:110, 1988

109. Gilbert JC, Onik GM, Hoddick WK, Rubinsky B. Real time ultrasonic monitoring of hepatic cryosurgery. Cryobiology 22:319, 1985

110. Onik G, Rubinsky B, Zemel R, et al. Ultrasound-guided hepatic cryosurgery in the treatment of metastatic colon carcinoma. Cancer 67:901, 1991

111. Zhou XD, Tang ZY, Yu YQ, et al. Clinical evaluation of cryosurgery in the treatment of primary liver cancer: report of 60 cases. Cancer 61:1889, 1988

112. Zhou XD, Tang ZY, Yu YQ, et al. The role of cryosurgery in the treatment of hepatic cancer: a report of 113 cases. J Cancer Res Clin Oncol 120:100, 1993

113. Stone MJ, Klintmalm GBG, Polter D, et al. Liver transplantation for hepatocellular carcinoma. Hepatology 18:218, 1993

114. Bismuth H, Chiche L, Adam R, et al. Liver resection versus transplantation for hepatocellular carcinoma in cirrhotic patients. Ann Surg 218:145, 1993

115. Yokoyama I, Sheahan DG, Carr B, et al. Clinicopathologic factors affecting patient survival and tumor recurrence after orthotopic liver transplantation for hepatocellular carcinoma. Transplant Proc 23:2194, 1991

116. Carr BI, Selby R, Madariaga J, Iwatsuki S, Starzl TE. Prolonged survival after liver transplantation and cancer chemotheraphy for advanced-stage hepatocellular carcinoma. Transplant Proc 25:1128, 1993

117. Spreafico C, Marchiano A, Regalia E, et al. Chemoembolization of hepatocellular carcinoma in patients who undergo liver transplantation. Radiology 192:687, 1994

118. Stone MJ, Klintmalm GBG, Polter D, et al. Neoadjuvant chemotherapy and liver transplantation for hepatocellular carcinoma: a pilot study in 20 patients. Gastroenterology 104:196, 1993

119. Tang ZY, Yu YQ, Xhou XD, et al. Cytoreduction and sequential resection: a hope for unresectable primary liver cancer. J Surg Oncol 47:27, 1991

120. Sitzmann JV, Order SE, Klein JL, et al. Conversion by new treatment modalities of nonresectable to resectable hepatocellular cancer. J Clin Oncol 5:1566, 1987

121. Sitzmann JV, Abrams R. Improved survival for hepatocellular cancer with combination surgery and multimodality treatment. Ann Surg 217:149, 1993

122. Nagasue N, Galizia G, Kohno H, et al. Adverse effects of preoperative hepatic artery chemoembolization for resectable hepatocellular carcinoma: a retrospective comparison of 138 liver resections. Surgery 106:81, 1989

123. Nakamura H, Liu T, Hori S, et al. Response to transcatheter oily chemoembolization in hepatocellular carcinoma 3 cm or less: a study in 50 patients who underwent surgery. Hepatogastroenterology 40:6, 1993

124. Higuchi T, Kikuchi M, Okazaki M. Hepatocellular carcinoma after transcatheter hepatic arterial embolization. Cancer 73:2259, 1994

125. Harada T, Matsuo K, Inoue T, et al. Is preoperative hepatic arterial chemoembolization safe and effective for hepatocellular carcinoma? Ann Surg 224:4, 1996

126. Lee KC, Kinoshita H, Hirohashi K, Kubo S, Iwasa R. Extension of surgical indications for hepatocellular carcinoma by portal vein embolization. World J Surg 17:109, 1993

127. Shimamura T, Nakajima Y, Une Y, et al. Efficacy and safety of preoperative percutaneous transhepatic portal embolization with absolute ethanol: a clinical study. Surgery 121:135, 1997

3

Chemotherapy
for Hepatocellular Carcinoma

DENNIE V. JONES JR.

Hepatocellular carcinoma (HCC) is one of the most common malignancies in the world, with approximately one million new cases recorded annually.[1] The Pacific rim of Asia and sub-Saharan Africa are regions of exceptionally high HCC prevalence secondary to chronic liver disease and cirrhosis, in turn secondary to hepatitis B or C (or both) viral infections and the ingestion of aflatoxin B.[2-4] HCC is relatively uncommon in North America and western Europe. However, with approximately 13,600 cases diagnosed annually in the United States and a 2:1 male predominance, it is estimated that HCC will be one of the top 10 causes of cancer death in American men in 1997.[5] Cirrhosis from virtually any cause may place a patient at risk for developing HCC. At present, only complete surgical resection with either partial hepatectomy or a liver transplant is potentially curative, but this procedure is possible in only a small subset of patients. Within the limits of the chemotherapeutic agents currently available, an increasing number of approaches are being investigated in an effort to increase patient survival and the quality of life.

Patient Assessment

Even though there have been substantial advances in hepatic surgery, an operative approach may not be feasible because of co-morbid disease or intra- or extrahepatic metastatic disease. In light of this situation, most lesions are not resectable for cure.

The evaluation of a patient with a suspected or biopsy-proved HCC for potential resection includes routine chemistries, with special attention to the "standard" liver function tests, such as serum bilirubin, transaminases, lactic dehydrogenase, and alkaline phosphatase; assessment of hepatic synthetic function (albumin, prothrombin time, partial thromboplastin time); and hepatitis virus serology, especially directed against the hepatitis B and C viruses. The serum α-fetoprotein (AFP) level was the first serologic marker available for the screening, detection, and follow-up of HCC; it is the most widely utilized "tumor marker" for HCC, but it is neither specific for HCC nor elevated in all cases of HCC. Another widely used marker is the assay for des-γ-carboxy prothrombin protein, which is induced by vitamin K absence (PIVKA-2). Although PIVKA-2 is elevated in most patients with HCC, it is also elevated in those with chronic hepatitis, metastatic neoplasms, or vitamin K deficiency. Other studies, such as the presence of serum fucosylated AFP, hepatocyte growth factor, and tumor P-glycoprotein levels, may also be prognostic but await confirmation in larger trials.[6-8]

In common with surgery, patients with advanced disease and a poor performance status often tolerate other therapeutic modalities poorly as well. Cirrhosis is a relative contraindication to a major liver resection, as the degree of functional impairment depends on the severity of the cirrhosis. Cirrhosis is the predominant cause of perioperative morbidity and mortality in patients who have undergone a hepatic resection.[9-13] Some authors cite a more than 10-fold increase in hepatic insufficiency after resection in patients with cirrhosis compared to patients with otherwise normal livers[11]; moreover, liver failure in patients with cirrhosis is usually fatal.[9,14]

Cirrhosis alone is not a contraindication to chemotherapy, though other coexistent conditions may mitigate against offering any particular patient palliative antineoplastic chemotherapy. Other poor prognostic features are male sex, age over 50 years, a poor performance status, duration of symptoms of less than 3 months, tumor rupture, tumor cell aneuploidy, a high DNA synthesis rate, hypocalcemia, and a high serum AFP level.[15]

Chemotherapy

Virtually every available cytotoxic chemotherapeutic agent has been administered to patients with HCC, as single agents and in combination regimens. To date there is no evidence that any systemically administered agent or regimen has reproducible response rates in excess of 20% in selected patients, and systemic therapy has no effect on survival rates or duration. As unresectable HCC is virtually, by definition, incurable, the substantial risks of chemotherapy must be carefully balanced against the potential gains to be made in palliation. At present, as there is no "standard" therapeutic regimen that can be recommended, it would be justifiable to offer most patients participation in a clinical trial or symptomatic management.

Among the patients who receive chemotherapy, those who respond to the therapy appear to have some modest survival benefit over those who do not; some patients survive beyond a year. As most do not respond to therapy, it has been impossible to demonstrate any benefit of therapy to the population of HCC patients as a whole. Additionally, most patients with unresectable HCC who undergo chemotherapy have advanced (stage 3 or 4) disease (Table 3.1).

TABLE 3.1. Tumor/nodes/metastasis (TNM) staging system for hepatocellular cancer

Primary tumor (T)

Tx	Primary tumor cannot be assessed
T0	No evidence of primary tumor
T1	Solitary tumor ≤2 cm in greatest dimension without vascular invasion
T2	Solitary tumor ≤2 cm in greatest dimension with vascular invasion *or* Multiple lesions in one lobe of the liver without vascular invasion, none >2 cm in greatest dimension *or* Solitary lesion >2 cm in greatest dimension without vascular invasion
T3	Solitary tumor >2 cm in greatest dimension with vascular invasion, *or* Multiple tumors limited to one lobe, none >2 cm in greatest dimension, with vascular invasion *or* Multiple tumors limited to one lobe, any >2 cm in greatest dimension, with or without vascular invasion
T4	Multiple tumors in more than one lobe or tumor(s) involve(s) a major branch or portal or hepatic vein(s)

Lymph nodes (N)

Nx	Regional lymph nodes cannot be assessed
N0	No regional lymph node metastases
N1	Regional lymph node metastases

Distant metastasis (M)

Mx	Presence of distant metastasis cannot be assessed
M0	No distant metastasis
M1	Distant metastasis

Stage grouping

1	T1	N0	M0
2	T2	N0	M0
3	T1	N1	M0
	T2	N1	M0
	T3	N0	M0
	T3	N1	M0
4A	T4	Any N	M0
4B	Any T	Any N	M1

Source: American Joint Commission on Cancer.

Systemic Chemotherapy

Of all of the neoplastic agents, doxorubicin was initially thought to have significant activity, though subsequent trials have failed to confirm single-agent response rates in excess of 20%.[16-18] Other agents alone or in combination, such as etoposide, cisplatin, mitoxantrone, 5-fluorouracil with leucovorin, epirubicin, liposomal doxorubicin, or AG-337 (Thymitaq), have failed to produce response rates that exceed 20–30%.[19-26]

Combination chemotherapy, though more active and more efficacious in many other neoplasms, provides little added benefit to patients with HCC. Most regimens are based on doxorubucin or 5-fluorouracil (or both). Slightly higher response rates have been reported, but the average response rate is still between 20% and 30%. Most of these studies are small and nonrandomized, often with fewer than 40 patients. When conducted in this fashion, it is usually impossible to demonstrate any survival impact such a therapy may have if applied to a larger population of unselected patients.

Hepatic Arterial Infusion Chemotherapy

The concept of a regional approach to the therapy of malignancy originated in 1950 when Klopp and associates[27] and Bierman and coworkers[28] independently began to infuse nitrogen mustard into the arterial supply of various neoplasms. Hepatic arterial chemotherapy by infusion was developed by Watkins and Sullivan[29] and Sullivan and Zurek.[30] A Teflon catheter was placed in the common hepatic artery, and 5-fluorouracil (5-FU) or 2-deoxy-5-fluorouridine (FUDR) was administered with the aid of an external infusion pump. Although this and other early systems were relatively labor-intensive and subject to multiple complications, subsequent advances in techniques and technology now make this method of administering therapy a viable option for many patients with HCC confined to the liver.

Regional chemotherapy for the treatment of HCC or isolated hepatic metastases is attractive for several reasons: There is a dual blood supply to the liver; the liver has a relatively high tolerance to most chemotherapeutic agents; and there are specific pharmacokinetic features of the drugs utilized most often. Approximately 1.5–2.0 liters of blood flows through the liver each minute, of which two-thirds is supplied by the portal vein.[31] The blood supply for micrometastases and clinically undetectable HCC is derived equally from the hepatic artery and portal vein. Primary and secondary macroscopic malignancies in the liver receive almost all of their blood supply from the hepatic artery.[32,33] Much of this evidence has been determined from animal autopsy data and has also been confirmed in humans.

Nearly all chemotherapeutic agents have a low therapeutic index[34]; and in light of the limited efficacy of most chemotherapeutic agents against most solid tumors, the primary goal of regional chemotherapy is to deliver a higher concentration and total dose of the drug to the tumor bed than can be achieved safely by a systemic infusion. As most antineoplastic agents exhibit steep dose-response curves,[34-36] the ability to deliver higher doses locally should increase their cytocidal efficacy. At the same time, it is hoped that this may be accomplished while minimizing the toxicity to uninvolved tissues. In the liver, it is possible because of the extensive hepatic extraction of the drugs currently used, such as the fluorinated pyrimidines (5-FU and FUDR); and the level of first-pass extraction is a significant factor in reducing systemic toxicity. Most of the agents used for hepatic arterial infusional (HAI) chemotherapy also have high total body clearance and short plasma half-lives. On the basis of their pharmacokinetic profiles, drugs such as cisplatin, mitomycin C, and BCNU are good agents, with a four- to eightfold increase in drug exposure to the tumor bed using the hepatic arterial versus the intravenous route of administration; however, the agents most often utilized for hepatic arterial chemotherapy, 5-FU and FUDR, have a 10-

fold and 400-fold increase in drug exposure, respectively, when given by HAI.[36] Because of the substantial amount of drug extraction, the concentration of drug within normal hepatocytes usually exceeds that found in tumor tissue, where uptake may be heterogeneous. For example, Sigurdson et al. documented that the liver/tumor ratio of the FUDR concentration in metastatic colorectal carcinoma cells was 2.35:1.00.[37]

In general, HAI is well tolerated, and the usual chemotherapy-related toxicity is uncommon. When administered by HAI, the fluoropyrimidines do not cause myelosuppression; and although mitomycin C, the nitrosoureas, and the anthracyclines may cause a decrease in the platelet or granulocyte counts, the level of myelosuppression is much less than that observed when the same drugs are administered systemically. Diarrhea, nausea and vomiting, and stomatitis are uncommon but may be noted in the presence of significant arteriovenous shunting.

Although the liver is capable of tolerating high doses of chemotherapeutic agents owing to its large functional reserve and high regenerative capacity, intrahepatic chemotherapy is associated with an increased risk of hepatobiliary toxicity. Possibly the most notable, especially for its lack of reversibility, is biliary sclerosis. This complication has been observed occasionally with mitomycin C[38] but is most often seen when FUDR is infused at dosages exceeding 0.3 mg/kg/day for 14 consecutive days or more or if there is an elevation in alkaline phosphatase levels without concomitant cessation of the infusion. An increase in the serum bilirubin level usually occurs later in the course of biliary sclerosis. Radiographically, the disease resembles sclerosing cholangitis; the biliary tree may appear normal on ultrasound scans, but the diagnosis can usually be made by endoscopic retrograde cholangiopancreatography (ERCP). Stricture formation is most commonly found at the bifurcation of the common hepatic duct into the left and right hepatic bile ducts. It is not totally unexpected, as the bile duct in the region of the hepatic bifurcation is perfused by branches of the hepatic artery, whereas the more distal comon bile duct is supplied by branches of the gastroduodenal and superior mesenteric arteries.[39] Histologically, there is extensive bile duct fibrosis and necrosis as well as cholestasis; there is little or no evidence of hepatitis.[35,38]

The cause of the chemotherapy-related biliary sclerosis is not known. Although, as noted above, the bile ducts receive their blood flow predominantly from the hepatic artery and thus are exposed to high levels of the chemotherapeutic agent(s), some lines of evidence suggest a potential role for ischemia.[40,41] Many efforts have been undertaken to reduce the incidence of biliary sclerosis. Von Roemling and Hrushesky noted a decrease in biliary toxicity when FUDR was administered in a circadian pattern, with two-thirds of the daily dose being delivered between 1500 and 2100 hours,[42] although this result could not be verified in a phase I-II trial by Patt and Mavligit.[43] Hohn et al. showed that decreasing the daily FUDR dose from 0.34 mg/kg/day to 0.2 mg/kg/day or less delays the onset of cholestasis but does not necessarily prevent it.[44] Kemeny and coworkers were unable to demonstrate any reduction in biliary sclerosis when FUDR was infused simultaneously with dexamethasone,[45] although the addition of dexamethasone allowed the use of higher FUDR dosages. The treatment group demonstrated an increased response rate (71% vs. 40%), with a trend toward increased survival and decreased bilirubin elevations. Stagg, et al. also reported less biliary toxicity with their regimen in which FUDR (0.1 mg/kg/day) is administered for days 1–7, followed by arterial boluses of 5-FU (15 mg/kg) administered on days 15, 22, and 29, with the cycle repeating on day 35.[46] Regardless of the regimen utilized, the key to reducing the incidence of biliary sclerosis is to monitor the patient closely, with the serum bilirubin, alkaline phosphatase, and transaminase levels being evaluated on a weekly basis. A threefold increase in alkaline phosphatase above the patient's baseline level is an indication to stop therapy. An increase in bilirubin is also an indication to withhold treatment until the level normalizes. If FUDR is to be restarted, it should be at a low dose (0.05 mg/kg/day); and if there is no resulting elevation in the alkaline phosphatase or bilirubin level, the dose may be slowly increased.[35,44]

Another liver-related toxicity associated with HAI chemotherapy is chemical hepatitis. Unlike biliary sclerosis, this problem is usually reversible but requires temporary discontinuation of therapy, especially if there is a threefold or more increase in serum transaminase levels. Hyperbilirubinemia occurs in one-fourth of these patients who develop chemical hepatitis, and the serum transaminase and the alkaline phosphatase levels remain slightly elevated in 37%.[35]

Another adverse effect is acalculous chemical cholecystitis, which occurred in one-third of patients treated in earlier trials.[47] It is due to the fact that the cystic artery usually originates from either the right or left hepatic artery. At resection the gallbladder appears fibrotic and hypovascular. It is now common to perform a prophylactic cholecystectomy at the time of catheter placement to avoid this problem.

Gastritis and gastroduodenal ulceration are other complications of HAI; they occur when there is perfusion of the stomach and duodenum due to inadequate ligation of vessels emanating from the hepatic artery or because of malpositioning of a percutaneously placed catheter. Abdominal pain consistent with gastroduodenitis has been observed in up to 56% of patients in several series, but most trials have not rigorously evaluated this symptom with endoscopy.[48–50] In the trials where it has been evaluated, 20–40% of patients develop endoscopically documented ulcerations.[50–53] The use of the usual medications utilized for peptic ulcer disease, antacids and histamine (H_2) receptor blocking agents, appear to have little or no impact on the development of the ulcers, although they may provide some symptomatic relief. The problem may be completely avoided by meticulous gastroduodenal devascularization[54]; following dissection and cannulation of the gastroduodenal artery, fluorescein is injected into the pump side port, and the stomach and duodenum are inspected under Woods lamp ultraviolet illumination.

Toxic or technical complications are usually not limiting factors to the use of HAI. Rather, the presence of extrahepatic disease is such a factor and can hardly be expected to respond to HAI. Additionally, significant intrahepatic or intralesional arteriovenous shunting in HCC patients decreases the likelihood of an optimal response, as chemotherapeutic agents effectively bypass the liver; in this setting there is often a concomitant increase in systemic toxicity. Finally, the ability to utilize HAI may rarely be compromised by an aberrant hepatic arterial supply that cannot be effectively cannulated.

To effect a higher response rate and in an effort to increase patient survival, HAI chemotherapy has been investigated as an alternative treatment strategy. The initial studies with HAI utilized external pump devices and often required hospitalization. The average rate of response was nearly doubled to 50%, although reported response rates varied from 25% to 75%.[55,56] There was a substantial rate of complications, such as catheter dislocation, arterial thrombosis, and sepsis. Improvements in the technical aspects of percutaneous catheter placement and in the pump devices have now made intraarterial therapy a less hazardous and more economically viable alternative. The internalized (implanted) pump has several advantages over the older, external pumps, primarily in that there has been a decrease in catheter-related infections. Additionally, patients are no longer required to wear bulky external pumps, such as the original "Chronofusor," so patient comfort and acceptance have been enhanced.[56]

When determining whether a percutaneous angiographically placed catheter with a bedside pump or a surgically implanted pump is more desirable, cost analysis is appropriate. Patt and Mavligit reported a cost comparison analysis of a 5-day infusion of hepatic arterial infusion of FUDR with a surgically implanted group versus an implanted port with an external pump versus percutaneous drug administration.[43] The cost of the completely per-cutaneous route of drug administration, including serial preinfusion angiography, hospitalization, medications, and at least 5 days of patient immobilization each month, was nearly twice as much for 12 monthly treatments as for a completely implanted pump or the external pump system. After the initial device placement, patients with pumps or ports do not require subsequent hospitalization; and it is possible for these patients to maintain a normal life style while receiving the outpatient infusion. Notably, Doci and colleagues found that implantable pumps have a median duration of patency of 28 months, whereas the implanted port and external pump were patent for a median 9 months.[57] The increase in catheter patency is due to continuous flow from the pump into the vessel, thereby decreasing the chance of vascular occlusion. Of course, catheter patency is not an issue for percutaneously placed catheters, but a full 12 months of therapy may not be possible owing to an increased incidence of arterial occlusion. An additional advantage of the totally implantable system is the avoidance of continuous skin perforation, which is required with the implanted port and percutaneous catheter, thereby diminishing the risk of infectious complications.

In patients with HCC confined to the liver, reported response rates tend to be greater, often in the range of 30–50%, when agents are administered intraarterially.[1,58–62] Haskell and colleagues noted that the response rate for HCC patients treated with HAI of 5-FU or FUDR was 32%, compared to approximately 10% when the same agents were administered intravenously.[63] Additionally, the median survival for HCC patients treated with HAI of fluoropyrimidines was 8 months, compared to only 3 months for those who received the same agents intravenously. Even a single agent such as cisplatin, which is relatively inactive in HCC patients when administered systemically, has reported response rates of 40–50% when administered regionally.[1] Patt and associates performed a retrospective analysis of patients with HCC who were treated with HAI of a combination of FUDR, doxorubicin, and mitomycin C and compared them to patients who received intravenous 5-FU and doxorubicin-containing regimens.[64] The patients in the two groups were similar to terms of median age, ethnicity, performance status, AFP levels, cirrhosis, hepatitis B virus exposure, and liver function. The median survival for patients who received intraarterial therapy was nearly twice that of those who received intravenous therapy (9 months vs. 5 months, respectively). As this randomized trial was not prospective and only two regimens were compared, it is impossible to state with certainty that either route, or any regimen, is truly superior, though the results are highly suggestive. Patt and colleagues later reported a 50% response rate in HCC patients treated with a combination of FUDR, leucovorin, doxorubicin, and cisplatin administered by HAI over 4 days, though the regimen was highly toxic to patients who were hepatitis B (HBV)- or hepatitis C (HCV)-positive; significant dose reductions were required in this group.[65] Patients who had no serologic evidence of HBV or HCV exposure had a longer survival.

Even though HAI therapy is associated with a greater therapeutic index than systemic therapy, systemic toxicities still occur. In an effort to determine if higher dosages of therapy could safely be administered intraarterially, Curley and colleagues performed a phase I study of percutaneous complete hepatic venous isolation and extracorporeal chemotherapy filtration.[66] A double-balloon catheter was placed in the inferior vena to capture the total hepatic venous outflow and then pump this blood through extracorporeal carbon filters to reduce the systemic blood doxorubicin levels to approximately 14% of the prefilter (hepatic venous) levels. The system was well tolerated, and the maximum tolerated dose of doxorubicin in the system was determined to be 120 mg/m^2. Several other groups have built on this experience. Maeda's group reported the use of HAI of epirubicin and two courses of hepatic venous isolation with dose-intensive doxorubicin (with doses up to 150 mg/m^2) in a 58-year-old woman with HCC. She achieved a complete response to the therapy.[67] In a larger study, Iwasaki and associates compared the results of hepatic venous isolation to hepatic arterial embolization and to HAI chemotherapy.[68] Superior 1- and 2-year survival rates were noted for the group treated with hepatic venous isolation; but with fewer than 15 patients per study arm it is difficult to determine what potential clinical impact these findings could have on a larger population of patients with unresectable HCC.

Hormonal Manipulation

Despite the possibility that the initiation and growth of HCC may depend on sex steroids, hormonal manipulation therapy has produced few if any objective responses. For example, despite the survival benefits suggested in several small studies using the antiestrogen tamoxifen in HCC patients,[69-71] subsequent larger studies failed to demonstrate any antitumor effect or survival benefit.[72-74] The tamoxifen dose utilized in the trial reported by Castells and associates, 20 mg/day,[73] was initially thought to be too low.[75] However, the estrogen receptor levels in HCC are usually low, and the dose of tamoxifen utilized should have been sufficient to cause receptor blockade. Additionally, evidence suggests that some HCCs are characterized by the production of a variant species of the estrogen receptor, lacking in exon 5, which binds estradiol poorly (if at all).[76,77] Villa and associates stated that the tumors that expressed the wild-type estrogen receptor responded to tamoxifen, whereas those that expressed the variant receptor responded preferentially to megestrol.[77] In contrast, Colleoni and coworkers found no objective responses to megestrol acetate in HCC patients.[78] A final suggestion is that tamoxifen may inhibit tumor growth by mechanisms other than estrogen receptor blockade, although higher concentrations may be required to achieve this effect.[75] Likewise, although the antiandrogen cyproterone acetate has inhibited the growth of the androgen-receptor-positive human HCC cell line (KYN-1/SM-10) xenografted into nude mice,[79] and Forbes and coworkers noted responses in 5 of 19 patients treated with cyproterone acetate,[80] attempts at therapy with ketoconazole have been unrewarding.[81]

Recombinant human interferon-α (IFNα) has been utilized in several trials. The Gastrointestinal Tumor Study Group administered IFNα to 30 patients with HCC and documented a 7% response rate.[82] Creagan and coworkers administered IFNα with doxorubicin to seven patients with a variety of solid tumors and noted a partial response in the one patient with HCC.[83] Lai et al. conducted a randomized trial of doxorubicin versus two schedules of IFNα in HCC patients and reported a 10% response rate with IFNα but no responses with doxorubicin.[84] There was no statistical difference between the median survival of the two groups (doxorubicin 4.8 weeks, IFNα 8.3 weeks). An interesting finding was noted in a study of HCC patients by Patt and colleagues, where a combination of 5-FU and recombinant human IFNα produced measurable antitumor responses in patients with low serum AFP levels.[85] This regimen was essentially inactive in patients with serum AFP levels in excess of 50 ng/dl or in those whose tumors had a diameter of more than 10 cm.

Immunotherapy

Several authors have attempted to use biologic response-modifying agents, cytokines and adoptive immunotherapy or both in HCC patients to effect a response. Most of the larger studies have included a few patients with HCC among a larger group of patients with metastatic disease. Hazama and associates reported the results of a combination of chemotherapy and biologic response modifiers in a cohort of nine patients with unresectable HCC.[86] Patients received interleukin-2 (IL-2), OK-432, and doxorubicin via an implantable pump into the hepatic artery; they also received cyclophosphamide, OK-432, and famotidine by systemic intravenous infusion. Transient fevers and hypotension were noted, but there was no evidence of substantial organ dysfunction. Of these nine patients, three achieved a complete response and two others a minor response. Han treated five HCC patients with systemic IL-2 and either autologous or homologous lymphokine activated killer (LAK) cells administered through the hepatic artery.[87] Three patients were noted to have a partial response. Matsuhashi and associates treated five HCC patients with a combination of hepatic arterial infusion of IL-2 and LAK cells and noted partial responses in two of the patients.[88] Fagan and colleagues reported the intraarterial administration of Il-2 and LAK cells in two patients with HCC and an intralesional injection of IL-2 in a third.[89] Although all three patients experienced at least a transient improvement in their performance status and a decrease in their serum AFP levels, no objective tumor responses were noted. Komatsu et al. treated nine HCC patients with a combination of IL-2 and LAK cells administered into the hepatic artery and observed one partial response.[90]

Adjuvant Therapies

In light of the poor long-term survival rates reported by most surgical trials after resection of HCC, there have been several small studies on postsurgical adjuvant therapy. For example, Yamamoto and colleagues reported the results of randomized controlled administration of 1-hexylcarbamoyl-5-fluorouracil in 67 patients following resection of HCC.[91] Even though a significant survival benefit was noted among patients who received adjuvant treatment compared to controls, the number of evaluable patients ($n = 55$) was small; these results await confirmation in a larger controlled trial. In a separate study, Takenaka and associates assigned 48 HCC patients who had undergone hepatic resection to three therapy groups: (1) no chemotherapy; (2) oral 5-FU derivatives (tegafur with uracil, or 1-hexylcarbamoyl-5-fluorouracil); or (3) HAI of Lipiodol with epirubicin.[92] Though the numbers of patients in each group were small, the 3-year disease-free survival in the group receiving hepatic arterial therapy was significantly higher than that for patients who received no further therapy. Patients treated with oral fluoropyrimidine therapy had disese-free survival that fell between the HAI and the no-treatment groups. Olthoff et al. treated 25 HCC patients who had undergone orthotopic liver transplantation with a 6-month course of intravenous 5-FU, doxorubicin, and cisplatin and noted an improved 3-year survival (46% vs. 5.8%) compared to historic controls.[93]

As HCCs produce both the retinoic acid receptor and the retinoid X receptor, attempts have been made to affect the disease through the use of retinoids. Despite a negative experience reported by the Southwest Oncology Group with [trans]-retinoic acid in HCC patients,[94] Muto and associates prospectively studied 89 patients with HCC randomized to either adjuvant polyprenoic acid or a placebo.[95] All patients had been previously treated with surgical resection or percutaneous ethanol injection. With a median follow-up of 38 months, 27% of the patients who had received polyprenoic acid experienced a disease recurrence or a new HCC, whereas those who had received placebo had a 49% incidence of disease recurrence or a second primary HCC. As with the trial by Yamamoto et al.,[91] these results are promising but must be confirmed in a larger clincial trial.

Conclusions

It is obvious that other than surgical resection for properly selected patients there is no standard therapy for HCC. There are myriad options for patients with unresectable disease limited to the liver, but none has yet been proved superior. The choice of treatment strategy depends on the condition of the patient and the experience of the health care team in each institution. Unfortunately, the outlook for those patients with extrahepatic disease remains bleak. Although much of the investigation into new agents and therapeutic strategies should continue, perhaps the best utilization of time, money, and effort would be directed at eradicating the potential etiologic factors that account for most cases of HCC: HBV vaccination programs, improvement in grain storage and handling facilities to reduce contamination by *Aspergillus* species, easier access to treatment programs for the alcoholic patient, and developing more effective strategies for screening high risk populations. These measures would have the greatest impact on reducing the large-scale suffering caused by HCC around the globe. For this disease an "ounce of prevention" would be well worth more than a "pound of cure."

References

1. Carr BI, Flickinger JC, Lotze MT. Hepatobiliary cancers. In: DeVita VT, Hellman S, Rosenberg SA (eds) Cancer; Principles and Practice of Oncology, 5th ed. Philadelphia, Lippincott-Raven, 1997, pp. 1087–1114
2. Beasley RP. Hepatitis B virus as the etiologic agent in hepatocellular carcinoma—epidemiologic considerations. Hepatology 2(suppl):21S, 1982

3. Kew MC, Rossouw E, Hodkinsson J, et al. Hepatitis B virus status of Southern African blacks with hepatocellular carcinoma: comparison between rural and urban populations. Hepatology 3:65, 1983

4. Tsukuma H, Hiyama T, Tanaka S, et al. Risk factors for hepatocellular carcinoma among patients with chronic liver disease. N Engl J Med 328:1797, 1993

5. Parker SL, Tong T, Bolden S, Wingo PA. Cancer statistics, 1007. CA Cancer J Clin. 47:5, 1997

6. Yamashita F, Tanaka M, Satomura S, Tanikawa K. Prognostic significance of Lens culinaris agglutinin A-reactive α-fetoprotein in small hepatocellular carcinomas. Gastroenterology 111:996, 1996

7. Yamazaki H, Oi H, Matsumoto K, et al. Biphasic changes in serum hepatocyte growth factor after transarterial chemoembolization therapy for hepatocellular carcinoma. Cytokine 8:178, 1996

8. Soini Y, Virkajärvi N, Raunio H, Pääkkö P. Expression of P-glycoprotein in hepatocellular carcinoma: a potential marker of prognosis. J Clin Pathol 49:470, 1996

9. Wong J, Choi TK. Primary liver cell cancer—Asian experience. In: Blumgart LH (ed) Surgery of the Liver and Biliary Tract. New York, Churchill Livingstone, 1988, pp.1135–1151

10. Ong GB. Techniques and therapies for primary and metastatic liver cancer. In: Hickey RC (ed) Current Problems in Cancer, Vol 2. Chicago, Year Book, 1977, pp. 1–48

11. Lin TY. Resectional therapy for primary malignant hepatic tumors. In: Murphy GP (ed) International Advances in Surgical Oncology. New York, Liss, 1979, pp. 25–54

12. Garrison RN, Cryer HM, Howard DA, Polk HC Jr. Clarification of risk factors for abdominal operations in patients with hepatic cirrhosis. Ann Surg 199: 648, 1984

13. Okuda K, Obata H, Nakajima Y, et al. Prognosis of primary hepatocellular carcinoma. Hepatology 4:3S, 1984

14. Tsuzuki T, Ogata Y, Iida S, Shimazu M. Hepatic resection in 125 patients. Arch Surg 119:1025, 1984

15. Dalton RR, Eisenberg BL. Surgical management of recurrent liver tumors. Semin Oncol 20:493, 1993

16. Sciarrino E, Simonetti R, LeMoli S, et al. Adriamycin treatment for hepatocellular carcinoma: experience with 109 patients. Cancer 56:2751, 1985

17. Chlebowski rT, Brzechwa-Adjukiewica A, Cowden A, et al. Doxorubicin (75 mg/m^2) for 2: clinical and pharmacokinetic results. Cancer Treat Rep 68:487, 1984

18. Ihde DC, Kane RC, Cohen MN, et al. Adriamycin therapy in American patients with hepatocellular carcinoma. Cancer Treat Rep 61:1385, 1977

19. Bing-hui Y, Zhao-you T. Randomized clinical trial of cisplatin in the treatment of hepatocellular carcinoma. In: Zhao-you T, Meng-chao W, Sui-sheng X (eds) Primary Liver Cancer. New York, Springer, 1989, pp. 434–437

20. Okada S, Okazaki N, Nose H, et al. A phase 2 study of cisplatin in patients with HCC. Oncology 50:22, 1993

21. Falkson G, Moertel CG, Lavin P, Pretorius FJ, Carbone PP. Chemotherapy studies in primary liver cancer: a prospective randomized trial. Cancer 42:2149, 1978

22. Melia WM, Johnson PJ, Williams R. Induction of remission in hepatocellular

carcinoma: a comparison of etoposide (VP16) with adriamycin. Cancer 51:206, 1983

23. Shiu WCT. Primary liver cancer in Hong Kong. Cancr Chemother Pharmacol 31(suppl 1):S143, 1992

24. Porta C, Moroni M, Nastasi G, Arcangeli G. 5-Fluorouracil and d,I-leucovorin calcium are active to treat unresectable hepatocellular carcinoma patients: preliminary results of a phase II study. Oncology 52:487, 1995

25. Khoo KS, Au E, Koo WH, et al. Phase II study of NSC 620212-doxorubicin HCI liposome injection (Lipodox) in hepatocellular carcinoma (HCC) [abstract 546]. Proc Am Soc Clin Oncol 15:226, 1996

26. Stuart KE, Hajdenberg J, Cohn A, et al. A phase II trial of Thymitaq™ (AG337) in patients wit h hepatocellular carcinoma (HCC) [abstract 449]. Proc Am Soc Clin Oncol 15:202, 1996

27. Klopp CT, Alford TL, Bateman J, Berry GN, Winship T. Fractionated intra-arterial cancer chemotherapy with methyl-bis-amine hydrochloride: a preliminary report. Ann Surg 132:811, 1950

28. Bierman HR, Byron RL, Miller FR, et al. Effects of intra-arterial administration of nitrogen mustard. Am J Med 8:535, 1950

29. Watkins E Jr, Sullivan RD. Cancer chemotherapy by prolonged arterial infusion. Surg Gynecol Obst 118:3, 1964

30. Sullivan RD, Zurek WZ. Chemotherapy for liver cancer by protracted ambulatory infusion. JAMA 194:481, 1965

31. Aeberhard P. Intraarterial chemotherapy with pump. Antibiot Chemother 210:41, 1988

32. Honjo I, Matsumura H. Vascular distribution of hepatic tumors. Rev Int Hepatol 15:681, 1965

33. Ackerman NB. The blood supply of experimental liver metastases. IV. Changes in vascularity with increasing tumor growth. Surgery 75:589, 1975

34. Frei E III, Canellos GP. Dose: a critical factor in cancer chemotherapy. Am J Med 69:585, 1980

35. Kemeny N, Schneider A. Regional treatment of hepatic metastases and hepatocellular carcinoma. Curr Probl Cancer 13:197, 1989

36. Ensminger WD, Gyves JW. Clinical pharmacology of hepatic arterial chemotherapy. Semin Oncol 10:176, 1983

37. Sigurdson ER, Ridge JA, Daly JM. Fluorodeoxyuridine uptake by human colorectal hepatic metastases after hepatic artery infusion. Surgery 100:285, 1986

38. Hohn DC, Shea WJ, Gemlo BT, et al. Complications and toxicities of hepatic arterial chemotherapy. Contr Oncol 29:169, 1988

39. Northover JM, Terblanche J. A new look at the arterial supply of the bile duct in man and its surgical implications. Br J Surg 66:379, 1979

40. Doppman JL, Girton ME. Bile duct scarring following ethanol embolization of the hepatic artery: an experimental study in monkeys. Radiology 152:621, 1984

41. Pettave, J. Gardiol D, Bergier N, Schnyder P. Necrosis of main bile ducts caused by hepatic artery infusion of 5-fluore-2deoxyuridine. Reg Cancer Treat 1?83, 1988

42. Von Roemling R, Hrushesky WJM. Determination of therapeutic index of floxuridine by its circadian infusion pattern. J Natl Cancer Inst 82:386, 1990

43. Patt YZ, Mavligit GM. Arterial chemotherapy in the management of colorectal cancer: an overview. Semin Oncol 18:478, 1991

44. Hohn DC, Rayner AA, Economou JS, et al. Toxicities and complications of implanted pump hepatic arterial and intravenous floxuridine infusion. Cancer 57:465, 1986

45. Kemeny N, Seiter K, Niedzwiecki D, et al. A randomized trial of intrahepatic infusion of fluorodeoxyuridine with dexamethasone versus fluorodeoxyuridine alone in the treatment of metastatic colorectal cancer. Cancer 69:327, 1992

46. Stagg RJ, Venook AP, Chase JL, et al. Alternating hepatic intraarterial FUDR and 5FU: a less toxic regimen for treatment of liver metastases from colorectal cancer. J Natl Cancer Inst 8:423, 1991

47. Kemeny MM, Goldberg D, Beatty JD, et al. Results of a prospective randomized trial of continuous regional chemotherapy and hepatic resection as treatment of hepatic metastases from colorectal primaries. Cancer 57:492, 1986

48. Ensminger WD. Intra-arterial therapy of hepatic metastases. In: Howell SB (ed) Intra-arterial and Intracavitary Cancer Chemotherapy. Boston, Martinus Nijhoff, 1984, PP. 71–76.

49. Niederhuber JE, Ensminger WD, Gyves JW, et al. Regional chemotheapy of colorectal cancer to the liver. Cancer 53:1336, 1984

50. Shepard KV, Levin B, Karl RC, et al. Therapy for metastatic colorectal cancer with hepatic artery infusion chemotherapy using a subcutaneous implanted pump. J Clin Oncol 3:161, 1985

51. Weiss GR, Garnick MB, Osteen RT, et al. Long-term hepatic arterial infusion of 5-fluorodeoxyuridine for liver metastases using an implantable infusion pump. J Clin Oncol 1:337, 1983

52. Ramming KP, O'Toole K. The use of the implantable chemoinfusion pump in the treatment of hepatic metastases of colorectal cancer. Arch Surg 121:1400, 1986

53. Cohen AM, Kaufman SD, Wood RC, et al. Regional hepatic chemotherapy using an implantable drug infusion pump. Am J Surg 145:529, 1983

54. Hohn DC, Melnick J, Stagg R, et al. Biliary sclerosis in patients receiving hepatic arterial infusions of floxuridine. J Clin Oncol 3:98, 1985

55. Smiley S, Schouten J, Change A, et al. Intrahepatic arterial infusion with 5-FU for liver metastases of colorectal carcinoma. Proc ASCO 22:391, 1981

56. Reed ML, Vaitkevicius VK, Al-Sarraf M, et al. The practicality of chronic hepatic artery infusion therapy of primary and metastatic hepatic malignancies. Cancer 47:402, 1981

57. Doci R, Bignami R, Quagliuolo V, et al. Continuous hepatic arterial infusion with 5-fluorodeoxyuridine for treatment of colorectal metastases. Reg Cancer Treat 3:3, 1990

58. Al-Sharraf M, Leo TS, Kithier K, et al. Primary liver cancer. Cancer 33:574, 1974

59. Yanagi I, Koga A, Okuda K, et al. The study of continuous arterial infusion chemotherapy with CDDP and 5-FU in patients with hepatocellular carcinoma. Gan To Kagaku Ryoho [Jpn J Cancer Chemother] 22:1508, 1995

60. Une Y, Shinamura T, Kamiyama T, et al. Effects of chemotherapy after hepatectomy in hepatic cancer patients. Gan To Kagaku Ryoho [Jpn J Cancer Chemother] 22:1037, 1995

61. Toyoda H, Nakano S, Kumada T, et al. The efficacy of continuous local arterial infusion of 5-fluorouracil and cisplatin through an implanted reservoir for severe advanced hepatocellular carcinoma. Oncology 52:295, 1995

62. Okusaka T, Okada S, Ishii H, et al. Phase II trial of zinostatin stimalamer (SMANCS) with or without embolization using gelatin sponge for hepatocellular carcinoma (HCC) [abstract 440]. Proc Am Soc Clin Oncol 15:200, 1996

63. Haskell CM, Lavey RS, Ramming KP. Liver. In: Haskell CM (ed) Cancer Treatment. 4th ed. Philadelphia, Saunders, 1995, p. 512

64. Patt YZ, Claghorn L, Charnsangavej C, et al. Hepatocellular cancer: a retrospective analysis of treatments to manage disease confined to the liver. Cancer 61:1884, 1988

65. Patt YZ, Charnsangavej C, Yoffe B, et al. Hepatic arterial infusion of floxuridine, leucovorin, doxorubicin, and cisplatin for hepatocellular carcinoma; effects of hepatitis B and C viral infection on drug toxicity and patient survival. J Clin Oncol 12: 1204, 1994

66. Curley SA, Newman RA, Dougherty TB, et al. Complete hepatic venous isolation and extracorporeal chemofiltration as treatment for human hepatocellular carcinoma: a phase I study. Ann Surg Oncol 1:389, 1994

67. Kitagawa T, Ku Y, Maeda I, et al. A case of advanced hepatoma cured by repeated percutaneous isolated liver perfusion using hepatic venous isolation and charcoal hemoperfusion. Gan To Kagaku Ryoho [Jpn J Cancer Chemother] 23:1592, 1996

68. Iwasaki T, Ku Y, Tominaga M, et al. The effect of high-dose intraarterial chemotherapy with percutaneous hepatic venous isolation and charcoal hemoperfusion (HVI.CHP) for unresectable multiple hepatocellular carcinoma—comparison with other therapeutic modalities. Gan To Kagaku Ryoho [Jpn J Cancer Chemother] 23:1426, 1996

69. Farinati F, Salvagnini M, de Maria N, et al. Unresectable hepatocellular carcinoma: a prospective controlled trial with tamoxifen. J Hepatol 11:297, 1990

70. Martines-Cerezo FJ, Tomás A, Donos L, et al. Controlled trial of tamoxifen in patients with advanced hepatocellular carcinoma. J Hepatol 20:702, 1994

71. Elba S, Giannuzzi V, Misciagna G, Manghisi OG. Randomized controlled trial of tamoxifen versus placebo in inoperable hepatocellular carcinoma. Ital J Gastroenterol 48:876, 1994

72. Melia WM, Johnson PJ, Williams R. Controlled clinical trial of doxorubicin and tamoxifen versus doxorubicin alone in hepatocellular carcinoma. Cancer Treat Rev 71:1213, 1987

73. Castells A, Bruix J, Brú C, et al. Treatment of hepatocellular carcinoma with tamoxifen: a double-blind placebo-controlled trial in 120 patients. Gastroenterology 109:917, 1995

74. Engstrom PF, Levin B, Moertel CG, Shott A. A phase II trial of tamoxifen in hepatocellular carcinoma. Cancer 65:2641, 1990

75. Farinati F. Tamoxifen treatment in hepatocellular carcinoma [letter]. Gastroenterology 111:272, 1996

76. Villa E, Dugani A, Fantoni E, et al. Type of estrogen receptor determines response to antiestrogen therapy. Cancer Res 56:3883, 1996

77. Villa E, Camellini L, Dugani A, Buttafoco A, Manenti F. Variant liver estrogen and response to tamoxifen [letter]. Gastroenterology 111:271, 1996

78. Colleoni M, Nelli P, Vicario G, Mastropasqua G, Manente P. Megestrol acetate in unresectable hepatocellular carcinoma. Tumori 81:351, 1995

79. Nagasue N, Yu L, Yamaguchi M, et al. Inhibition of growth and induction of

TGF-β_1 in human hepatocellular carcinoma with androgen receptor by cyproterone acetate in male nude mice. J Hepatol 25:554, 1996

80. Forbes A. Wilkinson ML, Iqbal MJ, Johnson PJ, Williams R. Response to cyproterone acetate treatment in primary hepatocellular carcinoma is related to fall in free 5α-dihydrotestosterone. Eur J Cancer Clin Oncol 23:295, 1987

81. Gupta S, Korula J. Failure of ketoconazole as anti-androgen therapy in nonresectable primary hepatocellular carcinoma. J Clin Gastroenterol 10:651, 1988

82. Gastrointestinal Tumor Study Group. A prospective trial of recombinant human interferon alpha 2B in previously untreated patients with hepatocellular carcinoma. Cancer 66:135, 1990

83. Creagan ET, Long HJ, Frytak S, Moertel CG. Recombinant leucocyte A interferon with doxorubicin: a phase I study in advanced solid neoplasms and implications for hepatocellular carcinoma. Cancer 61:19, 1988

84. Lai C-L, Wu P-C, Lok AS-F, et al. Recombinant α_2-interferon is superior to doxorubicin for inoperable hepatocellular carcinoma: a prospective randomised trial. Br J Cancer 60:928, 1989

85. Patt YZ, Yoffe B, Charnsangavej C, et al. Low serum alpha fetoprotein level in patients with hepatocellular carcinoma as a predictor of response to 5FU and interferon alpha 2b. Cancer 72:2574, 1993

86. Hazama S, Oka M, Shimizu R, et al. Intra-arterial combination immunotherapy in hepatocellular carcinoma. Gan To Kagaku Ryoho [Jpn J Cancer Chemother] 17:1638, 1990

87. Han FG. Treatment of advanced liver cancer by autologous and/or homologous LAK cells combined with human natural IL-2. Chin J Oncol 13:145, 1991

88. Matsuhashi N, Moriyama T, Nakamura I, et al. Adoptive immunotherapy of primary and metastatic liver cancer via hepatic artery catheter. Eur J Cancer 26:1106, 1990

89. Fagan EA, Pulley M, Limb A, et al. Adoptive immunotherapy administered via the hepatic artery and intralesional interleukin-2 in hepatocellular carcinoma. Cancer Treat Rev 16:151, 1989

90. Komatsu T, Yamauchi K, Furukawa T, Obata H. Transcatheter arterial injection of autologous lymphokine-activated killer (LAK) cells into patients with liver cancers. J Clin Immunol 10:167, 1990

91. Yamamoto M, Arii S, Sugahara K, Tobe T. Adjuvant oral chemotherapy to prevent recurrence after curative resection for hepatocellular carcinoma. Br J Surg 83:336, 1996

92. Takenaka K, Yoshida K, Nishizaki T, et al. Postoperative prophylactic lipiodolization reduces the intrahepatic recurrence of hepatocellular carcinoma. Am A Surg 169:400, 1995

93. Olthoff KM, Rosove MH, Shackleton CR, et al. Adjuvant chemotherapy improves survival after liver transplantation for hepatocellular carcinoma. Ann Surg 221:734, 1995

94. Meyskens FL Jr, Nguyen B, Jacobson J, Macdonald J. Phase II trial of b-transretinoic acid (TRA) in primary hepatomas (SWOG 9157) [abstract]. Proc Am Soc Clin Oncol 15:229, 1996

95. Muto Y, Moriwaki H, Ninomiya M, et al. Prevention of second primary tumors by an acyclic retinoid, polyprenoic acid, in patients with hepatocellular carcinoma. N Engl J Med 334:1561, 1996

4

Use of Chemoradiation for Management of Cholangiocarcinoma

Tyvin A. Rich

External beam irradiation (ExBRT) for management of biliary tract cancers has been used most often for palliation of localized symptoms of pain, bleeding, and obstruction and less frequently as radical treatment for patients with unresectable disease. Adjuvant irradiation has been given either before or after surgical resection in an effort to reduce local recurrence. In either situation, high-dose ExBRT is required and should be given with precise treatment planning and multiple beams. Conformal irradiation is a new technique used at a few institutions that may improve the results because higher total ExBRT doses can be given safely. Another way to deliver higher-dose radiation in patients with drainage access to the biliary tree is with endoluminl radioactive implants, which can be combined with ExBRT to deliver highly localized treatment.

The combined approach with ExBRT and concurrent chemotherapy (chemoradiation) has been investigated. Chemoradiation has been used mainly in the postoperative setting after the patient has been staged surgically. Data on the use of preoperative chemoradiation are available that parallel the development of this treatment approach for other gastrointestinal malignancies; hence the technique should be explored further.

Staging and Patterns of Failure After Surgical Resection

Assessment of the anatomic extent of disease prior to irradiation is accomplished by cholangiography, computed tomography (CT), and magnetic resonance imaging (MRI), which are described elsewhere in this volume. Radiographic information is crucial for successful radiotherapy planning because of the adjacent location of multiple radiosensitive structures.

A surgical report describing the anatomic extent of disease is also a necessary part of successful treatment planning. Another useful surgical technique is the placement of radiopaque clips for treatment planning even during the era of CT planning, as precise delineation of the tumor is often difficult to image within the porta hepatis. Surgery also provides the best means of histologic diagnosis; but when surgical staging is not available, a diagnosis can be obtained by CT-guided needle biopsy or by brushings of the biliary tree obtained by radiographic or endoscopic methods.

Jaundice can be relieved by internal or external catheter drainage or by surgical intervention. All of these means of drainage have been combined successfully with external irradiation. Because the diagnosis and palliation of jaundice can be frequently established without surgical intervention, there may be uncertainly when staging the anatomic extent of disease.

Radiotherapy for tumors of the biliary ducts and gallbladder requires an understanding of the pathways of tumor spread. The submucosal lymphatics within the biliary ductal system provide a pathway for regional spread to the lymphatics of the porta hepatitis, pancreaticoduodenal region, celiac axis, superior mesenteric vessels and the upper paraaortic region.[1-4]

Direct tumor invasion of the liver, porta hepatis blood vessels, or the pancreas is frequently associated with unresectable disease. Residual microscopic or gross disease may remain after surgery because of anatomic constraints for en bloc resection. The frequency of this problem is illustrated in the review of major surgical series, which shows that residual disease remaining after resection is related to the anatomic site of the tumor. For example, the percentage of patients with positive surgical margins was 76% in those with perihilar cancers but only 10% in those with distal biliary disease.[2] Similar findings are seen in other surgical series and indicate that surgical cure is significantly correlated with the ability to achieve a curative resection and with the extent of the resection (Table 4.1). The status of surgical margins and residual disease also appears to be related to overall survival for patients with biliary tract cancers. One implication of these data is that a reduction in the rate of R-1 and R-2 resections (those with microscopic

TABLE 4.1. Recent results of surgical treatment of cholangiocarcinoma (selected series)

Institution	Anatomic location	Positive margins (%)	Lymph nodes positive	5-year survival (%)
Johns Hopkins University Hospital[2]	Intrahepatic ($m = 9$)	22	None	~45
	Perihilar ($m = 109$)	74	6/45[a] (13%)	~12
	Distal bile duct ($m = 73$)	10	35/67[a] (52%)	~30
Mayo Clinic[1] (curative resections only)	Proximal ($m = 13$)			~50
	Mid-duct ($m = 14$)			~30
	Distal ($m = 22$)			~45
Medizinische Hochschule, Hannover[3]	Proximal ($m = 125$)			42 (stage I/II) 21 (stage IV)

[a]Lymph node status available for only a subgroup.

or macroscopic disease remaining after resection, respectively) may improve local control as well as affect survival favorably.

In patients undergoing resection, tumor transection or ductal instrumentation through gross tumor increases the risk of diffuse peritoneal seeding or surgical scar implantation.[5] Locoregional failure also appears to be correlated with transmural tumor spread, irrespective of tumor grade, as the local failure rate increased from 36% to 64% for patients with disease confined to the wall of the bile duct versus those with transmural disease. Other risk factors for local failure are positive lymph node status, perineural or microvascular invasion, and direct tumor extension into the liver.

Irradiation Alone: Rationale and Techniques

The treatment planning for cancers in this region must respect normal tissue tolerances of the stomach, small intestine, kidney, and spinal cord. Modest doses of radiation (45–50 Gy) can be achieved by ExBRT with or without a boost using fixed multiple-field or rotational-field treatment.[6] The use of an endoluminal radioactive impant is used for palliation or as a boost after ExBRT, although in the first situation it does not provide effective treatment for bulky disease.[6,7] A typical ExBRT CT treatment plan is shown in Figure 4.1. The field arrangement covers the primary tumor site, porta hepatis, celiac axis, and paraaortic lymph notes. ExBRT to 45–50 Gy can be delivered with this approach and may be followed by a more complex treatment plan. Complex treatment planning to the biliary tree with precision therapy can be achieved while limiting the dose to the normal liver and the small intestine. High doses can now be achieved more safely with the use of conformal ExBRT, a technique that tailors the irradiation portal to the disease process with the aid of three-dimensional computerized treatment planning. For treatment of unresectable bile duct cancers, the use of ExBRT doses of more than 45–55 Gy achieves local palliation and results in median survival times ranging from 10 to 12 months.[8,9]

The utility of a postoperative dose of 50 Gy following resection of an extrahepatic bile duct tumor has been tested prospectively against surgical resection alone at Johns Hopkins University Hospital, and no benefit of adjuvant radiation treatment was shown.[10] This negative study may have been a result of the use of a modest total radiation dose. Because ExBRT doses of more than 50 Gy can result in unacceptable levels of intestinal damage, it is necessary that we evaluate methods to increase the dose without producing increased morbidity.

One specialized technique used in conjunction with ExBRT is electron beam intraoperative radiotherapy boost (EB-IORT).[11] This technique concentrates irradiation directly in the tumor bed, and the uninvolved liver and gastrointestinal tract are moved aside during surgery. In patients with resected biliary cancers, EB-IORT alone resulted in an improved survival rate com-

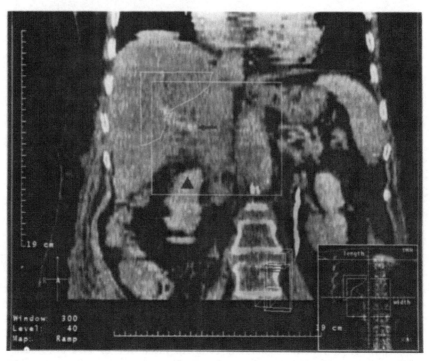

FIGURE 4.1-A.

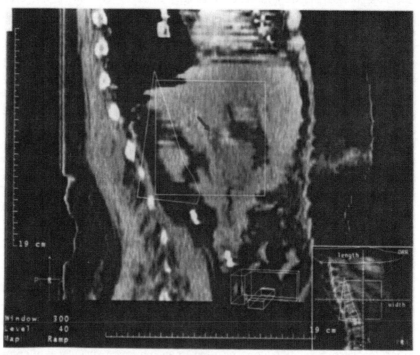

FIGURE 4.1-B.

pared to those treated with surgery alone.[12] In other studies from North America, EB-IORT boost has been used in combination with ExBRT.[5,13] The Mayo Clinic reported survivals of 23 and 6 months, respectively, for two patients with unresectable bile duct cancer after treatment with a 15- to 20-Gy intraoperative electron boost (with 9–15 MeV).[5] In a larger study from Rush-Presbyterian St. Luke's Medical center in Chicago, nine patients with advanced proximal biliary cancers were treated with EB-IORT.[13] Patients were considered for IORT if they had residual gross or microscopic disease confined to the region of the porta hepatis or if there was adjacent hepatic involvement. The field size was 7–10 cm in diameter, and the IORT dose was 10–22 Gy. Additional external beam irradiation was undertaken in five patients. The patients treated with EB-IORT were compared with concurrent groups treated without radiation or with external beam irradiation with or without iridium‾192 endoluminal boost irradiation. There was a significant improvement in the median survival rate for patients receiving high-dose radiation, regardless of boost technique, compared with those who were not irradiated (11–13 months versus 4.6 months, respectively).

An alternative specialized treatment technique is endoluminal irradiation, which has been used principally for palliation or as a boost after surgical resection and ExBRT.[14] Endoluminal does have ranged from 15 to 35 Gy when combined with external beam irradiation (usually 45–50 Gy); alternatively, endoluminal doses of up to 50–60 Gy have been used alone. The dose reference point may vary from 0.5 to 1.0 cm from the central catheter. The total nominal doses of external beam plus boost radiation are thus more than 60–70 Gy to the tumor; although this range exceeds the tolerance of the liver and small intestine, the highest doses are confined to a small volume and do not affect these organs. The treatment can also be given with high-dose rate iridium‾192 (selection HDR 192Ir; Nucletron, Columbia, MD) implants in a fractionated treatment schedule of 4 Gy/day x 5 days. The fractionated high-dose rate treatment, along with the favorable dose distribution obtained with endoluminal therapy, may also decrease late-occurring duodenitis. For patients in whom there are technical or medical limitations for fractionated therapy, a single 20-Gy boost with the high-dose technique can be used.

The median survival times for patients treated with endoluminal irradiation alone can range from 10 to 17 months, and the high rate of durable relief of jaundice indicates that good palliation can be achieved in these

FIGURE 4.1. (A) CT simulation radiograph showing coverage of the porta hepatis. There is contrast in the portal vein (arrow) that is visualized on this reconstructed image. The anterior field is designed to cover the paraaortic lymph nodes at this anatomic level by crossing over the midline. Note the coverage of the upper pole of the right kidney (arrowhead). (B) Lateral CT simulation radiograph corresponding to the anterior field shown in (A). The field is centered on the porta hepatis (arrow). A block was placed posteriorly to shield the kidney.

patients. Several long-term survivors have been reported after treatment with total gross excision and total ExBRT doses of more than 60 Gy delivered with a combination of ExBRT and specialized boost. Although a few survive more than 3–4 years, most patients fail with local disease progression.

Total ExBRT doses for biliary tract cancers are limited by the volume of irradiation imposed by the adjacent normal tissues. Whole-liver irradiation with doses higher than 30 Gy may result in radiation hepatitis and fatality.[15] For treatment of intrahepatic biliary tract cancers, the total dose to the whole liver is still limited to 30 Gy or less, but partial volumes of the liver can be treated with higher doses depending on the location and focality of the primary disease site.[16] Even with modest doses of whole-liver ExBRT (20–30 Gy), radiation hepatitis can occur (defined as a syndrome of elevated serum alkaline phosphatase, transaminases, and bilirubin levels; decreased platelet count; and clinically evident nonmalignant ascites). The time course of radiation hepatitis varies, and the biochemical changes are frequently reversible. With severe cases the histologic picture shows hepatocyte damage consistent with an acute cellular necrosis and central venous thrombosis. These changes occur in the centrolobular region with sinusoidal dilatation and congestion and dilatation of the centrolobular veins. Atrophic changes in centrolobular hepatic cords and thickening of the central vein walls are classic. The cellular mechanism for radiation hepatitis is characterized by endothelial lesions with fibrinous deposits that trap erythrocytes and platelets.[17] Collagen condenses and replaces the fibrin, leading to venous obstruction.

Because the predominant pattern of tumor recurrence for extrahepatic biliary cancers includes regional lymph nodes and liver metastasis, there is a rationale for the use of prophylactic liver or upper abdominal irradiation. The use of wide-field irradiation for localized biliary tract cancers has also been fostered by the apparent success of whole-abdomen irradiation for ovarian cancer and the pilot-feasibility studies on the treatment of advanced pancreatic cancer.[18] In these pilot studies, regional irradiation to the pancreas and surrounding lympth nodes was combined with prophylactic hepatic irradiation. Bolus 5-fluorouracil (5-FU) (500 mg/m^2/day) was given at the beginning and end of a course of hepatic irradiation. Treatment to the liver began 4 weeks after commencing pancreatic irradiation and delivered 23.4 Gy in 13 fractions over 2.5 weeks. The entire liver was encompassed within the irradiation portal as determined by CT scan. A phase II study was also performed and showed that the incidence of hepatic metastasis was reduced from an expected 50% or more to 28%.[19] These nonrandomized trials suggest that prophylactic upper-abdominal therapy should be studied further.

The tolerance of the whole liver to ExBRT is considered to be 30 Gy, but the tolerated radiation dose is lower when chemoradiation is used to treat the whole liver. When ExBRT is used with concomitant chemotherapy, doses of 20–25 Gy delivered over 2–3 weeks are considered safe.[20, 21] The type, number, and method of administration of chemotherapeutic agents used with ExBRT also affects tolerance. For example, with systemic chemotherapy consisting of 5-FU and mitomycin, a radiation dose of only 19.5 Gy resulted in fulminant radiation hepatitis.[22] With the use of protracted infusional 5-FU (300 mg/m^2/day) and ExBRT to a dose of 23.4 Gy, there was an increased incidence of radiation hepatitis compared to that seen with the use of intermittent high-dose 5-FU infusion (1000 mg/m^2).[23] Although there is some suggestion that radiation hepatitis seen at low doses represents a hypersensitivity reaction, it is wise to exercise caution and to undertake prophylactic hepatic irradiation only in the context of a research protocol.

Similarly, caution is necessary when using hepatic intraarterial infusion chemotherapy and whole-liver irradiation where the tolerated radiation doses have been reduced to 15–18 Gy.[24] The underlying mechanism of cellular injury here is primary vasculitis of the small hepatic vessels, which creates a venoocclusive or a Budd-Chiari-like syndrome.[25] The response of some patients to treatment with prednisone supports a vasculitis-like mechanism and should be kept in mind as a therapeutic intervention.

Complications with an endoluminal boost technique for bile duct cancers have been related mainly to cholangitis, which occurs to some degree in nearly all patients. Septic cholangitis and death occur in fewer than 15% of these patient, as antibiotic therapy is usually effective. Prophylactic antibiotics are not recommended because flora colonizing the catheter tract become drug-resistant. A better approach to reducing sepsis is to remove the drainage catheter whenever there is cholangiographic evidence of duct patency after treatment. Other reported complications when EB-IORT has been used as a boost technique include duodenitis, portal vein thrombosis, and dense periportal fibrosis.

Combination ExBRT and Chemotherapy

High-dose ExBRT plus chemotherapy has been used to treat hepatobiliary cancers based on the success of combined-modality therapy for treatment of other gastrointestinal malignancies.[26] Single-agent intravenous 5-FU infusional chemotherapy used during ExBRT to treat multiple gastrointestinal tumor types and sites can result in objective response rates of 10–20% of patients with extrahepatic biliary tract cancers.[27] In other cases, higher response rates after intraarterial infusion of 5-FU probably reflect the higher doses of chemotherapy delivered to the porta hepatis and liver.[28] Some have used floxuridine (FUDR) for hepatic arterial infusion because of its short half-life and its high rate of first-pass hepatic extraction, resulting in a 400-fold increase in hepatic drug exposure. The use of FUDR by hepatic artery infusion with concurrent irradiation has been explored in protocols at the University of Michigan. Because of the biliary sclerosis seen with this drug when infused through the hepatic artery, its combination with irradiation to treat biliary and hepatic cancers must be approached with caution. Conformal ExBRT doses of 60–65 Gy have been employed in an experimental protocol that treated patients with hepatobiliary cancers; the results suggested that disease-free survival rates may be improved over those of historical controls or of patients treated with less aggressive doses of ExBRT.[16]

In contrast to the regional intraarterial infusion given with irradiation, trials with protracted systemic intravenous infusion of 5-FU combined with ExBRT doses of 60–65 Gy in patients with gastrointestinal cancers have been reported from the University of Texas M. D. Anderson Cancer Center.[26,29] 5-FU by continuous intravenous infusion was given to patients with biliary tract cancers to the 5-FU was present with each fraction of ExBRT.[29] Although a few patients received bolus 5-FU (6 patients), low-dose 5-FU by continuous infusion (5-FU-CI) was delivered to most (23 patients). The median 5-FU dose was 2.75 g in 3 days for those treated with bolus administration and 15.5 g in 29 days for those given 5-FU-CI in doses of 250–300 mg/m^2/day throughout the course of ExBRT. The median radiation doses for bolus and continuous-infusion patients wee 44.0 Gy and 54.2 Gy, respectively. All radiation doses were given as 1.8–2.0 Gy/fraction 5 days per week. Transcatheter endoluminal implants were used in selected patients, as was intraoperative electron beam irradiation for those with suspected residual disease in the resected tumor bed. Similar infusional chemoradiation treatment was used in a multicenter study by the Eastern Cooperative Oncology Group where a 5-FU dose of 250 mg/m^2 was found to be well tolerated.[30]

Of note are the results of a subgroup of patients in the M.D. Anderson series who received preoperative infusional 5-FU chemoradiation (K.M. McMasters et al., Chapter 6). In all nine patients undergoing surgical resection there were histologically negative margins. In three patients there was a complete pathologic response in the primary tumor; and in another no evidence or residual cancer was found in the bile duct, but there was microscopic residual disease in a single lymph node. Three other patients also showed marked treatment effect histologically with only microscopic foci of viable tumor. In four surviving patients there is no evidence of disease after followup of 6–80 months. This pilot study is encouraging, as these data suggest that preoperative infusional 5-FU chemoradiation appears to have significant antitumor activity against biliary tract cancers; moreover, the toxicity of the treatment was low, and the operative morbidity was not increased in patients treated with preoperative infusional chemoradiation.

The complications seen during 5-FU chemoradiation included increased acute gastrointestinal symptoms of diarrhea, nausea, vomiting, and some nongastrointestinal complications of mucositis and hand–foot syndrome. These acute complications have been easily managed by antiemetics and anticholinergics in most patients. Cessation of chemotherapy was required in fewer than 20% of the patients.Late complications have been recorded in eight patients who had duodenal bleeding, most often secondary to radiation duodenitis. Septic cholangitis occurred in five patients.

Conclusions

The use of irradiation for management of cholangiocarcinoma is evolving. The data available today suggest that irradiation alone can aid in local control after resection or as the sole treatment modality when doses of more than 50 Gy are used. A new, interesting approach is the use of combined multimodality therapy for cholangiocarcinoma. Preliminary data suggest that the use of preoperative chemoradiation to cytoreduce these cancers prior to surgical resection should be examined further.

References

1. Nagorney DM, Donohue JH, Farnell MB, Schleck CD, Illustrup DM. Outcomes after curative resections of cholangiocarcinoma. Arch Surg 128:871, 1993
2. Nakeeb A, Pitt HA, Sohn TA, et al. Cholangiocarcinoma: a spectrum of intrahepatic, perihilar, and distal tumors. Ann Surg 4:463, 1996
3. Pichlmayr R, Weimann A, Klempnauer J, et al. Surgical treatment in proximal bile duct cancer: a single-center experience. Ann Surg 224:628, 1996
4. Ahrendt SA, Cameron JL, Pitt HA. Current management of patients with perihilar cholangiocarcinoma. Adv Surg 30:427, 1997
5. Buskirk SJ, Gunderson LL, Adson MA, et al. Analysis of failure following curative irradiation of gallbladder and extrahepatic bile duct carcinoma. Int J Radiat Oncol Biol Phys 10:2013, 1984
6. Rich TA. Treatment planning for tumors of the gastrointestinal tract. In: Paliwal BR, Griem ML (eds) Syllabus: A Categorical Course in Radiation Therapy Treatment Planning. RSNA Division of Editorial and Publishing Services, Oak Brook, IL, 1986, pp. 47–55
7. Johnson DW, Safai C, Goffinet DR. Malignant obstructive jaundice: treatment with external-beam and intracavitary radiotherapy. Int J Radiat Oncol Biol Phys 11:411, 1985
8. Mittal B, Deutsch M, Iwatsuki S. Primary cancers of extrahepatic biliary passages. Int J Radiat Oncol Biol Phys 11:849 1985
9. Kopelson G, Galdabini J, Warshaw AL, et al. Patterns of failure after curative surgery for extra-hepatic biliary tract carcinoma: implications for adjuvant therapy. Int J Radiat Oncol Biol Phys 7:413, 1981
10. Pitt HA, Nakeeb A, Abrams R, et al. Perihilar cholangiocarcinoma: post-operative radiotherapy does not improve survival. Ann Surg 221:788, 1995
11. Rich TA. Intraoperative radiotherapy: a review. Radiother Oncol 6:207, 1986
12. Todoroki T, Iwasaki Y, Orii K, et al. Resection combined with intraoperative radiation therapy (IORT) for stage IV (TNM) gallbladder carcinoma. World J Surg 15:357, 1991
13. Deziel DJ, Kiel KD, Kramer TS, et al. Intraoperative radiation therapy in biliary tract cancer. Am Surg 54:402, 1988
14. Nunnerley HB. Interventional radiology and internal radiotherapy for bile duct tumors. In: Preece PE, Cuschieri A, Rosin RD (eds) Cancer of the Bile Ducts and Pancreas. Philadelphia, Saunders, 1989, p. 93

15. Ingold JA, Reed GB, Kaplan HS, Bagshaw MA. Radiation hepatitis. AJR 93:200, 1965

16. Robertson JM, Lawrence TS, Dworzanin LM, et al. Treatment of primary hepatobiliary cancers with conformal radiation therapy and regional chemotherapy. J Clin Oncol 11:1286, 1993

17. Fajardo LF, Colby TV. Pathogenesis of veno-occlusive disease liver disease after radiation. Arch Pathol Lab Med 104:584, 1980

18. Komaki R, Hansen R, Cox JD, et al. Phase I-II study of prophylactic hepatic irradiation with local irradiation and systemic chemotherapy for adenocarcinoma of the pancreas. Int J Radiat Oncol Biol Phys 15:1447, 1988

19. Komaki R, Wadler S, Peters T, et al. High dose local irradiation plus prophylactic hepatic irradiation and chemotherapy for inoperable carcinoma of the pancreas: a preliminary report of a multi-institutional trial (RTOG protocol 88-01). Cancer 69:2807, 1992

20. Kun LE, Camitta BM. Hepatopathy following irradiation and adriamycin. Cancer 42:81, 1978

21. Haddad E, LeBourgeois JP, Kuentz M, Lobo P. Liver complications in lymphomas treated with a combination of chemotherapy and radiotherapy: preliminary results. Int J Radiat Oncol Biol Phys 9:1313, 1983

22. McCracken JD, Weatherall TJ, Oishi N. Adjuvant intrahepatic chemotherapy with mitomycin and 5-FU combined with hepatic irradiation in high-risk patients with carcinoma of the colon: a Southwest Oncology Group phase II study. Cancer Treat Rep 69:129, 1985

23. Evans DB, Abbruzzese JL, Cleary KR, et al. Preoperative chemoradiation for adenocarcinoma of the pancreas: excessive toxicity of prophylactic hepatic irradiation. Int J Radiat Oncol Biol Phys 33:913, 1995

24. Lokich J, Kinsella T, Perri J. Concomitant hepatic irradiation and intraarterial fluorinated pyrimidine therapy. Cancer 48:2569, 1981

25. Cassady JR, Carabell SC, Jaffe N. Chemotherapy-irradiation related hepatic dysfunction in patients with Wilm's tumor. Front Radiat Ther Oncol 13:147, 1979

26. Rich TA. Chemoradiation for gastrointestinal cancer. Front Radiat Ther Oncol 10:115, 1992

27. Falkson G. MacIntyre JM, Moertel CG. Eastern Cooperative Oncology Group experience with chemotherapy for inoperable gallbladder and bile duct cancer. Cancer 54:965, 1984

28. Smith GW, Bukowski RM, Hewlett JS, et al. Hepatic artery infusion of 5-fluorouracil and mitomycin C in cholangiocarcinoma and gallbladder carcinoma. Cancer 54:1513, 1984

29. Rich TA. Chemoradiation or accelerated fractionation: basic considerations. J Inf Chemo 1:2, 1992

30. Whittington R, Neuberg D, Tester WJ, Benson AB III, Haller DG. Protracted intravenous fluorouracil infusion with radiation therapy in the management of localized pancreaticobiliary carcinoma: a phase I Eastern Cooperative Oncology Group trial. J Clin Oncol 13:227, 1995

5

Alternative Treatment Approaches to Early Stage or Unresectable Hepatocellular Carcinoma Confined to the Liver

Francesco Izzo, Francesco Fiore, Carlo de Werra, and Steven A. Curley

As noted in Chapter 2, most patients diagnosed with hepatocellular cancer (HCC) are not candidates for resection. In some patients unresectability is based on the presence of extrahepatic metastasis at the time of diagnosis. Many more patients with HCC confined to the liver are not candidates for resection because of large tumor size, multicentricity, adjacency or direct invasion to major blood vessels, or concomitant cirrhosis with inadequate functional hepatic reserve.

In contrast, there is a subset of HCC patients with early-stage disease who may be candidates for alternative treatment approaches. These patients may have a small, solitary tumor situated deep in the liver that would require resection of a significant proportion of unaffected parenchyma. Many patients with cirrhosis do not have adequate functional hepatic reserve to tolerate the necessary hepatic resection. Some patients refuse resection and prefer to be treated with another approach. In any event, patients with early-stage disease should be treated with curative intent. Alternative liver-directed treatment approaches for potential cure or palliation, as appropriate, should be considered for patients with HCC confined to the liver. Terminal liver failure or a disorder related to liver dysfunction is the cause of death for most patients who succumb to HCC. Therefore, control of tumor in the liver is a major priority.

Direct Intratumoral Injection

Countries with a moderate or high incidence of HCC have developed screening programs for high risk populations, particularly patients infected with hepatitis B (HBV) or hepatitis C (HCV) virus.[1,2] Screening ultrasonography has detected an increased number of patients with asymptomatic HCCs with a diameter of 4 cm or less. Unfortunately, a significant proportion of patients with these relatively small tumors are not candidates for surgical resection because of the severity of their coexisting cirrhosis. As a result, ultrasound-guided percutaneous ethanol injection (PEI) of the liver tumors has been used for both palliative and curative treatment.

Injection of absolute ethanol into a tumor produces tumor cell cytotoxicity and necrosis of the tumor mass. HCCs larger than 5 cm in diameter usually cannot be treated with curative intent using PEI alone because of the diffusion characteristics of the ethanol and the toxicity associated with the amount of ethanol necessary to treat large tumors.[3,4] PEI is used to treat solitary lesions less than 5 cm in diameter or two to three hepatic tumors each less than 4 cm in diameter. Patients must have adequate coagulation studies and platelet counts, which may preclude PEI in some patients with Child's class C cirrhosis. PEI is performed as an outpatient procedure under ultrasound guidance (Fig. 5.1), and each lesion is injected with an average of 4–10 ml of absolute ethanol during two or three treatments each week to a total of six to eight treatments.[3,5]

Ultrasound-guided PEI was used to treat 27 HCCs in 23 patients in Taiwan.[3] All patients had histologic evidence of cirrhosis, but the clinical severity of the cirrhosis was not defined. All of the tumors were less than 4 cm in diameter at the onset of PEI. After PEI treatments were completed in the 15 patients with elevated serum α-fetoprotein (AFP) levels, the AFP levels returned to normal in 13 of the patients. Of the 23 patients, 6 underwent liver resection after completion of PEI, and there was no viable tumor in 4 of the 6. All 23 patients treated with PEI were alive at the time of the report, with only an 18-month follow-up.

A study of 207 HCC patients treated with PEI was performed in Italy.[6,7] The treated tumors were all less than 5 cm in diameter and were solitary in 162 patients and multiple in 45. The clinical severity of cirrhosis was Child's class A in 136 patients, class B in 54, and class C in 17. For the 162 patients with solitary. tumors, the 1-year survival following PEI was 90% and the 3-year survival 63%.[7] For the 45 patients with multiple tumors the 1-year survival was also 90%, but the 3-year survival was only 31%. The severity of cirrhosis was a significant prognostic indicator of long-term survival following PEI; the 3-year survival rates for patients with Child's class A, B, and C cirrhosis were 76%, 42%, and 0%, respectively. It was reported that 2485 treatments were performed in the 207 patients with no treatment—related mortality and a minimal morbidity rate. Transient pain at the injection site is common in patients treated with PEI, but the more serious complications of intraperitoneal hemorrhage, hepatic insufficiency, bile duct necrosis, hepatic infarction, and transient hypotension are infrequent. The same group has reported the survival results in 746 cirrhotic HCC patients, predominantly Child's class A or B, treated by PEI.[8] This large study confirms that PEI can produce long-term survival in approximately one-half of the patients with a small, solitary HCC.

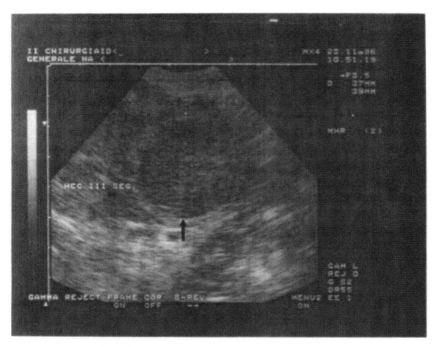

FIGURE 5.1. Transabdominal ultrasonography image demonstrating a 3.5 × 3.5 cm hepatocellular cancer (HCC) in segment III of the liver (arrow). This solitary, encapsulated tumor in a patient with Child's class B cirrhosis was treated successfully with several outpatient sessions of percutaneous ethanol injection.

A prospective, nonrandomized study in Spain compared surgical resection and PEI in patients with solitary HCCs less than 4 cm in diameter.[9] Surgical resection was performed in 33 patients (30 patients with Child's class A, 3 patients with class B), and PEI was performed on 30 patients (10 patients with Child's class A, 16 patients with class B, 4 patients with class C). The tumor recurrence rate 2 years after treatment was 45% in the surgical group and 60% in the PEI group. Despite the higher incidence of tumor recurrence in the PEI group, the 3- and 4-year survival rates of PEI-treated patients (55% and 34%, respectively) were not significantly different from those of the surgically treated patients (44% and 44%, respectively).

It appears that transarterial embolization followed by PEI may be an effective combination to treat unresectable HCC.[10] In 15 patients with solitary, large (3–9 cm in diameter) HCCs treated with this combination, all patients were alive at least 1 year after completion of the treatments, and there was complete necrosis of the treated tumors in the four patients who subsequently underwent surgical resection. The volume of ethanol that can be injected without severe pain or hypotension is limited using a percutaneous approach. However, the volume of ethanol that can be injected into a

HCC during laparotomy under general anesthesia can exceed 100 ml.[11] This "one-shot" technique can saturate a HCC thorougly with ethanol and can be used for multifocal tumors or lesions up to 10 cm in diameter. Finally, ethanol injection can be used in emergency situations as a sclerosant to control bleeding from ruptured HCCs.[12]

Curley et al. have reported a novel approach to direct intratumoral injection therapy.[13] The treatment uses a collagen matrix gel mixed with the chemotherapeutic agent cisplatin. The collagen matrix gel functions as a drug delivery vehicle that enhances tumor cell exposure to the chemotheraphy drug while limiting peak systemic exposure to it. Complete necrosis of rabbit hepatic VX-2 tumors occurred in the preclinical studies of this treatment. The promising preclinical studies led to a pilot clinical trial of 15 patients with unresectable liver tumors. All of the patients had at least 50% reduction in the volume of the treated tumors, with seven patients having a more than 90% reduction.[14] A multiinstitution phase II trial in patients with unresectable HCC opened in 1997.

Hepatic Artery Chemoembolization

Other attempts have been made to increase the activity of locoregionally administered treatments by prolonging the duration of contact between tumor tissue and the chemotherapy drugs. Intraarterially administered oily contrast medium (Lipiodol, ethiodol) is deposited selectively within HCCs and remains within the tumor for several months (Figs. 5.2, 5.3).[15] These substances also may act as carriers for chemotherapeutic agents or radioactive iodine (^{131}I).[16] A variety of chemotherapeutic agents have been co-administered with Lipiodol to treat HCC, including doxorubicin,[17] fluorodeoxyuridine (FUDR),[18] and cisplatin.[19] In most of the trials 50–90% of the patients had a decrease in serum AFP levels, and 1- and 5-year survival rates were 54–85% and 3–34%, respectively.[20–24] A randomized, controlled multicenter clinical trial studied lipiodol transcatheter arterial embolization in the presence versus the absence of doxorubicin for treating unresectable HCC.[25] The 3-year survival rates for the two groups were 33.6% and 34.9%, respectively, indicating that embolization of the tumor microcirculation is the most important factor in tumor control by Lipiodol; addition of the chemotherapy drug did not improve survival.

FIGURE 5.2. Transfemoral arteriography in a patient with a large, unresectable hepatocellular cancer (HCC) in the right lobe of the liver. (A) Celiac arteriogram demonstrating the large hypervascular HCC in the right lobe of the liver (arrow). (B) Selective catheterization of the right hepatic artery again indicates the hypervascular HCC (arrow) seen following iodinated contrast injection. (C) The HCC was treated with hepatic arterial chemoembolization using iodized oil (Lipiodol). The postembolization radiograph shows retention of the iodized oil in the right lobe HCC.

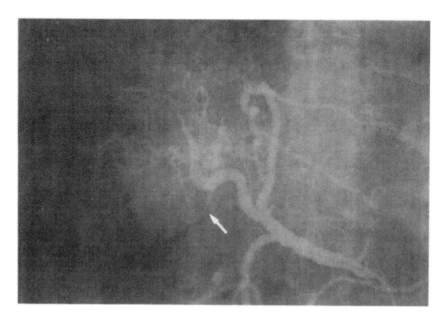

FIGURE 5.2-A.

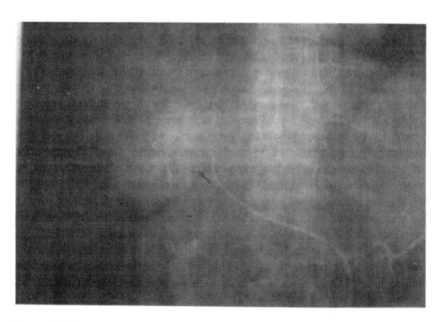

FIGURE 5.2-B.

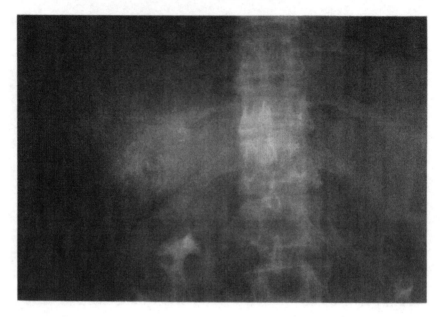

FIGURE 5.2-C.

Gelfoam powder (40–50 μm) or particles (250–589 μm) occlude the hepatic arterial circulation transiently. Gelfoam was co-administered with doxorubicin, mitomycin C, and cisplatin; an objective antitumor response rate of 24% and a 68% decrease in the serum AFP level was observed.[26] In a nonrandomized trial comparing intraarterial infusion of a combination of 5-fluorouracil (5-FU), cytosine arabinoside, and mitomycin C with hepatic arterial chemoembolization using Gelfoam mixed with mitomycin C and doxorubicin, the 1-, 2-, and 3-year survival rates were 22%, 9%, and 4%, respectively, for the intraarterial infusion group compared with 67%, 37%, and 22%, respectively, for the Gelfoam chemoembolization combination.[27] Thus the effect of transient vascular occlusion may potentiate the effects of chemotherapy, but more controlled trials are needed to define optimal interactions.

Hepatic arterial chemoembolization has been reported to prolong survival in uncontrolled retrospective studies of patients with HCC deemed unresectable based on anatomic or physiologic constraints.[26,28–31] HCC patients with tumors initially considered unresectable have undergone curative resection after tumor down-staging with hepatic arterial chemoembolization.[28,32] Only 10–20% of HCC patients with unresectable disease are down-staged sufficiently by chemoembolization to consider surgical excision of the residual disease.

There are significant risks associated with arterial chemoembolization in HCC patients. Hepatic failure, the most devastating complication of this treatment, manifests as jaundice, ascites, or encephalopathy. A significant proportion of the patients who develop hepatic failure after chemoembol-

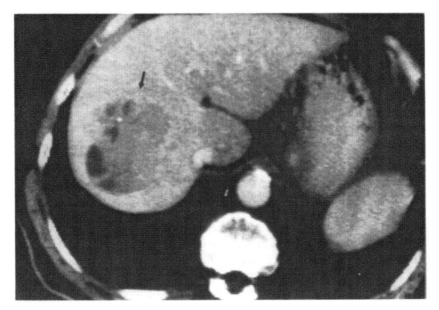

FIGURE 5.3-A.

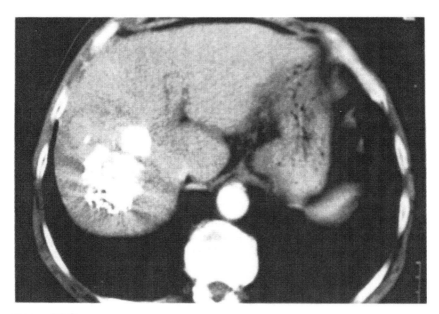

FIGURE 5.3-B.

FIGURE 5.3. CT scans from a patient with a large hepatocellular cancer (HCC) involving the right lobe of the liver. (A) CT performed prior to hepatic arterial chemoembolization with iodized oil (Lipiodol) demonstrates a large mass in the right lobe of the liver (arrow). (B) CT scan performed following hepatic arterial chemoembolization with iodized oil shows a somewhat inhomogeneous uptake of the iodized oil within the tumor.

ization do not survive these complications. The incidence of hepatic failure is usually inversely related to the functional hepatic reserve at the time of chemoembolization; for example, most investigators report a mortality rate of less than 5% after chemoembolization in noncirrhotic HCC patients.[26,28] Bismuth et al. reported that the incidence of hepatic failure after hepatic arterial chemoembolization correlated with the severity of cirrhosis in their patient population.[28] Jaundice or ascites following chemoembolization occurred in 62% of Brousse grade C cirrhotics compared to only 15% in grade A cirrhotics. Additionally, the overall morbidity (37.0% vs. 2.8%) and mortality (12.5% vs. 1.4%) rates were significantly higher for grade C than for grade A cirrhotics. Almost all patients develop a postembolization syndrome consisting of fever, right upper quadrant abdominal pain, adynamic ileus, and elevated serum liver function tests.[33] These signs and symptoms are usually self-limiting, and the patients can be treated with supportive measures including intravenous fluid administration, antiemetics, and patient-controlled analgesia. Liver abscess in the necrotic tumor develops in fewer than 10% of all patients, and the incidence of this complication can be reduced to less than 1% by routine use of prophylactic broad-spectrum intravenous antiboitics.[33]

Heat Ablation

As noted in Chapter 2, cryoablation has been applied to the treatment of HCC localized to the liver. Studies have demonstrated that primary or metastatic liver tumors must be cooled to at least -35°C throughout the entire tumor to achieve a reliable tumor cell kill. This low temperature is difficult to achieve at the periphery of tumors larger than 5 cm in diameter, when the tumor abuts a major intrahepatic branch of the portal vein or hepatic veins or if it lies near the inferior vena cava. Furthermore, the cryoprobes used for ablation are 3–20 mm in diameter, and significant hemorrhage from the probe tract can occur.

Tumor cells are also killed by heating tumor tissue. Cytotoxicity is produced in both normal and tumor cells by localized application of heat with temperatures that exceed 50°C.[34–36] A number of techniques have been evaluated that produce necrosis in solid tumors through local heat application, but the three techniques with the most clinical promise are radiofrequency, laser, and microwave ablation.

Radiofrequency Ablation

Radiofrequency electrocautery devices have been used for more than 70 years to achieve direct tissue ablation, usually for hemostasis during surgical procedures. Advances in electrocautery technology led to the development of monopolar and bipolar tissue ablation.[34] Only tissue through which radiofrequency electrical current passes directly is heated above a cytotoxic cellular temperature. The tissue temperature in the tumor to be ablated can be controlled between 50° and 100°C by increasing the radiofrequency power and current delivered. For monopolar tumor ablation, a needle electrode is placed in the tumor via a percutaneous or intraoperative approach, and an indifferent dispersive electrode pad is applied to the patient's outer skin surface, much like the grounding pads used for hemostatic electrocautery during surgical procedures. For bipolar ablation two needle electrodes are placed 2–4 cm apart in the tumor, and the current is passed across these two needles, thereby obviating the need for a dispersive grounding electrode pad. The geometry of the radiofrequency current pathway around the ablation electrodes creates a relatively uniform zone of radiant/conductive heat within the first few millimeters of electrode–tissue interface. The conductive heat emitted from the tissue uniformly radiates out from the electrode; and if the impedance is relatively low, a dynamic expanding sphere of ablated tissue is created. The final size of the sphere of heat-ablated tissue is proportional to the square of the radiofrequency current, also known as the radiofrequency power density. The radiofrequency power/current delivered via a monopolar electrode decreases in proportion to the square of the distance from the electrode. Therefore the tissue temperature falls rapidly with increasing distance away from the electrode.

The decrease in tissue heating with increasing distance away from the electrode results in only 1.0–1.5 cm spheres of tumor tissue ablation when using monopolar simple needle electrodes.[35,36] The zone of tissue necrosis can be increased to 2.0–3.0 cm by the use of bipolar needle electrodes.[37] New monopolar and bipolar needles (16–18 gauge diameter) have been developed with hook electrodes that can be deployed from the needle tip into the tumor. These deployed hooks create a series of electrodes with a diameter up to 4 cm, across which the radiofrequency current can be passed. Using a radiofrequency current generator with a 20–90 watt power output for 5–10 minutes, a 4.0–5.0 cm diameter tumor can be ablated with the hook electrodes fully deployed.

Radiofrequency ablation has been used to treat patients with HCC. The needle electrodes can be placed in the tumor percutaneously using computed tomography (CT) or ultrasound guidance. Using this percutaneous approach, Rossi et al. showed that HCCs up to 3 cm in diameter could be ablated.[38] CT scans obtained following radiofrequency ablation demonstrate zones of tissue necrosis early and then a cavitary lesion within the liver parenchyma 1–2 months after treatment. Long-term follow-up on these patients is not yet available, but this percutaneous approach can be used to ablate a small, solitary HCC with a single treatment and may thus have several advantages over percutaneous ethanol injection. We have also used radiofrequency ablation to treat both HCC and metastatic liver tumors.[39] We performed this treatment under laparoscopic guidance or intraoperatively during a full laparotomy. In this manner, using intraoperative ultrasound guidance, it is possible to ablate large tumors (6–8 cm in diameter) by moving the needle electrodes to different areas within the tumor and then sequentially ablating these areas (Fig. 5.4). We performed radiofrequency ablation of 28 HCCs in 24 patients between July 1, 1996, and March 31, 1997. The treatment was well tolerated by the patients with no significant morbidity and no treatment-related deaths. There has been no hemorrhage from the 16-gauge needle electrode tracts. With more experience, radiofrequency ablation may come to have several advantages over cryoablation for treatment of primary and metastatic liver malignancies.

Laser Ablation

Laser fibers can be inserted into liver tumors using a percutaneous or intra-operative aproach. The side-firing laser fibers have been shown to produce rapid heating of the tissue surrounding the laser tip.[40] There is complete tissue vaporization a few millimeters from the laser tip, followed by concentric zones of tissue necrosis from heat injury leading to zones of tissue hyperemia without cell death farther away from the laser tip. The rapid heat production by the laser fiber has limited the utility of this instrument because the tissue coagulum that is rapidly produced limits further propagation of heat through the tumor tissue. Laser treatment has been applied to patients with malignant liver tumors. Although this treatment was found to be safe, the laser fiber can effectively produce only 1–2 cm diameter zones of tumor necrosis.[41] The relatively small zones of tumor tissue necrosis have limited the utility of laser ablation of hepatic malignancies.

Microwave Ablation

Microwave probes have been used to produce heat ablation of liver tumors. Microwave produces dielectric heat and tissue necrosis by rapidly heating the intracellular water. Current methodology employs 1 mm diameter probes placed directly into the tumor; these probes produce necrosis of small areas, and the tumor can be ablated only by moving the probe at 5- to 10-mm intervals to treat progressive regions within the tumor. Each small zone of tissue necrosis is produced using a 70-90 watt power output for 30 seconds.

A single series of 19 HCC patients treated with microwave heat ablation has been reported.[42] All 19 patients had cirrhosis. Analysis of the microwave treatment efficacy and survival in this study was compromised in that 14 patients also were treated with hepatic arterial chemoembolization. Nonetheless, the authors treated lesions 1.5–9.0 cm in diameter. Six patients with solitary HCCs were treated, four of whom are alive without evidence of recurrent disease 14–64 months after treatment. The other two patients with solitary tumors died due to recurrent HCC within the liver. In nine patients two to five tumors were treated; six of these patients are alive without evidence of recurrent disease 14–47 months after microwave ablation; three have died of recurrent HCC. The final four patients had more than six tumors treated with microwave ablation; all of these patients died with recurrent HCC in the liver.

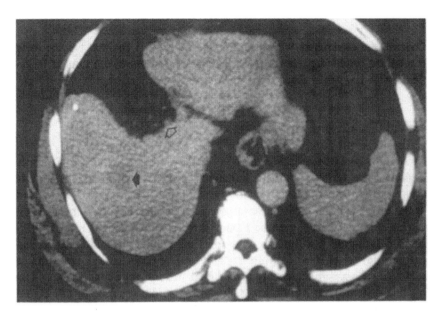

FIGURE 5.4-A.

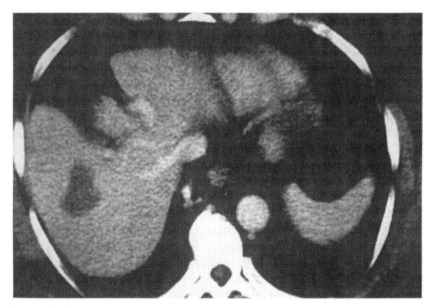

FIGURE 5.4-B.

FIGURE 5.4. CT scans from a patient with an intrahepatic recurrence of hepatocellular cancer (HCC) in the right lobe of the liver. (A) CT performed prior to intraoperative radiofrequency ablation of the HCC shows the recurrent tumor (solid arrow) and the site of the previous liver resection (open arrow). (B) CT performed 1 month after intraoperative radiofrequency ablation demonstrates complete necrosis of the HCC.

Comment

Overall, the experience with heat ablation of HCC is limited, but the early results are promising. Hence these techniques to control the tumors in patients with liver-only disease warrant further investigation.

Novel Treatment Approaches

Cytotoxic chemotherapeutic agents in standard doses have not significantly improved the survival of HCC patients. The efficacy of chemotherapeutic drugs is poor in part because of the systemic dose-limiting toxicity related to the drugs and the intrinsic resistance of HCC to many anticancer drugs. Curley et al. performed a phase I study that combined hepatic arterial infusion of high-dose doxorubicin with complete hepatic venous isolation and extracorporeal chemofiltration.[43] Complete hepatic venous isolation is achieved with a percutaneously placed dual-balloon vena cava catheter. Using this system it was possible to deliver doxorubicin at a dose of 120 mg/m^2 with minimal hepatic toxicity and limited systemic side effects. Systemic toxicity was limited because hepatic venous blood was pumped across carbon filters before returning it to the patients; this chemofiltration produced an 83% reduction in systemic doxorubicin levels compared to hepatic venous levels. Although this was a phase I study, 7 of the 10 patients had a reduction in the size of their HCCs, and two of the lesions were converted from unresectable to resectable. This system also has been investigated for arterial delivery of combination chemotherapy treatments or cytotoxic chemotherapeutic drugs combined with agents that block P-glycoprotein and reverse the multidrug resistance phenotype.[44] Additional studies of this treatment approach are being performed to define safe and effective drug combinations, dosages, and treatment intervals.

Improved treatment programs for HCC may depend ultimately on strategies that do not rely on cytotoxic chemotherapeutic drugs or ionizing radiation. Immunotherapy and cytokines have been used in preliminary evaluations to treat unresectable HCC. In small pilot trials, immunomodulatory agents such as thymosin have produced objective tumor reduction in more than half of the treated patients.[45] The mechanism of action of thymosin against HCC cells has been investigated. It was observed that thymosin is not directly cytotoxic against HCC cells, but it activates Kupffer cells to release monokines, such as tumor necrosis factor, that produce cytotoxicity against the HCC cells.[46] Cytokine receptors also have been used experimentally to target the treatment of human HCC.[47] In this study a human HCC line that overexpresses the interleukin-6 (IL-6) receptor was implanted into nude mice. Chimeric molecules composed of IL-6 fused to *Pseudomonas* exotoxin were administered to the tumor-bearing animals; they significantly retarded the growth rate of the tumors.

New treatments for solid human tumors such as HCC will evolve from advances in our understanding of genetic and epigenetic events during tumorigenesis and progression to metastatic disease. Normal hepatocytes express a specific cell surface receptor for asialoglycoproteins; and when these receptors bind an asialoglycoprotein ligand, the receptor–ligand complex is internalized and degraded in cytoplasmic lysosome.[48] Many HCC cells no longer express the receptors for asialoglycoprotein, and this alteration in the plasma membrane receptors has been used to deliver cytoprotective agents bound to asialoglycoproteins, which are internalized and released in normal hepatocytes but which are not available to the malignant cells.[48-50] High-affinity ligands for the asialoglycoprotein receptor also can be conjugated to DNA, which capable of directly transcription in hepatocytes.[51] This gene transfer technique potentially could be used to correct genetic defects that occur during hepatocarcinogenesis related to viral infections, environmental toxins, or other chronic liver diseases. Conversely, other targeting strategies may be used to correct genetic defects in hepatocytes that already have undergone malignant transformation. Isolated infusion techniques have been used to expose hepatocytes to a retroviral vector to mediate gene transfer into the cells.[52] Another targeting technique is intravenous injection of specific gene expression plasmids in cationic liposome complexes.[53] These liposomes can be taken up nonspecifically into a variety of organ sites or can be modified to include ligands that in theory are recognized by specific normal or malignant cell types, thereby delivering the desired gene product to the target organ and normal or cancer cells. Finally, targeted delivery of toxins to HCC cells may be achieved by linking the toxin to tumor-specific antibodies.[54]

Cytokine-based immunotherapy has not produced a marked antitumor response or improved the survival of patients with most human solid malignancies. Immunotherapy still may have a role in improving the treatment of malignancies such as HCC by direct gene transfer that induces cell—mediated immunity against the specific gene products, thereby providing an immunotherapeutic response against the tumor.[55] As knowledge accrues regarding human hepatocarcinogenesis and the specific genetic and molecular aberrations that occur during this process, the techniques to correct the genetic defects and to develop novel molecular pharmacologic manipulations can be refined to improve the outcome of patients with HCC.

References

1. Curley SA, Izzo F, DeBellis M, Cremona F, Parisi V. Identification and screening of 416 patients with chronic hepatitis at high risk to develop hepatocellular cancer. Ann Surg 222:375, 1995
2. Izzo F, Cremona F, Ruffolo F, et al. Outcome of 67 hepatocellular cancer patients detected during screening of 1,125 chronic hepatitis patients. Ann Surg (in press)
3. Sheu JC, Sung JL, Huang HT, et al. Intratumor injection of absolute ethanol under

ultrasound guidance for the treatment of small hepatocellular carcinoma. Hepatogastroenterology 34:255, 1987

4. Vilana R, Bruix J, Bru C, et al. Tumor size determines the efficacy of percutaneous ethanol injection for the treatment of the small hepatocellular carcinoma. Hepatology 16:353, 1992

5. Sheu JC, Huang GT, Chen DS, et al. Small hepatocellular carcinoma: intratumor ethanol treatment using new needle and guidance systems. Radiology 163:43, 1987

6. Livraghi T, Salmi A, Bolondi L, et al. Small hepatocellular carcinoma: percutaneous alcohol injection: results in 23 patients. Radiology 168:313, 1988

7. Livraghi T, Bolondi L, Lazzaroni S, et al. Percutaneous ethanol injection in the treatment of hepatocellular carcinoma in cirrhosis. Cancer 69:925, 1992

8. Livraghi T, Giorgio A, Marin G, et al. Hepatocellular carcinoma and cirrhosis in 746 patients: long term results of hepatocellular ethanol injection. Radiology 197:101, 1995

9. Castells A, Bruix J, Bru C, et al. Treatment of small hepatocellular carcinoma in cirrhotic patients: a cohort study comparing surgical resection and percutaneous ethanol injection. Hepatology 18:1121, 1993

10. Tanaka K, Okazaki H, Nakamura S, et al. Hepatocellular carcinoma: treatment with a combination therapy of transcatheter arterial embolization and percutaneous ethanol injection. Radiology 179:713, 1991

11. Livraghi T, Lazzaroni S, Pellicani S, et al. Percutaneous ethanol injection of hepatic tumors: single—session therapy with general anesthesia. AJR 161:1065, 1993

12. Chung SCS, Lee TW, Kwok SPY, Li AKC. Injection of alcohol to control bleeding from ruptured hepatomas. Br M J 301:421 1990

13. Curley SA, Fuhrman GM, Siddik ZH, et al. Direct intratumoral injection of a novel collagen matrix gel and cisplatin effectively controls experimental live tumors. Cancer Res Ther Control 4:247, 1995

14. Curley SA, Abramson N, Benson AB, et al. Phase I study of intradose-CDDP in patients with primary and metastatic liver tumors. Hepatology 20:279A, 1994

15. Dusheiko GM, Hobbs KE, Dick R, Burroughs AK, Treatment of small hepatocellular carcinoma. Lancet 340:285, 1992

16. Vetter D, Wenger JJ, Bergier JM, et al. Transcatheter oily chemoembolization in the management of advances hepatocellular carcinoma in cirrhosis: results of a Western comparative study in 60 patients. Hepatology 13:427, 1991

17. Kirk S, Blumgart R, Craig B, et al. Irresectable hepatoma treated by intrahepatic iodized oil doxorubicin hydrochloride: initial results. Surgery 109:694, 1991

18. Hamashita Y, Takahashi M, Bussaka H, et al. Intraarterial infusion of 5-fluoro-2-deoxyuridine-C8 dissolved in a lymphographic agent in malignant liver tumors. Cancer 64:2437, 1989

19. Konno T, Maeda H, Ikwai K, et al. Effect of arterial administration of high molecular weight anticancer agents SMANCS with lipid lymphographic agent on hepatoma: a preliminary report. Eur J Cancer Clin Oncol 19:1053, 1983

20. Ravoet C, Bleiberg H, Gerard B. Non-surgical treatment of hepatocarcinoma. J Surg Oncol Suppl 3:104, 1993

21. Konno T, Kai Y, Yamashita R, Nagamitsu A, Kimura M. Targeted chemotherapy for unresectable primary and metastatic liver cancer. Acta Oncol 33:133, 1994

22. Urata K, Matsumata T, Kamakura T, Hasuo K, Sugimachi K. Lipiodolization for unresectable carcinoma: an analysis of 205 patients using univariate and multivariate analysis. J Surg Oncol 56:54, 1994

23. Rossi C, Isceri S, Pagliacci M, Galaverini MC, Corinaldesi A. Chemoembolization of hepatocarcinoma: six years' experience. Radiol Med (Torino) 89:835, 1995

24. Chung JW, Park JH, Han JK, Choi BI, Han MC. Hepatocellular carcinoma and portal vein invasion: results of treatment with transcatheter oily chemoembolization. AJR 165:315, 1995

25. Kawai S, Okamura J, Ogawa M, et al. Prospective and randomized clinical trial for the treatment of hepatocellular carcinoma: a comparision of lipiodol transcatheter arterial embolization with and without adriamycin. Cancer Chemother Pharmacol 31(suppl 1):S1, 1992

26. Venook AP, Stagg RJ, Lewis BJ, et al.Chemoembolization for hepatocellular carcinoma. J Clin Oncol 8:1108, 1990

27. Hirai K, Kawazoe Y, Yamashita K, et al. Arterial chemotherapy and transcatheter arterial embolization therapy for non-resectable hepatocellular carcinoma. Cancer Chemother Pharmacol 23:537, 1989

28. Bismuth H, Morino M, Sherlock D, et al. Primary treatment of hepatocellular carcinoma by arterial chemoembolization. Am J Surg 163:387, 1992

29. Lin DY, Liaw YF, Lee TY, Lai CH. Hepatic arterial embolization in patients with unresectable hepatoma: a randomized controlled trial. Gastroenterology 94:453, 1988

30. Clouse ME. Hepatic artery embolization for bleeding and tumors. Surg Clin North Am 69:419, 1989

31. Yamada Y, Sato M, Kawabata M, et al. Hepatic artery embolization in 120 patients with unresectable hepatoma. Radiology 55:148, 1993

32. Hwang T-L, Chen MF, Lee T-Y, et al. Resection of hepatocellular carcinoma after transcatheter arterial embolization. Arch Surg 122:756, 1987

33. Berger DH, Carrasco H, Hohn DC, Curley SA. Hepatic artery chemoembolization or embolization for primary and metastatic liver tumors: post-treatment management and complications. J Surg Oncol 60:116, 1995

34. Sanchez H, vanSonnenberg E, D'agostine H, et al. Percutaneous tissue ablation by radiofrequency thermal energy as a preliminary to tumor ablation. Minim Invasive Ther 2:299, 1993

35. McGahan JP, Browning PD, Brock JM, Tesluk H. Hepatic ablation using radiofrequency electocautery. Invest Radiol 25:267, 1990

36. Rossi S, Fornari F, Paties C, Buscarini L. Thermal lesions induced by 480KHz localized current field in guinea pig and in pig livers. Tumori 76:54, 1990

37. Curley SA, Davidson BS, Fleming RYD, et al. Laparoscopically-guided bipolar radiofrequency ablation of areas of porcine liver. Surg Endosc 11:729, 1997

38. Rossi S, Di Stasi M, Buscarini E, et al. Percutaneous radiofrequency interstitial thermal ablation in the treatment of small hepatocellular carcinoma. Cancer J Sci Am 1:73 1995

39. Izzo F, Di Muria A, Ruffolo F, Parisi V, Curley SA. Intraoperative use of radiofrequency interstitial tissue ablation to treat primary and metastatic liver tumors: a pilot study. J Exp Clin Cancer Res 16:330, 1997

40. Bosman S, Phoa SS, Bosma A, Van Gemerr MJC. Effect of percutaneous interstitial thermal laser on normal liver of pigs: sonographic and histopathological correlations. Br J Surg 78:572, 1991

41. Nelsoe CP, Torp-Pedersen S, Burcharth F, et al. Interstitial hyperthermia of colorectal liver metastases with an US-guided Nd-Yag laser with a diffuser tip: a pilot clinical study. Radiology 187:333, 1993

42. Sato M, Watanabe Y, Ueda S, et al. Microwave coagulation therapy for hepatocellular carcinoma. Gastroenterology 110:1507, 1996
43. Curley SA, Stone DL, Newman RA, et al. A novel system to treat human hepatocellular cancer: a phase I study. Ann Surg Oncol 1:389, 1994
44. Fuhrman GM, Cromeens DM, Newman RA, et al. Hepatic arterial infusion of verapamil and doxorubicin with complete hepatic venous isolation and extracorporeal chemofiltration: pharmacologic evaluation of reduction in systemic drug exposure and assessment of hepatic toxicity. Surg Oncol 3:17, 1994
45. Palmieri G, Cimmino L, Gravina A, et al. Thymostimulin treatment of hepatocellular carcinoma: preliminary data. In: Proceedings of the First International Conference on Hepatobiliary Tumors, Vol. 1, 1992, p. 52
46. Balch G, Izzo F, Chiao P, Klostergaard J, Curley SA. Thymostimulin (TP-1) activates Kupffer cells to produce cytotoxicity against human hepatocellular cells. Ann Surg Oncol 4:149, 1997
47. Siegall CB, Kreitman RJ, Fitzgerald DJ, Pastan I. Antitumor effects of interleukin 6-*Pseudomonas* exotoxin chimeric molecules against the human hepatocellular carcinoma. PLC/PRF/5 in mice. Cancer Res 51:2831, 1991
48. Wu GY, Wu CH Stockert RJ. Model for specific rescue of normal hepatocytes during methotrexate treatment of hepatic malignancy. Pro Natl Acad Sci USA 80:3078, 1983
49. Wu GY, Keegan-Rogers V, Franklin S, et al. Targeted antagonism of galactosamine toxicity in normal rate hepatocytes *in vitro*. J Biol Chem 263:4719, 1988
50. Keegan-Rogers V, Wu GY. Targeted protection of hepatocytes from galactosamine toxicity in vivo. Cancer Chemother Pharmacol 26:93, 1990
51. Wilson JM, Grossman M, Wu CH, et al. Hepatocyte-directed gene transfer *in vivo* leads to transient improvement of hypercholesterolemia in low density lipoportein receptor-deficient rabbits. J Biol Chem 267:963, 1992
52. Ferry N, Duplessis O, Houssin D, et al. Retroviral-mediated gene transfer into hepatocytes *in vivo*. Proc Natl Acad Sci USA 88:8377 1991
53. Zhu N, Liggitt D, Liu Y, Debs R. Systemic gene expression after intravenous DNA delivery into adult mice. Science 261:209, 1993
54. Masuda K, Takahashi K, Hirano K, Takagishi Y. Selective antitumor effect of thioether-linked immunotoxins composed of gelonin and monoclonal antibody to alpha-fetoprotein or its (ab')$_2$ fragment. Tumoru Biol 15:175, 1994
55. Plautz GE, Yang ZY, Wu BY, et al. Immunotherapy of malignancy by *in vivo* gene transfer into tumors. Proc Natl Acad Sci USA 90:4645, 1993

6

Treatment of Cholangiocarcinoma

KELLY M. MCMASTERS AND STEVEN A. CURLEY

Cholangiocarcinomas, malignant tumors that arise from the intrahepatic or extrahepatic bile ducts, are rare, comprising fewer than 10% of primary malignancies of the liver.[1] There are only about 4000 new cases of cholangiocarcinoma per year in the United States, being diagnosed most frequently during the fifth and sixth decades of life.[2] The prognosis for patients with this disease remains dismal despite advances in the operative and nonoperative management.[3-7]

Classification

Most classification systems have distinguished intrahepatic from extrahepatic cholangiocarcinomas. Extrahepatic cholangiocarcinomas are then often classified as proximal third, middle third, or distal third lesions. A simple, clinically useful classification system has been proposed recently by the group at Johns Hopkins University. Using this system, cholangiocarcinomas are classified as intrahepatic, perihilar, or distal (Fig. 6.1).[8]

Intrahepatic cholangiocarcinomas are defined as those confined to the liver that do not involve the extrahepatic biliary tree, do not present with obstructive jaundice, and have no evidence of a primary tumor elsewhere. Approximately 6% of cholangiocarcinomas are intrahepatic. These tumors are managed, when possible, by liver resection.

Perihilar tumors are those that involve or require resection of the hepatic duct bifurcation (Klatskin tumors). Perihilar tumors may cause obstructive jaundice early in the course of the disease, when the primary tumor is still small. Cholangiocarcinomas that involve the hepatic duct bifurcation and also have a significant intrahepatic component are considered perihilar tumors. Approximately 67% of cholangiocarcinomas are perihilar. These tumors, when resectable, are managed by resection of the hepatic duct confluence with or without concomitant liver resection. Knowledge of the Bismuth-Corlette classification[9] is also helpful for clinical decision-making for perihilar tumors (Fig. 6.2).

Distal cholangiocarcinomas are those that arise in the mid or distal bile duct. They are potentially amenable to pancreaticoduodenectomy. Obstruc-

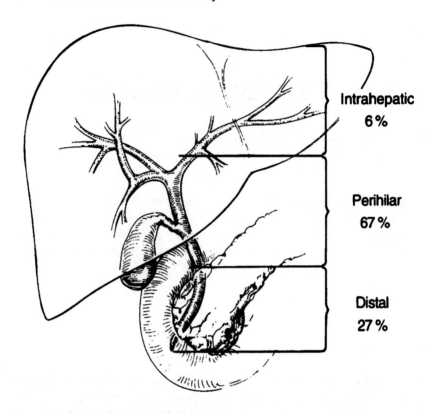

FIGURE 6.1. Distribution of 294 cholangiocarcinomas into intrahepatic, perihilar, and distal subgroups. (From Nakeeb et al.,[8] with permission).

TYPE I	TYPE II	TYPE IIIa	TYPE IIIb	TYPE IV

FIGURE 6.2. Bismuth-Corlette[9] classification of hilar cholangiocarcinoma. Types I and II can be resected with excision of the extrahepatic bile duct with or without the hilar plate and caudate lobe. Types IIIa and IIIb can be resected with the addition of an en bloc right or left hepatic lobectomy, respectively. Type IV is, by definition, unresectable. (From Blumgart and Stain,[4] with permission).

tive jaundice is usually present, and distal cholangiocarcinomas may be mistaken for adenocarcinoma of the pancreatic head. Approximately 27% of cholangiocarcinomas are distal.

Some tumors are diffuse and can involve extensive portions of the intrahepatic and extrahepatic bile ducts.

Clinical Features

Intrahepatic cholangiocarcinomas usually reach a large size before becoming clinically evident. Patients with these large peripheral hepatic tumors may present with hepatomegaly and an upper abdominal mass, abdominal and back pain, and weight loss.[2] Jaundice and ascites are late and usually preterminal sequelae in patients with large intrahepatic cholangiocarcinomas.

Patients with extrahepatic (perihilar and distal) cholangiocarcinoma usually present with painless jaundice. Patients also may report concomitant onset of fatigue, pruritus, fever, vague abdominal pain, anorexia, and weight loss.

Laboratory Studies

Serum alkaline phosphatase levels are elevated in more than 90% of patients with cholangiocarcinoma.[2] Serum bilirubin also is elevated in most cholangiocarcinoma patients, particularly those with a tumor arising in the central portion of the liver or the extrahepatic hilar bile ducts.[3] Mild anemia occurs occasionally, but other serum laboratory studies are usually normal. In contrast to hepatocellular carcinoma, serum α-fetoprotein (AFP) levels are abnormal in fewer than 5% of cholangiocarcinoma patients.[2] There is an increase in serum carcinoembryonic antigen (CEA) levels in 40–60% of cholangiocarcinoma patients.[2,10] Another tumor marker, CA 19-9, is elevated in more than 80% of patients with cholangiocarcinoma.[10] One study showed that the serum tumor marker CA 19-9 had an 89% sensitivity and 86% specificity for diagnosing cholangiocarcinoma in patients with sclerosing cholangitis.[11] Combining serum CA 19-9 levels with serum CEA levels may further increase the diagnostic accuracy for detecting cholangiocarcinoma in patients with sclerosing cholangitis.[12]

Intrahepatic Cholangiocarcinoma

Diagnosis

Intrahepatic cholangiocarcinoma usually can be visualized as a mass by ultrasonography or computed tomography (CT). Needle biopsy of the lesion under ultrasound or CT guidance usually is helpful for determining the diagnosis.

Treatment

Resection

Most patients with intrahepatic cholangiocarcinoma present with large tumors and usually have evidence of regional lymph node, pulmonary, or bone metastases at the time of diagnosis. In patients who present with jaundice from large intrahepatic cholangiocarcinomas, death usually ensues within a year of diagnosis. Rarely, small peripheral cholangiocarcinomas that are detected before they metastasize or cause jaundice may be resected with resultant long-term survival.[13-16] A study of 19 patients who underwent resection of intrahepatic cholangiocarcinoma demonstrated that patients with no porta hepatis lymph node metastases had a 3-year survival rate of 64% compared to 0% for patients with nodal metastases.[17] A larger cohort of 32 patients who underwent resection of intrahepatic cholangiocarcinomas confirmed the negative prognostic impact of regional lymph node metastases and large size (> 5 cm diameter) of the primary tumor.[18] Another series demonstrated a 5-year survival rate of 44% for patients with resected intrahepatic cholangiocarcinoma.[8]

Liver Transplantation

Orthotopic liver transplantation has been described in patients with intrahepatic cholangiocarcinoma.[18-20] The 1-year survival in series prior to 1990 was 29.4%, with only two of the patients undergoing liver transplantation alive 5 years after the transplant. Almost 90% of the patients who survived at least 90 days after the liver transplant died from recurrent cholangiocarcinoma, frequently at extrahepatic sites. In small series patients have had 5-year posttransplantation survival rates up to 53%.[19,20] The improved survival is based on careful selection of cholangiocarcinoma patients for liver transplantation—specifically by not giving transplants to patients with lymph node metastases or invasion of major intra- or extrahepatic blood vessels.

Extrahepatic (Perihilar and Distal) Cholangiocarcinoma

Fardel first described a primary malignancy of the extrahepatic biliary tract in 1890.[21] A 1957 report described three patients with small adenocarcinomas involving the confluence of the left and right hepatic ducts.[22] Such primary cholangiocarcinomas arising at the bifurcation of the extrahepatic biliary tree are known commonly as Klatskin's tumors, following Klatskin's report in 1965 of a large series of patients with these lesions.[23]

Diagnosis

The diagnosis of pancreatic cancer is often the first consideration in patients presenting with painless jaundice. For this reason, a CT scan of the abdomen may be the first radiologic study obtained. Patients with painless jaundice due to pancreatic cancer may or may not have a mass in the head of the pancreas evident on a CT scan. They do, however, have dilation of the extrahepatic biliary tree and gallbladder. In contrast, a diagnosis of hilar cholangiocarcinoma should be suspected in the patient with painless jaundice whose CT scan demonstrates dilated intrahepatic bile ducts with a normal gallbladder and extrahepatic biliary tree. High-resolution, thin-section CT scans can provide information on the location of an obstructing tumor and on the extent of involvement of the liver and porta hepatis structures by the tumor (Figs. 6.3–6.6).

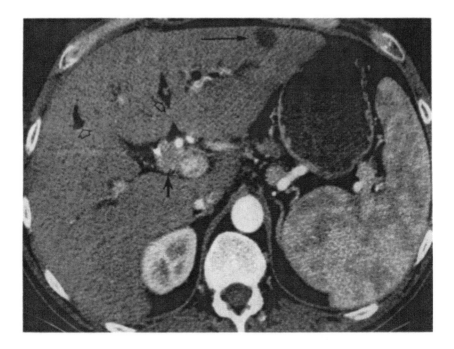

Figure 6.3. High-resolution, thin-section CT scan in a patient with obstructive jaundice. The scan demonstrates a tumor (solid arrow) at the hepatic hilum lying anterior and lateral to the portal vein. Dilated intrahepatic bile ducts (open arrow) and a liver metastasis (long arrow) are seen. Biopsy of the hilar tumor confirmed the diagnosis of cholangiocarcinoma.

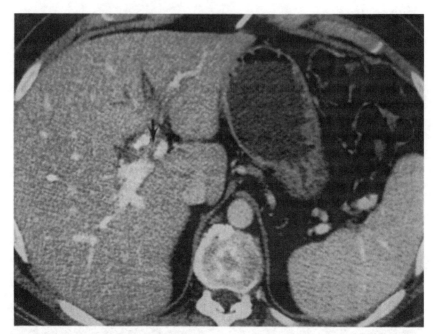

FIGURE 6.4. High-resolution, thin-section CT scan of a patient with obstructive jaundice. The scan demonstrates a tumor at the confluence of the left and right hepatic bile ducts compressing the portal vein (arrow). Biopsy of the hilar tumor confirmed the diagnosis of cholangiocarcinoma.

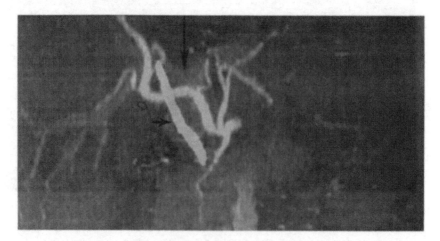

FIGURE 6.5. Vascular reconstruction of the hepatic arteries and portal vein from a bolus contrast injection spiral CT scan from a patient with hilar cholangiocarcinoma. There is no evidence of vascular invasion on this image, which was confirmed at the time of resection. A biliary stent (solid arrow) is seen overlying the right hepatic artery (open arrow). The portal vein is also evident (long arrow).

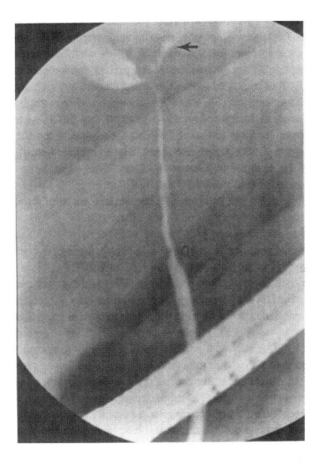

FIGURE 6.6. Endoscopic retrograde cholangiopancreatography (ERCP) showing a long stricture of the extrahepatic bile duct extending from the confluence of the left and right hepatic ducts (solid arrow) to the top of the duodenum (open arrow). Brushings obtained at the time of ERCP confirmed a diagnosis of cholangiocarcinoma.

Ultrasonography is the simplest noninvasive study for the jaundiced patient. It is not uncommon to find a patient who has jaundice and weight loss due to gallstones. The absence of gallstones on ultrasound examination changes the nature of the clinical investigation. Like the CT scan, ultrasonography can demonstrate a nondilated gallbladder and common bile duct associated with dilated intrahepatic ducts.[24] Additionally, as gray-scale ultrasonography has improved, the diagnosis of cholangiocarcinoma is supported by finding a hilar bile duct mass in between 65–90% of patients.[25,26] Ultrasonography and CT scans also are useful for determining preoperatively the presence of intrahepatic tumor due to direct extension or metastases, portal vein invasion by tumor, and enlarged periportal lymph nodes suggesting nodal metastases.[26,27]

Cholangiography identifies the area(s) of stricture and dilation within the bile duct system. Percutaneous transhepatic cholangiography (PTC) and endoscopic retrograde cholangiopancreatography (ERCP) are useful for assessing patients with extrahepatic biliary obstruction. A prospective, randomized comparison of PTC and ERCP in jaundiced patients revealed that the two techniques had similar diagnostic accuracy.[28] PTC was 100% accurate at demonstrating obstruction at the confluence of the left and right hepatic ducts, and ERCP had an accuracy of 92% demonstrating these lesions. ERCP has the additional benefit of providing a pancreatogram. A normal pancreatogram helps to exclude a small carcinoma of the head of the pancreas as a cause of biliary obstruction. Some investigators have recommended combined PTC and ERCP to establish the extent of the lesion in the bile ducts, but such concomitant studies are helpful only in selected patients with complete obstruction of the biliary tree.[29]

Cytologic specimens can be obtained at the time of PTC and ERCP. The presence of malignant cells in bile or bile duct brushings is confirmed in approximately 50% of patients undergoing PTC or ERCP.[25]

The final radiologic study to consider is celiac and superior mesenteric arteriography with late-phase portography. Arteriography in patients with hilar cholangiocarcinoma can be important because extensive encasement of the hepatic arteries or portal vein precludes curative resection. Combining the findings on cholangiography with vascular involvement by tumor on arteriography has been found to have better than 80% accuracy in predicting unresectability.[30] An occasional patient does have compression or displacement of vascular structures rather than true malignant invasion or encasement. We obtain arteriographic studies in fewer than 10% of our patients because a high-resolution, thin-section CT scan with intravenous bolus contrast administration can demonstrate hepatic artery and portal vein involvement by a hilar tumor, obviating the need for more invasive angiographic studies.

Difficult Diagnosis

For patients with a bile duct stricture suspected to be malignant on cholangiography but with inconclusive or negative cytologic studies, a real diagnostic dilemma exists. Because the differential diagnosis includes benign stricture, sclerosing cholangitis, Caroli syndrome, lymphoma, and other rare disorders, it is imperative to obtain an accurate diagnosis. For example, sclerosing cholangitis can be focal in nature and mimic perihilar cholangiocarcinoma. A careful history and physical examination may suggest inflammatory bowel disease and possibly associated sclerosing cholangitis. If markedly elevated, the CEA and CA 19-9 levels can be helpful in suggesting cholangiocarcinoma but are in no way diagnostic.[10–12]

If a perihilar or pancreatic head mass is demonstrated on ultrasonography, CT, or magnetic resonance imaging (MRI), it is usually possible to perform an image-directed needle biopsy of this area. However, it is still difficult to obtain a diagnosis preoperatively in a significant number of cases.

It is a mistake to assume that a stricture is benign because the cytology is negative for tumor cells. False-negative cytologic specimens from ERCP, PTC, and needle biopsies are common in patients subsequently confirmed to have hilar cholangiocarcinomas.

In some cases, ERCP can be performed with the "mother-daughter" scope to visualize the lumen of the common bile duct and to obtain directed biopsy specimens. Endoscopic ultrasonography occasionally identifies a mass that was not seen on the CT scan. For distal lesions, it may be possible to perform directed needle biopsies using endoscopic ultrasonography. If the diagnosis is still not clear, surgical exploration is indicated in patients who are candidates for resection. Stent placement and close follow-up are undertaken in high risk patients so long as the patient and physician both understand the risk of cancer. Because it is sometimes impossible to differentiate a benign bile duct stricture from a malignant one despite all of the above tests, the decision to manage this problem operatively or nonoperatively requires considerable clinical judgment.

Unfortunately, it may be difficult to differentiate benign from malignant processes even at operation. Laparoscopy is probably a prudent first step and may spare patients with liver metastases or carcinomatosis an unnecessary laparotomy. It takes little time to insert a single camera port for diagnostic laparoscopy, even if only to view the peritoneal and liver surfaces. Enlarged lymph nodes can be biopsied laparoscopically if it might alter patient management. If laparoscopy reveals no obvious tumor, laparotomy is necessary.

The abdomen is explored through a right subcostal incision, which is extended to a bilateral subcostal incision if necessary. A generous Kocher maneuver is performed. The porta hepatis is palpated for tumor, and any abnormal lymph nodes are sent for frozen section histologic examination. If necessary, the porta hepatis is dissected to expose the hepatic duct bifurcation.

Even with the area of the stricture in the surgeon's hand at laparotomy, it is sometimes impossible to determine a benign from a malignant stricture. In this case there are two basic options. One may choose to perform resection only in the face of a tissue diagnosis of cancer. In this case a diligent attempt at intraoperative diagnosis is undertaken. Biopsies are performed of any suspicious areas. If the stricture is in the distal common bile duct, transduodenal core needle biopsies of the pancreatic head may be done. Even if a discrete mass is palpated, it is often not diagnostic. It is sometimes helpful to insert the choledochoscope into the cystic duct stump after cholecystectomy or directly into the common bile duct through a choledochotomy. Under direct vision through the choledochoscope, it may be possible to biopsy the area of suspected tumor and to determine the extent of tumor involvement. If these maneuvers fail to diagnose cancer, a choledo-choenterostomy or hepaticojejunostomy may be performed, or it is preferable in some cases to manage the stricture by stenting. Even in the best of hands, some strictures that were thought to be benign are misdiagnosed using this approach.

The second intraoperative option is to perform a resection in the absence of a tissue diagnosis of malignancy. For perihilar lesions, the hepatic duct bifurcation is resected. A frozen section diagnosis should be obtained, as well as an assessment of the proximal and distal bile duct margins. Hepaticojejunostomy is performed, with or without stent placement. Distal strictures are approached in a similar manner, but resection of these lesions requires a pancreaticoduodenectomy. The controversy over whether to proceed with pancreaticoduodenectomy without a confirmed diagnosis of cancer rages on; we believe that resection without a tissue diagnosis is warranted for patients who present with jaundice and a low density mass in the head of the pancreas on dynamic CT scan. Although an occasional patient undergoes resection for a benign condition (pancreatitis), most of the time the clinical suspicion of malignancy is confirmed. For patients with a stricture in the distal common duct and no associated mass, the decision is somewhat more difficult. In patients who are acceptable candidates for major operation, pancreaticoduodenectomy should be considered, as there is simply no other way to be certain that the stricture is related to a benign process.

Treatment

Surgery

Curative resection and palliation are the possible goals of operation for extrahepatic cholangiocarcinomas. Because the lesions in most patients with unresectable perihilar tumors can be effectively palliated by PTC- or ERCP-placed stents, operative procedures to provide drainage of the hepatic ducts are not employed as frequently as in the past. Operation is not necessary for palliation in most patients with unresectable perihilar or distal bile duct tumors.

Curative resection of perihilar cholangiocarcinoma involves resection of the common and hepatic ducts with negative proximal and distal margins. Liver resection is necessary in some cases to achieve negative margins. Regional lymphadenectomy is performed by resecting the portal lymph nodes en bloc with the bile duct. Hepaticojejunostomy is done with or without stent placement. Although it is not necessary to stent most anastomoses, it is sometimes prudent to perform a stented Roux-en-Y hepaticojejunostomy with a "chimney" to provide access to the anastomosis for dilation and stent placement in the event of stricture or recurrence (Fig. 6.7). Stented hepaticojejunostomy also allows access to the remaining biliary tree for delivery of brachytherapy.[32]

Surgical bypass for relief of biliary obstruction in patients with unresectable tumors can be accomplished by segment III bypass or, rarely, segment V bypass. Operative intubation techniques offer an alternative to ERCP- or PTC-placed stents but have no advantage over the less invasive methods. Technical aspects of these procedures have been described in detail.[3,4,6]

Resection of perihilar cholangiocarcinoma affords the patient the best chance for significant survival, although 5-year survival rates after resection of perihilar cancers are 40% in the most hopeful reports and 10% or less in other accounts. Almost all patients who die after a seemingly curative resection of the extrahepatic bile ducts do so as a result of recurrent tumor.[3–8]

The patterns of failure after curative extrahepatic bile duct resection for hilar cholangiocarcinoma have been described in a few series of patients (Table 6.1).[33] Locoregional tumor recurrence developed in a high percentage of patients, with failure in the liver (62%), tumor bed (42%), and regional lymph nodes (20%). The caudate lobe is the most frequent site of liver recurrence. Regional lymph nodes include porta hepatis, retroduodenal, and perigastric node groups along the gastrohepatic ligament. Distant metastasis developed in most patients who exhibited a locoregional recurrence but was the site of first failure in only 24%.

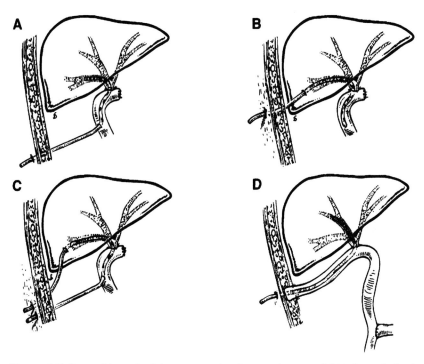

FIGURE 6.7. Stented hepaticojejunostomy. A tube may be passed (A) through the jejunum; (B) through the liver; or (C) as a U tube. (D) Alternatively, a "chimney" may be created by bringing the blind end of the jejunal loop through the abdominal wall to the subcutaneous tissue or by suturing it to the abdominal wall in a subfascial location. The anastomosis is stented with a transjejunal tube, which is brought out through the abdominal wall. The end of the jejunum is marked with a metal ring or clips to allow radiologic access at a later time when the tube has been removed. In this way percutaneous access of the jejunal loop can provide an avenue for subsequent dilation, stent placement, or even passage of the choledochoscope. (Adapted from Blumgart and Baer,[31] with permission).

TABLE 6.1. Sites of tumor recurrence after curative resection of proximal perihilar cholangiocarcinomas

Site	Frequency (%)
Liver	62
Tumor bed	42
Regional lymph nodes	20
Peritoneum	16
Lungs	71
Bone	31
Skin and subcutaneous tissue	7

Detailed anatomic studies have offered an explanation for the high incidence of liver and local recurrence following resection of a hilar cholangiocarcinoma. In a series of 26 patients undergoing surgery for hilar cholangiocarcinoma, direct invasion of hepatic parenchyma at the hilum was noted in 12 patients (46.2%), with 11 patients (42.3%) also having carcinoma extending into the bile ducts draining the caudate lobe or directly invading the caudate lobe parenchyma.[34] A study of 106 adult human cadavers showed that 97.2% had bile ducts draining the caudate lobe that entered directly into the main left hepatic duct, right hepatic duct, or both.[35] These caudate lobe bile ducts frequently enter the main left or right hepatic ducts within 1 cm of the proper hepatic duct. Thus, a carcinoma arising at the confluence of the right and left hepatic ducts need not be large to extend into the bile ducts draining the caudate lobe.

Because cholangiocarcinoma is known to spread along the wall of the bile ducts and because the caudate lobe and hepatic hilum are frequent sites of tumor recurrence following extrahepatic duct resection, a number of surgeons now recommend more aggressive resections to include the caudate lobe and hepatic hilar parenchyma.[35–41] The improved equipment and understanding of techniques requisite for a safe liver resection allow performance of aggressive extended resections with little or no increase in operative morbidity and mortality. The median survival associated with a more radical surgical approach has varied from 10 to 37 months, with 5-year survival rates of 20–44% and 10-year survival rates as high as 14%.[35–41] These studies clearly show that liver resection is worthwhile only if completely tumor-negative resection margins can be attained because there were no 5-year survivors with positive resection margins.

Pancreaticoduodenectomy is performed for distal cholangiocarcinomas. Survival of patients undergoing resection of distal cholangiocarcinomas generally has been reported to exceed that of patients with resected perihilar tumors. In one series the 5-year survival rate for patients undergoing resection (pancreaticoduodenectomy) for distal cholangiocarcinoma was 28% versus 11% following resection of perihilar tumors.[8]

Adjuvant Radiation Therapy

Although several retrospective series have suggested a benefit for adjuvant radiation therapy after resection of perihilar cholangiocarcinoma,[42-48] the only prospective analysis indicated no advantage in terms of survival or quality of life for patients treated with radiation therapy.[49] In this prospective study, no concomitant chemotherapy to act as a radiation sensitizing agent was administered. Therefore the best available evidence does not support routine use of postoperative radiotherapy. However, anecdotal experience with successful high-dose brachytherapy or external beam chemoradiation therapy continues to appear in the medical literature and indicates that formal, prospective investigation of multimodality adjuvant therapy should be considered. There are certainly occasional patients with unresected cholangiocarcinoma or with incomplete resection who are long-term survivors following such multimodality treatment.

Adjuvant Chemotherapy

Unfortunately, no effective adjuvant chemotherapy regimens have been demonstrated to date.

Neoadjuvant Chemoradiation

Because of the disappointing results of postoperative radiation therapy, a neoadjuvant approach has been developed.[50] At the M. D. Anderson Cancer Center, nine patients with biopsy-proved extrahepatic cholangiocarcinoma have undergone preoperative (neoadjuvant) chemoradiation. Chemoradiation was delivered by concomitant administration of continuous-infusion 5-fluorouracil (5-FU) (300 mg/m^2/day, Monday through Friday) and external beam radiotherapy. External beam radiation was delivered Monday through Friday at a dose of 1.8 Gy/day to a total dose of 50.4 Gy (n = 5) or 45 Gy (n = 2). Two patients with tumors of the intrapancreatic portion of the common bile duct received a rapid fractionation regimen of 3.0 Gy/day to a total dose of 30 Gy, the biologic equivalent of the 50.4 Gy dose.[51]

Preoperative chemoradiation was generally well tolerated. The characteristics of the patients undergoing preoperative chemoradiation are summarized in Table 6.2. Six of the nine patients who underwent preoperative chemoradiation were thought to have unresectable disease at presentation: four based on radiographic images and two based on abdominal exploration at other institutions. Two patients with perihilar tumors received an additional 10-Gy boost of irradiation delivered postoperatively by iridium-192 wire brachytherapy. Three of the four patients with distal tumors received an external beam intraoperative radiation therapy (IORT) boost of 10 Gy to the area of the celiac axis and retroperitoneum. All nine of the patients who underwent preoperative chemoradiation had tumor-free resection margins. Three of the nine patients (33%) undergoing preoperative chemoradiation

TABLE 6.2. Characteristics of patients undergoing preoperative chemoradiation

Patient no.	Age (years)	Sex	Site	XRT Dose (Gy)	XRT boost (Gy)	Histologic response	First recurrence	Status	Survival (months)
1	56	M	Perihilar	50.4	None	II, moderate	None	NED	80
2	41	M	Perihilar	45	10 (¹⁹²I wire)	II, no residual primary tumor, microscopic tumor foci in two lymph nodes	None	NED	32
3	56	M	Perihilar	45	10 Gy ¹⁹²I Wire	II, moderate response	None	NED	25
4	68	M	Perihilar	50.4	None	IV, pathologic CR	None	NED	6
5	69	F	Perihilar	50.4	None	IV, pathologic CR	None	DNED	11
6	63	F	Distal	50.4	None	III, marked response	Unknown	DOD	26
7	75	M	Distal	50.4	10 (IORT)	IV, pathologic CR	Liver	DOD	12
8	58	M	Distal	30ᵃ	10 (IORT)	I, minimal response	Liver	DOD	11
9	50	M	Distal	30ᵃ	10 (IORT)	I, minimal response	Peritoneum	DOD	8

XRT = x-irradiation; CR = complete response; NED = no evidence of disease; DOD = dead of disease; DNED = patient died of massive myocardial infarction without evidence of recurrence.
All margins in these nine patients were negative.
ᵃRapid fractionation regimen.

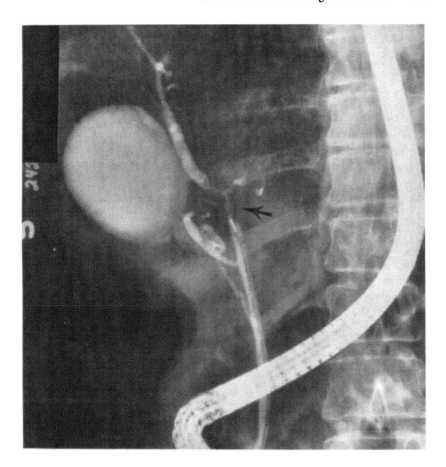

FIGURE 6.8-A.

FIGURE 6.8. Radiographic evaluation of a patient with a perihilar tumor who underwent preoperative chemoradiation with a pathologic complete response. (A) ERCP evaluation demonstrating a perihilar tumor (arrow). (B) Preoperative CT scan demonstrating a tumor mass (arrow) adjacent to the biliary stent. (C) CT scan following preoperative chemoradiation. Note the indistinct tumor margins and typical radiation effect.

had a pathologic complete response, with no evidence of tumor in the operative specimen (Fig. 6.8). A fourth patient had no evidence of viable primary tumor but was found to have microscopic metastases in two portal lymph nodes. The remaining five patients had varying degrees of histologic response.

Surgical complications in the preoperative chemoradiation group included three minor wound infections and one cardiac arrhythmia with transient pulmonary edema. There were no biliary anastomotic leaks or intraabdominal infections postoperatively.

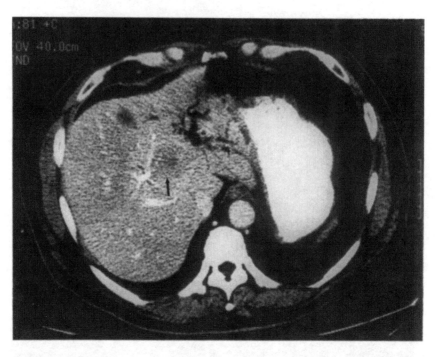

FIGURE 6.8-B.

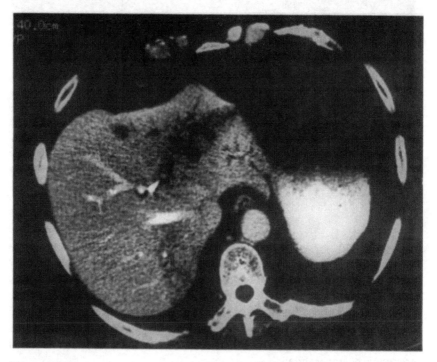

FIGURE 6.8-C.

Three of nine patients (33%) who underwent preoperative chemoradiation experienced a pathologic complete response. Two of these patients had perihilar tumors, one of the patients is alive and well 6 months after operation. The other patient died of a massive myocardial infarction 11 months after operation and had no evidence of recurrence at autopsy. The remaining complete responder had a distal lesion and died with extensive liver metastasis 12 months after resection. Another patient with a perihilar tumor had a complete pathologic response of the primary tumor but had microscopic disease in two lymph nodes; this patient is alive and free of disease at 32 months.

At this time, none of the five patients with perihilar cholangiocarcinoma treated with preoperative chemoradiation have experienced recurrence, although one has died of co-morbid disease. All had tumor-free resection margins. Although the number of patients is small, these data suggest that preoperative chemoradiation may increase the likelihood of obtaining negative resection margins in patients with perihilar cholangiocarcinoma. Whether this treatment leads to improved survival remains to be determined. Additional multicenter trials of preoperative chemoradiation are warranted.

Liver Transplantation

Total hepatectomy with immediate orthotopic liver transplantation has been described in 78 patients with hilar cholangiocarcinoma.[5,19,20] The 90-day mortality due to hemorrhage, sepsis, and graft rejection was 23.1%. Of the 60 patients who survived more than 3 months following transplantation, the median survival was 11 months. In this same group of 60 patients, the 5-year survival rate was 5.0%. For the patients who died more than 3 months after transplantation, death was due to tumor recurrence in 85.4%. Because of these poor results, most transplant centers no longer perform liver transplants in patients with hilar cholangiocarcinoma. Liver transplantation for hilar cholangiocarcinoma should be considered only as part of a prospective protocol evaluating multimodality treatment.

Treatment of Unresectable Cholangiocarcinoma

Chemotherapy

Given the high percentage of unresectable hilar cholangiocarcinomas, various chemotherapeutic regimens and radiotherapeutic regimens have been used in the hope of providing improved palliation and prolongation of survival. Unfortunately, reports describing chemotherapy or radiotherapy for hilar cholangiocarcinoma rarely describe the treatment results in more than 10–20 patients.

A 1988 review of systemic chemotherapy for bile duct cancer noted that 97 patients had been treated with nine different treatment programs.[52] Mitomycin C, doxorubicin, and 5-FU are the agents that have shown the greatest activity against cholangiocarcinoma. The collective partial response rate in the 97 patients was 29%, with no complete responses. The median survival of these patients receiving systemic chemotherapy ranged between 6 and 11 months. No reports since 1988 have indicated a better response rate with systemic chemotherapy. With no significant increase in survival and considering the quality-of-life issues related to chemotherapeutic toxicity, systemic chemotherapy has not demonstrated a distinct advantage in patients with hilar cholangiocarcinoma.

Regional chemotherapy by hepatic artery infusion has some potential advantages over systemic chemotherapy. The proximal bile duct receives its arterial blood supply from the hepatic artery, so an increased concentration of drug can be delivered directly to the region of the tumor, including the liver. By using drugs such as 5-FU and floxuridine, systemic exposure to drug is limited because of the high rate of hepatic extraction of these agents. There are reports of 46 hilar cholangiocarcinoma patients who have been treated by hepatic artery chemotherapy infusion.[52,53] The partial response rate for the entire group of patients was 43%, but there were no complete responses and no significant prolongation of survival. Hepatic artery infusion chemotherapy may have a palliative role in patients with hilar cholangiocarcinoma, but currently available drugs do not provide improved survival.

Radiotherapy

Radiotherapy for bile duct cancer is yet more confusing owing to the various types, doses, routes of administration, and association with resected and unresected tumors, all in small numbers of patients. Radiotherapy may be delivered by external beam, intraluminal brachytherapy, or intraoperatively. There are no convincing randomized prospective data to indicate that routine use of radiotherapy prolongs survival for patients with unresectable cholangiocarcinoma.[5,42-49] Whether radiotherapy in this setting provides palliation is debatable. Occasional long-term survivors following aggressive radiotherapy or chemoradiation alone, coupled with a significant complete pathologic response rate for neoadjuvant chemoradiation, make this an option worthy of study in carefully controlled clinical studies.

Prognostic Factors

In contrast to reports from two to three decades ago, most patients with extrahepatic cholangiocarcinoma now are diagnosed premortem. The most important factor affecting prognosis is the resectability of the tumor. Patients who undergo resection with curative intent have 3-year survival rates as high as 50% and 5-year survival rates between 10% and 44%.[54,55] Significant determinants of improved prognosis in patients undergoing curative resection include well differentiated tumors, absence of lymph node metastases, absence of direct tumor extension into the liver, papillary histology (versus nodular or sclerotic), a serum bilirubin level at presentation of less than 9 mg/dl, and a near-normal or normal performance status.[55] Palliative resection, surgical bypass procedures, and various types of intubation and drainage procedures are associated with 3-year survival rates of 0–4%.[56] Hilar cholangiocarcinomas have a poorer prognosis than do carcinomas arising in the middle or distal thirds of the extrahepatic bile duct, which is related directly to presentation of tumor at a more locally advanced stage with liver involvement by tumor and resultant lower resection rates.

Pathologic features of the bile duct cancer are predictors of outcome. The prognosis is affected adversely if the tumor infiltrates through the serosa of the bile duct, invades the liver directly, demonstrates vascular invasion, or has metastasized to regional lymph nodes.[57] Histologic type and grade also are important factors. Patients with the relatively unusual papillary bile duct adenocarcinoma have the most favorable prognosis, with 3-year survival rates up to 75%.[56,57] Patients with the more common nodular or sclerotic types of hilar cholangiocarcinoma have 3-year survival rates of less than 20%. Patients with well or moderately differentiated carcinomas have a 3-year survival rate of 21%, whereas no patient with a poorly differentiated carcinoma survived longer than 2 years.[57]

Conclusions

Cholangiocarcinoma is a rare disease with a poor prognosis. Conventional treatment cures few patients. It is clear that surgical resection with negative margins remains the only standard therapy that offers the possibility, albeit small, of cure. The role of multimodality therapy must be clarified, as there is no strong evidence to indicate that chemotherapy or radiation therapy is beneficial in most cases, either as an adjuvant or palliatively. Multicenter trials are necessary to test new treatment approaches for cholangiocarcinoma.

References

1. Anthony PP. Tumours and tumour-like lesions of the liver and biliary tract. In: MacSween RNM, Anthony PP, Scheuer PJ (eds) Pathology of the Liver, 2nd ed. Edinburgh, Churchill Livingstone, 1987, p. 574
2. Moto R, Kawarada Y. Diagnosis and treatment of cholangiocarcinoma and cystic adenocarcinoma of the liver. In: Okuda K, Ishak KG (eds) Neoplasms of the Liver. Tokyo, Springer, 1987, p.381
3. Pitt H, Dooley W, Yeo C, Cameron J. Malignancies of the biliary tract. Curr Probl Surg 32:1, 1995

4. Blumgart LH, Stain SC. Surgical treatment of cholangiocarcinoma. In: Sugarbaker P (ed) Hepatobiliary Cancer. Boston, Kluwer, 1994, pp.75–96
5. Curley SA, Levin B, Rich TA. Liver and bile ducts. In: Abeloff MD, Armitage JO, Lichter AS, Niederhuber JE (eds) Clinical Oncology. New York, Churchill Livingstone, 1995, pp. 1305–1372
6. Blumgart LH, Benjamin IS. Cancer of the bile ducts In: Blumgart LH (ed) Surgery of the Liver and Biliary Tract. Edinburgh, Churchill Livingstone, 1994, pp. 967–995
7. Vauthey J-N, Blumgart LH. Recent advances in the management of cholangiocarcinomas. Semin Liver Dis 14:109, 1994
8. Nakeeb A, Pitt HA, Sohn TA, et al. Cholangiocarcinoma: a spectrum of intrahepatic, perihilar, and distal tumors. Ann Surg 224:463, 1996
9. Bismuth H, Corlette MB. Intrahepatic cholangioenteric anastomosis in carcinoma of the hilus of the liver. Surg Gynecol Obstet 140:170, 1975
10. Jalanko H, Kuusela P, Roberts P, et al. Comparison of a new tumor marker, CA 19-9T, with a-fetoprotein and carcinoembryonic antigen in patients with upper gastrointestinal disease. J Clin Pathol 37:218, 1984
11. Nichols JC, Gores GJ, LaRusso NF, et al. Diagnostic role of serum CA 19-9 for cholangiocarcinoma in patients with primary sclerosing cholangitis. Mayo Clin Proc 68:874, 1993
12. Ramage JK, Donaghy A, Farrant JM, et al. Serum tumor markers for the diagnosis of cholangiocarcinoma in primary sclerosing cholangitis. Gastroenterology 108:865, 1995
13. Liver Cancer Study Group of Japan. Primary liver cancer in Japan. Cancer 54:1747, 1984
14. Liver Cancer Study Group of Japan. Primary liver cancer in Japan: sixth report. Cancer 60:1400, 1987
15. Okuda K. Liver Cancer Study Group of Japan. Primary liver cancers in Japan. Cancer 45:2663, 1980
16. Liguory C, Canard JM. Tumours of the biliary system. Clin Gastroenterol 12:269, 1983
17. Chou FF, Sheen-Chen SM, Chen CL, et al. Prognostic factors of resectable intrahepatic cholangiocarcinoma. J Surg Oncol 59:40, 1995
18. Pichlmayr R, Lamesch P, Weimann A, Tusch G, Ringe B. Surgical treatment of cholangiocellular carcinoma. World J Surg 19:83, 1995
19. Sansalone CV, Colella G, Caccamo L, et al. Orthotopic liver transplantation for primary biliary tumors: Milan multicenter experience. Transplant Proc 26:3561, 1994
20. Goldstein RM, Stone M, Tillery GW, et al. Is liver transplantation indicated for cholangiocarcinoma? Am J Surg 166:768, 1993
21. Fardel D. Malignant neoplasms of the extrahepatic biliary ducts. Ann Surg 76:205, 1922
22. Altemeier WA, Gall EA, Zinninger MM, et al. Sclerosing carcinoma of the major intrahepatic bile ducts. Arch Surg 75:450, 1957
23. Klatskin G. Adenocarcinoma of the hepatic duct at its bifurcation within the porta hepatis. Am J Med 38:241, 1965
24. Wheeler PG, Dawson JL, Nunnerly H, et al. Newer techniques in the diagnosis and treatment of proximal bile duct carcinoma: an analysis of 41 consecutive patients. Q J Med 50:247, 1981

25. Okuda K, Ohto M, Tsuchiya Y. The role of ultrasound, percutaneous transhepatic cholangiography, computed tomographic scanning, and magnetic resonance imaging in the preoperative assessment of bile duct cancer. World J Surg 12:18, 1988
26. Garber ST, Donald JJ, Lees WR. Cholangiocarcinoma: ultrasound features and correlation of tumor position with survival. Abdom Imaging 18:69, 1993
27. Neumaier CE, Bertolotto M, Perrone R, et al. Staging of hilar cholangiocarcinoma with ultrasound. J Clin Ultrasound 23:173, 1995
28. Elias E, Hamlyn AN, Jain S, et al. A randomized trial of percutaneous transhepatic cholangiography with the Chiba needle versus ERCP for bile duct visualization in jaundice. Gastroenterology 71:439, 1976
29. Tanaka M, Ogawa Y, Matsumoto S, et al. The role of endoscopic retrograde cholangiopancreatography in preoperative assessment of bile duct cancer. World J Surg 12:27, 1988
30. Voyles CR, Bowley NJ, Allison DJ, et al. Carcinoma of the proximal extrahepatic biliary tree, radiologic assessment and therapeutic alternatives. Ann Surg 197:188, 1983
31. Blumgart LH, Baer HU. Hilar and intrahepatic biliary-euteric anastomosis. In: Blumgart LH (ed) Surgery of the Liver and Biliary Tract. Edinburgh, Churchill Livingstone, 1994
32. Alexandre JH, Dehni N, Bouillot JL. Stented hepaticojejunostomies after resection for cholangiocarcinoma allow access for subsequent diagnosis and therapy. Am J Surg 169:428, 1995
33. Mittal B, Deutsch M, Iwatsuki S. Primary cancers of the extrahepatic biliary passages. Int J Radiat Oncol Biol Phys 11:849, 1985
34. Mizumoto R, Kawarada Y, Suzuki H. Surgical treatment of hilar carcinoma of the bile duct. Surg Gynecol Obstet 162:153, 1986
35. Mizumoto R, Suzuki H. Surgical anatomy of the hepatic hilum with special reference to the caudate lobe. World J Surg 12:2, 1988
36. Bengmark S, Ekberg H, Evander A, et al. Major liver resection for hilar cholangiocarcinoma. Ann Surg 207:120, 1988
37. Iwasaki Y, Okamura T, Ozaki A, et al. Surgical treatment for carcinoma at the confluence of the major hepatic ducts. Surg Gynecol Obstet 162:457, 1986
38. White TT. Skeletization resection and central hepatic resection in the treatment of bile duct cancer. World J Surg 12:48, 1988
39. Pinson CW, Rossi RL. Extended right hepatic lobectomy, left hepatic lobectomy, and skeletonization resection for proximal bile duct cancer. World J Surg 12:52, 1988
40. Washburn WK, Lewis WD, Jenkins RL. Aggressive surgical resection for cholangiocarcinoma. Arch Surg 130:270, 1995
41. Baer HU, Stain SC, Dennison AR, Eggers B, Blumgart LH. Improvements in survival by aggressive resections of hilar cholangiocarcinoma. Ann Surg 217:20, 1993
42. Cameron JL, Pitt HA, Zinner MJ, et al. Management of proximal cholangiocarcinomas by surgical resection and radiotherapy. Am J Surg 159:91, 1990
43. Schoenthaler R, Phillips TL, Castro J, et al. Carcinoma of the extrahepatic bile ducts: the University of California at San Francisco experience. Ann Surg 219:264, 1994
44. Buskirk SJ, Gunderson LL, Schild SE, et al. Analysis of failure after curative irradiation of extrahepatic bile duct carcinoma. Ann Surg 215:125, 1992

45. Alden ME, Mohiuddin M. The impact of radiation dose in combined external beam and intraluminal IR-192 brachytherapy for bile duct cancer. Int J Radiat Biol Phys 28:945, 1994

46. Tollenaar RA, vendeVeld CJ, Taat CW, et al. External radiotherapy and extrahepatic bile duct cancer. Eur J Surg 157:587, 1991

47. Gonzalez Gonzalez D, Gerard JP, Maners AW, et al. Results of radiation therapy in carcinoma of the proximal bile duct (Klatskin tumor). Semin Liver Dis 10:131, 1990

48. Hayes JK, Sapozink MD, Miller FJ. Definitive radiation therapy in bile duct carcinoma. Int J Radiat Oncol Biol Phys 15:735, 1988

49. Pitt HA, Nakeeb A, Abrams RA, et al. Perihilar cholangiocarcinoma: postoperative radiotherapy does not improve survival. Ann Surg 221:788, 1995

50. McMasters KM, Tuttle TM, Leach SD, et al. Neoadjuvant chemoradiation for extrahepatic cholangiocarcinoma. Am J Surg 174:605, 1997

51. Evans DB, Abbruzzese JL, Cleary KR et al. Rapid-fractionation pre-operative chemoradiation for malignant periampullary neoplasms. J R Coll Surg Edinb 40:319, 1995

52. Oberfield RA, Rossi RL. The role of chemotherapy in the treatment of bile duct cancer. World J Surg 12:105, 1988

53. Curley SA, Cameron JL: Hilar bile duct cancer: a diagnostic and therapeutic challenge. Cancer Bull 44:309, 1992.

54. Lai ECS, Tompkins RK, Roslyn JJ, et al. Proximal bile duct cancer: quality of survival. Ann Surg 205:111, 1987

55. Nagorney DM, Donohue JH, Farnell MB, et al. Outcomes after curative resections of cholangiocarcinoma. Arch Surg 128:871, 1993

56. Tompkins RK, Thomas D, Wile A, et al. Prognostic factors in bile duct carcinoma. Ann Surg 194:447, 1981

57. Ouchi K, Suzuki M, Hashimoto L, et al. Histologic findings and prognostic factors in carcinoma of the upper bile duct. Am J Surg 157:552, 1989

7

Diagnosis and Treatment of Primary Gallbladder Cancer

STEVEN A. CURLEY

Adenocarcinoma of the gallbladder is the fifth most common gastrointestinal malignancy. When compared with the worldwide incidence of hepatocellular cancer, gallbladder carcinoma accounts for fewer than 10% of the annual cases of primary hepatobiliary cancer. However, in countries such as the United States and those of western Europe with a low incidence of hepatocellular cancer, gallbladder carcinoma is relatively more prevalent. It was estimated that in the United States in 1997 there would be 6900 new cases of gallbladder cancer diagnosed compared to 12,000 cases of hepatocellular cancer.[1]

Autopsy and biliary tract operation data from 112,713 patients revealed that the average incidence of gallbladder carcinoma ranges from 0.55% to 1.91%.[2] Over the past three decades there appears to be a slight increase in the incidence of gallbladder carcinoma in Western countries, but this increase may be ascribed to more thorough reporting mechanisms rather than a true increase in incidence.[2] The peak incidence of gallbladder carcinoma occurs during the sixth and seventh decades of life. Unlike hepatocellular cancer and cholangiocarcinoma, gallbladder carcinoma has a higher incidence in women than men, with a ratio of approximately 3:1.[2] Gallbladder cancer develops more commonly in Hispanic populations than in Black and White populations.[3] This increased risk in Hispanic groups correlates with obesity, cholelithiasis, and dietary habits.

Gallbladder carcinoma is most prevalent in southwest American Indians, its incidence being six times higher than that in non-Indian populations. Gallbladder carcinoma has been found in 6% of southwest American Indians undergoing biliary tract surgery.[4] Gallbladder carcinoma is the second most common gastrointestinal malignancy in this population, with the youngest reported patient with gallbladder carcinoma an 11-year-old Navajo girl.[5]

Causative Factors

There are no apparent associations between gallbladder carcinoma and hepatitis B or C virus infection, cirrhosis, or mycotoxin exposure. Similarly, chemical hepatocarcinogens have not clearly been demonstrated to increase the risk of developing gallbladder carcinoma, although there are suggestions that workers exposed to carcinogenic substances such as methylcholanthrene and nitrosamines have a higher incidence and earlier onset of gallbladder carcinoma than do control populations.[6] Experimental studies indicate that animals exposed to hepatocarcinogens alone rarely form gallbladder carcinoma, but when the animals also were fed a gallstone-inducing diet, more than 50% developed gallbladder carcinoma.[7]

There is a significant association between gallstones and gallbladder carcinoma, with gallstones present in 74–92% of patients with gallbladder carcinoma.[8] The risk of developing gallbladder carcinoma increases directly with increasing gallstones size.[9] Patients with gallstones 2.0–2.9 cm in diameter have a 2.4 times higher relative risk of developing gallbladder carcinoma than those with no stones, whereas patients with gallstones larger than 3.0 cm in diameter have a 10.1 times higher risk of developing gallbladder carcinoma. Patients with long-standing chronic cholecystitis can develop calcification of the gallbladder wall, also known as porcelain gallbladder. It is possible that chronic inflammation or infection of the gallbladder increases the risk of developing gallbladder carcinoma, as 22% of patients with calcified gallbladders have gallbladder carcinoma.[10,11] Cholelithiasis and cholecystitis are more common in women, which in part may explain the higher incidence of gallbladder carcinoma in this gender group.[12] Gallbladder carcinomas stain weakly positive for estrogen receptors in fewer than 10% of cases, and estrogen does not appear to be a causative factor in this cancer.[13]

Gallstones or other factors that cause chronic inflammation of the gallbladder mucosa may induce a series of premalignant changes. If not treated with cholecystectomy, these premalignant lesions may progress to invasive gallbladder carcinoma. Epithelial dysplasia, atypical hyperplasia, and carcinoma *in situ* have been identified in the gallbladder mucosa of 83.0%, 13.5%, and 3.5%, respectively, of patients undergoing cholecystectomy for cholelithiasis or cholecystitis.[14] Areas of mucosal dysplasia can be observed in more than 90% of patients with invasive gallbladder carcinoma.[15] There also is evidence that adenomatous polyps arising from the gallbladder mucosa are premalignant lesions, because a review of 1605 cholecystectomies produced 11 benign adenomas, 7 adenomas with areas of malignant transformation, and 79 invasive gallbladder carcinomas.[16] Regions of residual adenomas were found in 20% of the cases of invasive gallbladder carcinoma.

Pathology

The gross appearance of gallbladder carcinoma varies depending on the stage of the disease and extent of spread. Early-stage lesions that have not infiltrated all layers of the gallbladder wall may be indistinguishable from chronic cholecystitis. On opening the gallbladder in these early-stage patients, gall-stones usually are present and there may be subtle mucosal abnormalities, such as plaque-like lesions or small ulcerations. Occasionally a sessile or pedunculated tumor is present, suggesting the diagnosis of gallbladder carcinoma.[17] More advanced gallbladder carcinomas are grossly evident by their infiltration into the liver or contiguous organs, such as the duodenum or stomach.[17] These tumors are white to gray on cut section and are firm. When associated with a calcified gallbladder, the carcinomas are extremely hard, difficult to section, and have a gritty consistency.

Microscopically, more than 90% of gallbladder carcinomas are adenocarcinomas, with the remaining lesions being adenosquamous carcinomas, anaplastic carcinomas, and rarely carcinoid tumors or embryonal rhabdomyosarcoma.[8] Carcinoma *in situ* is an early lesion with the malignant cellular characteristics involving only the mucosal layer of the gallbladder wall. Gallbladder adenocarcinomas generally have a predominant papillary or tubular arrangement of cells.[17] Papillary adenocarcinoma is characterized by an extended stroma covered by columnar cells. The tubular formations of tubular adenocarcinoma may be lined by tall columnar cells or cuboidal epithelium. Mucin production and signet ring cells are identified frequently in gallbladder adenocarcinomas.[17] More poorly differentiated carcinomas have solid sheets or nests of small, scattered cells infiltrating the stroma and destroying the normal gallbladder wall architecture. The hallmark of each of these types of invasive carcinoma is infiltration into the muscle and adventitial layers of the gallbladder wall. Vascular, lymphatic, and perineural invasion by the carcinoma can be demonstrated frequently.

Advanced local and regional disease is usually present at the time of diagnosis of gallbladder carcinoma. Only 10% of patients with this disease have cancer confined to the gallbladder wall.[8] Direct extension of the carcinoma into the gallbladder fossa of the liver is present in 69–83% of patients.[18] Direct invasion of the liver usually indicates the presence of other regional disease, because fewer than 12% of patients with liver involvement have no other sites of regional disease. Direct invasion of the extrahepatic biliary tract occurs in 57% of cases; the duodenum, stomach, or transverse colon are involved in 40%; and the pancreas is involved in 23%.[2] The hepatic artery or portal vein is encased by tumor in 15% of patients. Regional lymph node metastases in the cystic, choledochal, or pancreatioduedenal lymphatic drainage basins are present in 42–70% of patients.[18] Somewhat more distant lymph node metastases occur along the aorta or inferior vena cava in approximately 25% of cases. Importantly, lymph node metastases can occur in the absence of liver or other contiguous organ involvement by the gallbladder carcinoma.

Flow cytometry is not useful as a prognostic indicator of gallbladder cancer because 85% of these lesions are aneuploid or multiploid.[19] Primary gallbladder cancers with a high proliferative index are associated with a significantly higher incidence of lymph node metastasis and a poorer prognosis.[19] Similarly, mutations in the *p53* tumor suppressor gene are detected by immunohistochemistry more frequently in gallbladder cancer cases with transmural invasion or lymph node metastases; hence *p53* mutations are associated with a significantly worse prognosis.[20] It is not clear if such molecular alterations are independent indicators of outcome or only markers or progression to a more aggressive, metastatic phenotype.

The pattern of lymph node metastases from gallbladder carcinoma is predictable based on anatomic studies that have identified three pathways of lymphatic drainage of the gallbladder (Fig. 7.1).[21] The main pathway is the

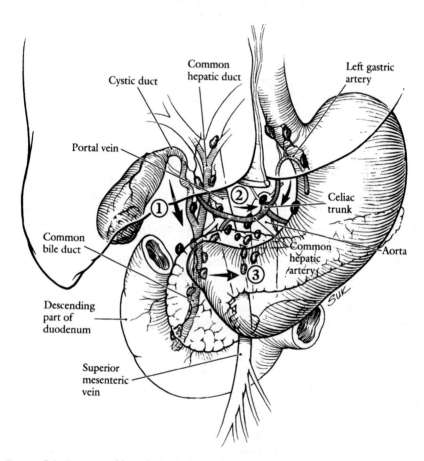

FIGURE 7.1. Patterns of lymphatic drainage from the gallbladder. The main pathway of lymphatic drainage and thus lymph node metastases from gallbladder cancer is the cholecystoretropancreatic nodes (1). This pathway drains from the gallbladder to nodes along the cystic duct and common bile duct and then to nodes posterior to the duodenum and pancreatic head. The cholecystoceliac pathway (2) runs from the gallbladder through the gastrohepatic ligament to celiac nodes. The third lymphatic drainage route is the cholecystomesenteric pathway (3), which courses from the gallbladder posterior to the pancreas to aortocaval nodes.

cholecystoretropancreatic pathway with lymphatic vessels on the anterior and posterior surface of the gallbladder that converge at a large retroportal lymph node. This principal retroportal lymph node communicates with choledochal and pancreaticoduodenal lymph nodes. The cholecystoceliac pathway consists of lymphatics from the anterior and posterior walls of the gallbladder that run to the left through the hepatoduodenal ligament to reach the celiac lymph nodes. The cholecystomesenteric pathway is comprised of lympatic channels that run to the left in front of the portal vein and then communicate with groups of pancreaticoduodenal lymph nodes or aorticocaval lymph nodes lying near the left renal vein.

Some patients with advanced gallbladder cancer develop carcinomatosis from intraperitoneal dissemination of cancer cells. The final pattern of spread of gallbladder carcinoma is related to vascular invasion. Noncontiguous liver, pulmonary, and bone metastases have been found in 66%, 24%, and 12% of gallbladder carcinoma patients, respectively.[18]

The staging systems used for gallbladder carcinoma are based on the pathologic characteristics of local invasion by the tumor and lymph node metastases. Before the American Joint Cancer Committee (AJCC) developed a tumor/node/metastasis (TNM) staging schema for gallbladder carcinoma, the Nevin staging system was used frequently.[22] Studies of gallbladder carcinoma performed in Japan generally apply the staging system of the Japanese Society of Biliary Surgery.[23] Most recent studies stage patients according to the TNM criteria. Carcinoma *in situ* corresponds to a $T_{1a}N_0M_0$ tumor in the AJCC staging system. The characteristics of these three staging systems are outlined in Tables 7.1 and 7.2.

Diagnosis

The most common symptoms and signs in patients with gallbladder carcinoma are nonspecific. Right upper quadrant abdominal pain, which may or may not be exacerbated by eating a fatty meal, is the predominant presenting complaint in 75–97% of patients.[2,8,24] Right upper quadrant abdominal tenderness is present in a slightly smaller percentage of patients. These symptoms and signs usually are ascribed to cholelithiasis or cholecystitis. Nausea, vomiting, and anorexia are present in 40–64% of patients; clinically evidence jaundice is present in 45%; and weight loss of more than 10% of normal body weight is noted in 37–77%.

Although 45% of patients obviously are jaundiced at presentation, 70% present with a serum bilirubin elevated at least two times normal.[24] Serum alkaline phosphatase levels are elevated in two-thirds of patients with gallbladder carcinoma. Elevated serum levels of alanine aminotransferase and aspartate aminotransferase are present in one-third of patients and are consistent with advanced hepatic invasion and metastases. Serum carcinoembryonic antigen (CEA) levels generally are measured only in patients diag-

TABLE 7.1. Three commonly used staging systems for gallbladder carcinoma

Stage	Nevin	Japanese Society of Biliary Surgery	TNM[a]
I	Cancer confined to the mucosa	Cancer confined to subserosal layers	$T_{1a}N_0M_0$ $T_{1b}N_0M_0$ $T_2N_0M_0$
II	Cancer involves the mucosa and muscularis	Direct invasion of the liver and/or bile duct, porta hepatis lymph node metastases	
III	Cancer extends through the serosa (all three layers of the gallbladder wall involved)	More extensive liver invasion by cancer, more extensive regional lymph node metastases (gastrohepatic, retropancreatic)	$T_1N_1M_0$ $T_2N_1M_0$ T_3anyNM_0
IV	Tumor through all three layers of the gallbladder wall with cystic lymph node metastasis	Liver, peritoneal, and/or distant organ metastases	T_4anyNM_0 $AnyTanyNM_1$
V	Tumor invades the liver by direct extension and/or metastasis to any distant organ	No stage V	No stage V

[a]American Joint Cancer Commission.

TABLE 7.2. TNM staging for gallbladder carcinoma

T	Primary tumor
T_x	Primary tumor cannot be assessed
T_1	Tumor invades mucosa or muscle layer
	T_{1a} Tumor invades mucosa
	T_{1b} Tumor invades muscle
T_2	Tumor invades perimuscular connective tissue; no extension beyond serosa or into liver
T_3	Tumor invades beyond serosa or into one adjacent organ or both (extension < 2 cm into liver)
T_4	Tumor extends > 2 cm into liver and/or into two or more adjacent organs (stomach, duodenum, colon, pancreas, omentum, extrahepatic bile ducts)
N	Regional lymph nodes
N_x	Regional lymph nodes cannot be assessed
N_0	No regional lymph node metastasis
N_1	Regional lymph node metastasis
	N_{1a} Metastasis in cystic duct, pericholedochal, and/or gastrohepatic lymph nodes
	N_{1b} Metastasis in peripancreatic, periduodenal, periportal, celiac, and/or superior mesenteric artery lymph nodes
M	Distant metastasis
M_x	Presence of distant metastasis cannot be assessed
M_0	No distant metastasis
M_1	Distant metastasis

nosed preoperatively with advanced stages of disease. In these patients with TNM stage III or IV disease, the serum CEA level is elevated in more than 80% of patients.[24] The incidence of elevated serum CEA levels in early-stage disease is not known. Serum levels of carbohydrate antigen 19-9 (CA19-9) are elevated in more than 90% of patients with gallbladder cancer.[25] Some benign conditions, including chronic cholelithiasis, can be associated with mild elevated serum CA19-9 levels, but levels over 1000 units/ml suggest the diagnosis of a pancreatic or biliary tract malignancy.

Before ultrasonography and computed tomography (CT) became widely available, the preoperative diagnosis rate for gallbladder carcinoma was only 8.6–16.3%.[2,26] Ultrasonography is the primary imaging study for symptomatic patients with presumed cholelithiasis or choledocholithiasis. High-resolution transabdominal ultrasonography can detect early-stage and locally advanced gallbladder carcinoma.[27] Early tumors as small as 5 mm can be recognized as a polypoid mass projecting into the gallbladder lumen or as a focal thickening of the gallbladder wall.[28] In patients with locally advanced gallbladder carcinoma, ultrasonography can demonstrate extrahepatic and intrahepatic bile duct obstruction, regional lymphadenopathy, direct hepatic extension of tumor, and hepatic metastases. Preoperative ultrasonography suggests the correct diagnosis in up to 75% of patients with gallbladder carcinoma.[29,30] CT scans are performed less frequently in patients with presumed benign biliary tract disease. However, if gallbladder carcinoma is suspected, CT findings can predict correctly the diagnosis in 88–95% of patients.[31–33] The CT characteristics of gallbladder carcinoma include diffuse or focal gallbladder wall thickness of more than 0.5 mm in 95% of patients, gallbladder wall contrast enhancement in 95%, an intraluminal mass in 90%, direct liver invasion by tumor in 85%, regional lymphadenopathy in 65%, concomitant cholelithiasis in 52%, dilated intrahepatic or extrahepatic bile ducts in 50%, noncontiguous liver metastases in 12%, invasion of contiguous gastrointestinal tract organs in 8%, and intraluminal gallbladder gas in 4%.[33] CT also can demonstrate calcification of the gallbladder wall (Fig. 7.2).

Resection

Historically, only 10–30% of patients with gallbladder cancer present with disease that can be resected with curative intent.[34–36] Most patients are not candidates for curative resection because of extensive locoregional disease, noncontiguous liver metastases, or distant metastases. Although it is clear that long-term survival can be achieved in some patients with resectable lesions, the extent of resection remains a controversial issue.

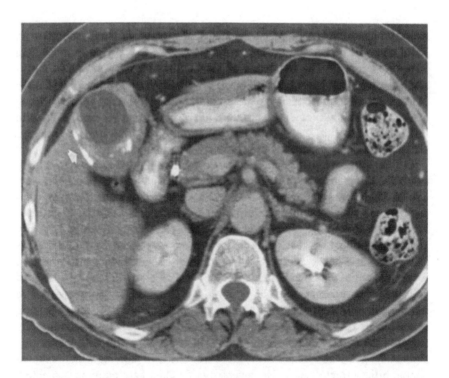

FIGURE 7.2. CT scan of the abdomen in a patient with gallbladder cancer. The scan demonstrates marked thickening and calcification (arrow) of the gallbladder wall.

Most surgeons consider simple cholecystectomy adequate treatment for gallbladder carcinoma confined to the mucosa ($T_{1a}N_0M_0$). The 5-year survival rate for patients undergoing simple cholecystectomy for disease confined to the mucosa ranges from 57% to 100%.[37-40] There is not universal agreement on simple cholecystectomy as the sole treatment for patients with $T_{1a}N_0M_0$ tumors, some authors recommend that extended cholecystectomy (cholecystectomy, wedge resection of the gallbladder fossa including a 3- to 5-cm margin of normal liver, and a cystic, pericholedochal, gastrohepatic, pancreaticoduodenal, and paraaortic lymphadenectomy) be performed to treat patients with these early-stage lesions.[41,42] These authors recommended that all gallbladders be opened at the time of cholecystectomy for frozen section evaluation of any suspicious areas in the mucosa. If an unsuspected gallbladder carcinoma is diagnosed by frozen section biopsy or if a $T_{1a}N_0M_0$ gallbladder carcinoma is diagnosed on final pathology, the authors advocated that an extended cholecystectomy by performed. The bias for this aggressive surgical treatment of $T_{1a}N_0M_0$ gallbladder carcinoma is based on the small number of cases of regional lymph node recurrences in patients treated with simple cholecystectomy alone. No rationale is provided for the liver resection because the small number of patients who did fail after simple cholecystectomy developed metastases in pericholedochal cystic lymph nodes and not in the liver. Furthermore, the incidence of subsequent lymph node metastases in $T_{1a}N_0M_0$ patients was less than 10% in the small groups of 32 and 36 patients, respectively.[41,42] The incidence of lymph node metastases was only 2.5% in a study of patients who underwent cholecystectomy and regional lymphadenectomy.[38] The mortality rate for extended resection ranged from 2% to 5%, and major postoperative morbidity occurred in 13–40%.[37-39,43] Therefore, in my view the morbidity and mortality associated with extended cholecystectomy for $T_{1a}N_0M_0$ lesions is excessive compared to the potential survival benefit that would occur in fewer than 3% of these early-stage patients.

There is a rationale for performing extended cholecystectomy in patients with T_{1b} tumors or AJCC TNM stage II and III gallbladder carcinomas that is based on an understanding of the patterns of spread of this cancer (Figs. 7.1, 7.3). The incidence of regional lymph node metastasis among 165 patients with T_{1b} gallbladder carcinoma was 15.6%, among the 867 patients with a T_2 primary lesion 56.1%, and among the 453 patients with T_3 tumors 74.4%.[38] The 5-year survival rate following extended cholecystectomy for AJCC stage II and III gallbladder carcinoma ranges from 7.5% to 37.0%.[37-39,41,43] AJCC stage II or III gallbladder carcinoma patients treated with simple cholecystectomy alone had a 0% five-year survival rate compared to a 29% five-year survival rate in those treated with extended cholecystectomy.[43] T_{1b} lesions are classified as stage I in the AJCC system; but, arguably, with a 15.6% incidence of regional lymph node metastases, there may be a long-term survival benefit in a significant number of these patients who undergo extended cholecystectomy.

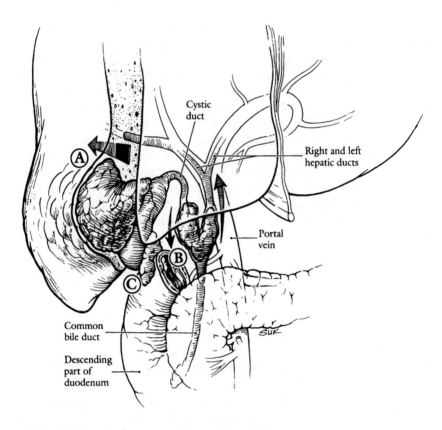

FIGURE 7.3. Regional patterns of spread by gallbladder cancer that can occur with or without lymph node metastases. The tumor may directly invade into the liver (A) or grow along the cystic duct into the extrahepatic bile ducts (B). Finally, locally advanced tumors may directly invade surrounding viscera, such as the colon, stomach, or duodenum (C).

All surgeons do not perform an en bloc resection of the extrahepatic bile duct as part of an extended cholecystectomy. Because gallbladder carcinoma is found to invade the extrahepatic bile duct in 57% of cases (Fig.7.3), with almost all of them occurring in patients with T_3 or T_4 tumors, an *en bloc* resection of the proper hepatic and common bile duct with Roux-en-Y hepaticojejunostomy should be included in an extended cholecystectomy for transmurally invasive tumors. This group includes cases where a clinically unsuspected gallbladder carcinoma is diagnosed pathologically following a simple cholecystectomy with a positive margin at the cystic duct. Generally, I prefer to perform a resection of segments IVB and V of the liver, with *en bloc* removal of the extrahepatic bile duct and regional lymphatics (Fig. 7.4).

Extremely radical operations have been proposed for patients with extensive $T_3N_1M_0$ or $T_4N_{0-1}M_0$ tumors, including hepatopancreaticoduodenectomy

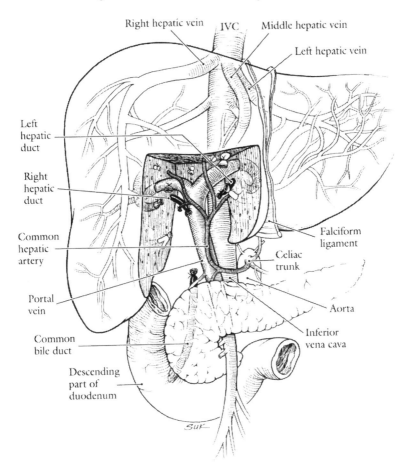

FIGURE 7.4. Resection of segments IVB and V associated with surgical excision of a gallbladder cancer. The anterior branch of the right portal vein and middle hepatic vein branches are ligated. The extrahepatic bile duct has also been resected, and biliary-enteric drainage is reestablished by anastomosing the right and left bile ducts to a Roux-en-Y limb of jejunum.

for locally advanced gallbladder carcinoma.[38,44] The operative mortality rate for this radical procedure is at least 15% with a more than 90% incidence of major morbidity. Resection of the portal vein, hepatic artery, or both with vascular reconstruction frequently is necessary to resect completely all gross malignant disease. The largest report of patients undergoing hepatopancreaticoduodenectomy for gallbladder carcinoma included 150 cases from Japan with a 5-year survival rate of 14%.[38] The patients who did not die from intraoperative or postoperative complications all succumbed to recurrent or metastatic carcinoma.

Others recommend routine right trisegmentectomy for gallbladder carcinoma, but there are no convincing data to suggest the superiority of this approach if a less radical hepatic resection can provide at least a 1-cm tumor-free margin.[45] In fact, a recent study of 106 patients who underwent extended cholecystectomy for gallbladder cancer that included only wedge resection of the gallbladder bed reported a 5-year survival rate of 52% for stage III and IV lesions with negative resection margins.[46] In contrast, patients who underwent noncurative, margin-positive resections had a 5% five-year survival rate.

One report advocated intraoperative frozen section evaluation of the gallbladder in patients with Mirizzi syndrome.[47] Mirizzi syndrome is obstructive jaundice caused by external compression of the common hepatic bile duct by a stone impacted in the neck of the gallbladder. It was found that 5 of 18 patients (27.8%) with Mirizzi syndrome had an unsuspected gallbladder cancer, in contrast to a 2% incidence of gallbladder cancer in patients with simple cholelithiasis.

It is estimated that 70,000 laparoscopic cholecystectomies are performed each year in the United States.[48] On average, gallbladder carcinoma is diagnosed in 2% of patients undergoing cholecystectomy for presumed benign biliary tract disease.[2] Thus approximately 1400 patients annually who undergo laparoscopic cholecystectomy could suffer inadvertent intraperitoneal dissemination of unsuspected gallbladder carcinoma. The spillage of tumor cells at the time of laparoscopic cholecystectomy has caused seeding of peritoneal surfaces and laparoscopy port sites in several patients.[49-55] This dissemination of tumor cells is an unfortunate occurrence because it may preclude a potentially curative open resection and limit the patient's long-term survival. We reviewed our experience with gallbladder cancer at the University of Texas M. D. Anderson Cancer Center and found no difference in the incidence of wound recurrence of tumor at laparoscopic port sites compared to open laparotomy incision sites.[56] This finding suggests that biologically aggressive gallbladder cancer cells can implant and grow at any surgical wound site.

Because of the large number of cholecystectomies being performed laparoscopically and the small but measurable risk of dissemination of tumor cells, it has been recommended that (1) unless the surgeon feels capable of performing a definitive extended cholecystectomy for gallbladder carcinoma, cases where gallbladder carcinoma is suspected preoperatively by clinical or radiologic criteria should be referred without laparoscopy, laparotomy, or percutaneous biopsy; and (2) if gallbladder carcinoma is suspected on visual inspection during an attempted laparoscopic cholecystectomy, either an open definitive operation should be performed or the operation should be terminated without biopsy and the patient referred for appropriate surgical therapy.[49] The surgical decision-making algorithm I use for gallbladder cancer patients is illustrated in Figure 7.5.

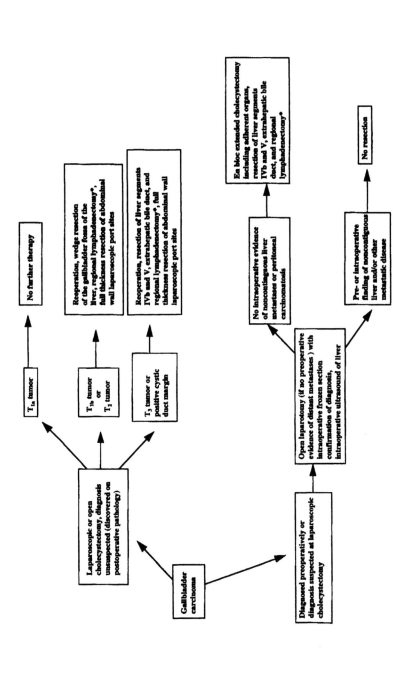

FIGURE 7.5. Algorithm to guide surgical decision-making for patients with gallbladder cancer. *Regional lymphadenectomy includes complete dissection and removal of the cystic, pericholedochal, pancreaticoduodenal, gastrohepatic, and paraaortic lymph nodes.

Palliation

Most patients with gallbladder carcinoma are diagnosed at an advanced, unresectable stage of disease. As for patients with hilar bile duct cancer, relief of symptomatic jaundice is a consideration. Patients with unresectable gallbladder carcinoma frequently have extensive involvement of the extrahepatic bile duct and may have bulky porta hepatis lymphadenopathy, which makes endoscopic placement of an internal stent difficult. When unresectable gallbladder carcinoma is diagnosed at the time of laparotomy, a surgical biliary bypass, such as an intrahepatic cholangioenteric anastomosis, can be performed and results in significant symptomatic relief in more than 90% of patients.[57] When the diagnosis is made based on radiographic and percutaneous biopsy findings, jaundie can be relieved by placing percutaneous transhepatic biliary catheters.

In contrast to patients with hilar bile duct carcinoma, where gastroduodenal obstruction is a relatively rare event, 30–50% of patients with advanced gallbladder carcinoma develop a clinically significant element of gastroduodenal obstruction.[58] It can be treated surgically with a bypass procedure (e.g., gastrojejunostomy) or by placement of a decompressing gas-trostomy tube and feeding jejunostomy tube. A percutaneous endoscopic gastrostomy tube also can be used to decompress the obstructed stomach in patients with advanced disease and limited expected survival time.

Chemotherapy

Studies that describe the results of chemotherapeutic treatment for unresectable or metastatic gallbladder carcinoma suffer from small numbers of patients and inclusion of those with hilar bile duct carcinoma.[59] A study of 53 patients with gallbladder carcinoma who received systemic chemotherapy with 5-fluorouracil (5-FU) or 5-FU plus other chemotherapeutic agents showed objective antitumor responses in 12% or fewer of the patients in each treatment arm.[60] Fluoropyrimidines combined with doxorubicin administered systemically have produced objective response rates of 30–40%.[61,62] Complete remission is rare and transient following such systemic chemotherapy regimens, and median survival is 11 months or less. The toxicities associated with these treatments are not insignificant, and survival is only a few months longer than that of patients who received no treatment.

Hepatic arterial infusion chemotherapy also has been described in small numbers of patients with locally advanced gallbladder carcinoma. Partial response rates of 55–60% and complete response rates of 9% have been reported.[63,64] However, the median duration of response was only 3 months, and all patients developed progressive disease. The median survival of 12 months with hepatic arterial infusion chemotherapy is not a significant improvement over the median survival for patients treated with intravenous chemotherapy. There may be less frequent and less severe systemic toxicity with hepatic arterial infusion chemotherapy, but the magnitude of this benefit is slight and does not justify routine use of this approach to treat unresectable gallbladder carcinoma. Currently, there are no particularly compelling cytotoxic chemotherapeutic agents to treat locally unresectable or metastatic primary hepatobiliary malignancies.

Radiation Therapy

Analyses of the patterns of failure after resection of gallbladder carcinoma revealed that local recurrence was the first (and in a significant number of cases the only) site of failure in more than one-half of the patients.[2,65] External beam radiation therapy to a total dose of 45 Gy can produce radiographic evidence of tumor reduction in 20–70% of these tumors and provide temporary relief of jaundice in up to 80% of patients.[66–88] In general, external beam radiation therapy is a palliative treatment. The median survival for locally advanced gallbladder carcinoma patients treated with radiation therapy is approximately 10 months.[65–68] Occasional long-term survivors are reported following treatment with higher doses of radiation or with administration of radiation-sensitizing chemotherapeutic agents such as 5-FU during external beam radiation therapy.[65] However, extrahepatic bile duct stricture has been reported in several of the long-term survivors treated with high doses of radiation.[69]

Intraoperative radiation therapy with a dose of 20–30 Gy has been delivered to treat unresectable gallbladder carcinoma.[70,71] Recanalization of obstructed extrahepatic bile ducts occurs in most patients treated with this technique. Intraoperative radiation therapy has not been associated with increased operative or postoperative morbidity in patients with unresectable tumors. The median survival of patients treated with intraoperative radiation therapy is less than 12 months, and this treatment modality appears to palliate biliary tract obstruction without significantly improving survival.

Multidisciplinary Approaches

Most patients who undergo an extended cholecystectomy or more radical resection for AJCC stage II, III, or IV gallbladder carcinoma develop tumor recurrence and die as a result of their disease. Nonrandomized studies and case reports have suggested that overall survival can be improved by administering adjuvant radiation therapy, chemotherapy, or both after resection of stage II, III, or IV tumors.[72–74] Unfortunately, the number of patients who have undergone postsurgical adjuvant treatment is small, and a variety of treatment regimens have been used. In a nonrandomized study, nine patients with stage IV gallbladder carcinoma were treated with complete surgical resection alone, and 17 patients were treated with complete resection combined with 20–30 Gy of postoperative external beam radiation. The surgical procedures performed in both groups of patients included extended cholecystectomy and a variety of more radical procedures, including hepatopancreaticoduodenectomy. There were no 3-year survivors among the nine patients treated with resection alone, but there was a 10.1% three-year survival rate among the 17 patients treated with resection and radiation therapy. Unfortunately, there are no randomized trials of patients with stage II and III gallbladder carcinoma treated with a coherent program of adjuvant therapy. Such trials are necessary to demonstrate an improvement in survival for patients who receive adjuvant therapies after a curative resection for gallbladder carcinoma.

References

1. Parker SL, Tong T, Bolden S, Wingo PA. Cancer statistics, 1997. CA Cancer J Clin 47:5, 1997
2. Piehler JM, Crichlow RW. Primary carcinoma of the gallbladder. Surg Gynecol Obstet 147:929, 1978
3. Strom BL, Soloway RD, Rios-Dalenz JL, et al. Risk factors for gallbladder cancer. Cancer 76:1747, 1995
4. Nelson BD, Porvaznik J, Benfield JR. Gallbladder disease in southwestern American Indians. Arch Surg 103:41, 1971
5. Rudolph R, Cohen JJ. Cancer of the gallbladder in an 11-year-old Navajo girl. J Pediatr Surg 7:66, 1972
6. Mancuso TF, Brennan MJ. Epidemiological considerations of cancer of the gallbladder, bile ducts, and salivary glands in the rubber industry. J Occup Med 12:333, 1970
7. Enomoto M, Naoe S, Harada M, et al. Carcinogenesis in extrahepatic bile duct and gallbladder; carcinogenic effect of N-hydroxy-2-acetamidofluorene in mice fed a "gallstone-inducing" diet. Jpn J Exp Med 44:37, 1974
8. Nagorney DM, McPherson GAD. Carcinoma of the gallbladder and extrahepatic bile ducts. Semin Oncol 15:106, 1988
9. Diehl AK. Gallstone size and the risk of gallbladder cancer. JAMA 250:2323, 1983
10. Polk HC. Carcinoma and the calcified gallbladder. Gastroenterology 50:582, 1966
11. Berk RN, Armbuster TG. Carcinoma of the porcelain gallbladder. Radiology 2:175, 1973
12. Parkash O. On the relationship of cholelithiasis to carcinoma of the gall-bladder and on the sex dependency of the carcinoma of the bile ducts. Digestion 12:129, 1975
13. Ko CY, Schmit P, Cheng L, Thompson JE. Estrogen receptors in gallbladder cancer: detection by an improved immunohistochemical assay. Am Surg 61:930, 1995

14. Albores-Saavedra J, Alcantra-Vazquez A, Cruz-Ortiz H, et al. The precursor lesions of invasive gallbladder carcinoma: hyperplasia, atypical hyperplasia, and carcinoma in situ. Cancer 45:919, 1980
15. Black WC. The morphogenesis of gallbladder carcinoma. In: Fenoglio CM, Wolff M (eds) Progress in Surgical Pathology. New York, Masson, 1980, p. 207
16. Kuzuka S, Tsubone M, Yasui A, et al. Relation of adenoma to carcinoma in the gallbladder. Cancer 50:2226, 1982
17. Sumiyoshi K, Nagai E, Chijiiwa K, Nakayama F. Pathology of carcinoma of the gallbladder. World J Surg 15:315, 1991
18. Fahim RB, McDonald JR, Richards JC, Ferris DO. Carcinoma of the gallbladder: a study of its modes of spread. Ann Surg 156:114, 1962
19. Mishizawa-Takano J-E, Ayabe H, Hatano K, Yamaguchi H, Tagawa U. Gallbladder cancer: a comparative study among clinicopathologic features, AgNORs, and DNA content analysis. Dig Dis Sci 41:840, 1996
20. Diamantis I, Karamitopoulou E, Perentes E, Zimmerman A. p53 protein immunoreactivity in extrahepatic bile duct and gallbladder cancer: correlation with tumor grade and survival. Hepatology 22:774, 1995
21. Ito M, Mishima Y, Sato T. An anatomical study of the lymphatic drainage of the gallbladder. Radiol Anat 13:89, 1991
22. Nevin JE, Moran TJ, Kay S, King R. Carcinoma of the gallbladder. Cancer 37:141, 1976
23. Japanese Society of Biliary Surgery. The General Rules for Surgical and Pathological Studies on Cancer of Biliary Tract, 2nd ed. Tokyo, Kanehara Syuppan, 1986
24. Carmo MD, Perpetuo MO, Valdivieso M, et al. Natural history study of gallbladder cancer. Cancer 42:330, 1978
25. Steinberg W. Clinical utility of the CA 19-9 tumor-associated antigen. Am J Gastroenterol 85:350, 1990
26. Tashiro S, Konno T, Mochinaga M, et al. Treatment of carcinoma of the gallbladder in Japan. Jpn J Surg 12:98, 1982
27. Koga A, Yamauchi S, Izumi Y, et al. Ultrasonographic detection of early and curable carcinoma of the gallbladder. Br J Surg 72:728, 1985
28. Wibbenmeyer LA, Sharafuddin MJA, Wolverson MK, et al. Sonographic diagnosis of unsuspected gallbladder cancer: imaging findings in comparison with benign gallbladder conditions. AJR 165:1169, 1995
29. Soiva M, Aro K, Pamilo M, et al. Ultrasonography in carcinoma of the gallbladder. Acta Radiol 28:711, 1987
30. Palma LD, Rizzatto G, Pozzi-Mucelli RS, Bazzoccbi M. Gray-scale ultrasonography in the evaluation of the carcinoma of the gallbladder. Br J Radiol 53:662, 1980
31. Itai Y, Araki T, Yoshihawa K, et al. Computed tomography of gallbladder carcinoma. Radiology 137:713, 1980
32. Chijiiwa K, Yumiyoshi K, Nakayama F. Impact of recent advances in hepatobiliary imaging techniques on the preoperative diagnosis of carcinoma of the gallbladder. World J Surg 15:322, 1991
33. Thorsen MK, Quiroz F, Lawson TL, et al. Primary biliary carcinoma: CT evaluation. Radiology 152:479, 1984

34. Hamrick RE, Liner J, Hastings PR, Cohn I. Primary carcinoma of the gallbladder. Ann Surg 195:270, 1982
35. Klamer TW, Max MH. Carcinoma of the gallbladder. Surg Gynecol Obstet 156:641, 1983
36. Barr LH. Carcinoma of the gallbladder. Am Surg 50:275, 1984
37. Gagner M, Rossi RL. Radical operations for carcinoma of the gallbladder: present status in North America. World J Surg 15:344, 1991
38. Ogura Y, Mizumoto R, Isaji S, et al. Radical operations for carcinoma of the gallbladder: present status in Japan. World J Surg 15:337, 1991
39. Gall FP, Kockerling F, Scheele J, et al. Radical operations for carcinoma of the gallbladder: present status in Germany. World J Surg 15:328, 1991
40. Yamaguchi K, Tsuneyoshi M. Subclinical gallbladder carcinoma. Am J Surg 163:382, 1992
41. Ouchi K, Owada Y, Matsuno S, Sato T. Prognostic factors in the surgical treatment of gallbladder carcinoma. Surgery 101:731, 1987
42. Bergdahl L. Gallbladder carcinoma first diagnosed at microscopic examination of gallbladders removed for presumed benign disease. Ann Surg 191:19, 1980
43. Donohoe JH, Nagorney DM, Grant CS, et al. Carcinoma of the gallbladder. Arch Surg 125:237, 1990
44. Nimura Y, Hayakaw N, Kamiya J, et al. Hepatopancreaticoduodenectomy for advanced carcinoma of the biliary tract. Heptaogastroenterology 38:170, 1991
45. Collier NA, Blumgart LH. Tumors of the gallbladder. In: Blumgart LH (ed) Surgery of the Liver and Biliary Tract, 2nd ed. New York, Churchill Livingstone, 19—, p. 955
46. Tsukada K, Hatakeyama K, Kurosaki I, et al. Outcome of radical surgery for carcinoma of the gallbladder according to the TNM stage. Surgery 120:816, 1996
47. Redaelli CA, Büchler MW, Schilling MK, et al. High coincidence of Mirizzi syndrome and gallbladder carcinoma. Surgery 121:58 1997
48. Grace PA, Quereshi A, Coleman J, et al. Reduced postoperative hospitalization after laparoscopic cholecystectomy. Br J Surg 78:160, 1991
49. Fong Y, Brennan MF, Turnbull A, et al. Gallbladder cancer discovered during laparoscopic surgery. Arch Surg 128:1054, 1993
50. Drouard F, Delamarre J, Capron J. Cutaneous seeding of gallbladder cancer after laparoscopic cholecytectomy. N Engl J Med 325:1316, 1991
51. Pezet D, Fondrinier E, Rotman N, et al. Pariental seeding of carcinoma of the gallbladder after laparoscopic cholecytectomy. Br J Surg 79:230, 1992
52. Kim H-J, Roy T. Unexpected gallbladder cancer with cutaneous seeding after laparoscopic cholecystectomy. South Med J 87:817, 1994
53. Weiss SM, Wengery PA, Harkavy SE. Incisional recurrence of gallbladder cancer after laparoscopic cholecystectomy. Gastrointest Endosc 40:244, 1994
54. Martinez J, Targarona EM, Balagué C, Peri Mi, Trias M. Port site metastasis: an unresolved problem in laparoscopic surgery. Int Surg 80:315, 1995
55. Clair DG, Lautz DB, Brooks DC. Rapid development of umbilical metastases after laparoscopic cholecytectomy for unsuspected gallbladder carcinoma. Surgery 113:355, 1993
56. Ricardo A, Feig BW, Ellis LM, et al Gallbladder cancer and trocar site recurrences: the facts regarding the myth. Am J Surg (in press)

57. Bismuth H, Castaing D, Traynor O. Resection or palliation: priority of surgery in the treatment of hilar cancer. World J Surg 12:39, 1988
58. Jones RS. Palliative operative procedures for carcinoma of the gallbladder. World J Surg 15:348, 1991
59. Kajanti M, Pyrhönen S. Epirubicin-sequential methotrexate-5-fluorouracil-leucovorin treatment in advanced cancer of the extrahepatic biliary system: a phase II study. Am J Clin Oncol 17:223, 1994
60. Falkson G, MacIntyre JM, Moertel CG. Eastern Cooperative Oncology Group experience with chemotherapy for inoperable gallbladder and bile duct cancer. Cancer 54:965, 1984
61. Hall SW, Benjamin RS, Murphy WK, et al. Adriamycin, BCNU, FTORAFUR chemotherapy of pancreatic and biliary tract cancer. Cancer 44:2008, 1979
62. Harvey JH, Smith FP, Schein PS. 5-Fluorouracil, mitomycin, and doxorubicin (FAM) in carcinoma of the biliary tract. J Clin Oncol 2:1245, 1984
63. Smith GW, Bukowski RM, Hewlett JS, Groppe CW. Hepatic artery infusion of 5-fluorouracil and mitomycin C in cholangiocarcinoma and gallbladder carcinoma. Cancer 54:1513, 1984
64. Kairaluoma MI, Leinonen A, Niemela R, et al. Superselective intra-arterial chemotherapy with mitomycin C in liver and gallbladder cancer. Eur J Surg Oncol 14:45, 1988
65. Buskirk SJ, Gunderson LL, Adson MA, et al. Analysis of failure following curative irradiation of gallbladder and extrahepatic bile duct carcinoma. Int J Radiat Oncol Biol Phys 10:2013, 1984
66. Smoron GL. Radiation therapy of carcinoma of gallbladder and biliary tract. Cancer 40:1422, 1977
67. Pilepich MV, Lambert PM. Radiotherapy of carcinomas of the extrahepatic biliary system. Radiology 127:767, 1978
68. Kopelson G, Harisiadis L, Tretter P, Chang CH. The role of radiation therapy in cancer of the extra-hepatic biliary system: an analysis of thirteen patients and a review of the literature of the effectiveness of surgery, chemotherapy and radiotherapy. Int J Radiat Oncol Biol Phys 2:883, 1977
69. Martenson JA, Gunderson LL, Buskirk SJ, et al. Hepatic duct stricture after radical radiation therapy for biliary cancer: recurrence or fibrosis: Mayo Clin Proc 61:530, 1986
70. Busse PM, Cady B, Bothe A, et al. Intraoperative radiation therapy for carcinoma of the gallbladder. World J Surg 15:352, 1991
71. Todoroki T, Iwasaki Y, Okamura T, et al. Intraoperative radiotherapy for advanced carcinoma of the biliary system. Cancer 46:2179, 1980
72. Morrow CE, Sutherland DER, Florack G, et al. Primary gallbladder carcinoma: significance of subserosal lesions and results of aggressive surgical treatment and adjuvant chemotherapy. Surgery 94:709, 1983
73. Athlin LEA, Domellof LKH, Bergman FO. Advanced gallbladder carcinoma: a case report and review of the literature. Eur J Surg Oncol 17:449, 1987
74. Kraybill WG, Lee H, Picus J, et al. Multidisciplinary treatment of biliary tract cancers. J Surg Oncol 55:239, 1994
75. Todoroki T, Iwasaki Y, Orii K, et al. Resection combined with intraoperative radiation therapy (IORT) for stage IV (TNM) gallbladder carcinoma. World J Surg 15:357, 1991

8

Hepatic Resection
for Colorectal Cancer Metastases

CHARLES R. SHUMATE

Achievement of long-term disease-free survival with surgical resection of metastases requires a single, predictable site of dissemination of the primary cancer. This situation occurs in a small but significant proportion of patients with recurrent colorectal carcinoma. In an ideal setting, treatment for primary or metastatic malignancy provides a high probability for complete response and a reasonable opportunity for long-term disease-free survival, it also has minimal side effects. Numerous methods have been advocated for the treatment of colorectal cancer liver metastases, but unfortunately none satisfies all of these criteria for an ideal treatment. Systemic chemotherapy, regional chemotherapy, cryotherapy, and surgical resection have advocates, but when multiple treatment methods are endorsed for the same problem it suggests that no one method is appropriate for all patients or that substantial treatment response is lacking.

Surgical resection of colorectal liver metastases in patients with liver-only disease provides long-term survival in a significant number of patients. Surgical morbidity and mortality rates are low, long-term side effects seldom occur, and the immediate response is complete. Nonetheless, controversy exists regarding the use of hepatic resection because of a lack of randomized prospective clinical trials and a sense of nihilism among some members of the medical community concerning the use of an invasive surgical treatment for metastatic disease. Complete resolution of these issues may not be possible. In my view, we should continue to offer resection to patients who are physiologically able to tolerate hepatic surgery and meet specific criteria known to be associated with long-term survival.

Successful resection of colorectal cancer liver metastases has evolved primarily since the 1960s. This deliberate evolution has depended on increased knowledge of the natural history of patients with untreated colorectal cancer liver metastases, better disease staging evaluation via technologic advancements in diagnostic imaging, and improvements in surgical techniques and critical care that permit safe partial hepatectomy. Hughes and colleagues contributed much to our understanding of the role of the surgeon in altering the natural history of colorectal cancer liver metastases.[1] Their study demonstrated that patients treated with only surgical resection of colorectal cancer liver metastases had an approximately 33% five-year over-all survival rate and a 25% five-year disease-free survival rate. The develop-ment and subsequent improvements of computed tomography (CT) coupled with intraoperative application of diagnostic ultrasonography permit accu-rate assessment of the extent of disease and have aided in patient selection and determination of the type of liver resection to be performed. Appropri-ate patient selection for liver resection will be improved further with the ongoing advances in diagnostic technology.

Historically, surgeons were hesitant to perform elective hepatic surgery because of their concern about uncontrollable hemorrhage and resultant pa-tient demise. Operative mortality rates for liver resection were as high as 50% during the mid 1960s but have dropped to 5% or less as indicated by a review of recent series.[2] The lessons learned from other surgical disciplines, improved anesthetic and post-operative management, and increased experi-ence with liver resection have combined to improve the operative morbidity and mortality rates. The value and impact of new instruments and their wide-spread application must also be emphasized. Intraoperative ultrasonography and ultrasonic dissectors are two examples of equipment that has been used in re-cent years to enhance surgical precision and control during hepatic surgery.

Patient outcome results from partial hepatectomy depend on the experience and knowledge, particularly of anatomy, of the surgeon. Many pitfalls and poor patient outcomes await the uneducated and inexperienced. Operating within a solid organ is more difficult than working at its periphery. The external surface of the liver has few landmarks to guide surgeons through the maze of intertwin-ing hepatic and portal vessel branches below the surface. Surgeons who choose to venture into hepatic surgery must have a thorough understanding of the po-tential anatomic variations and the safe management of these variations, and they must have adequate support staff and resources in the operating room and hospital. Medical oncologists and primary care physicians should identify quali-fied surgeons in their geographic areas for referral of patients with resectable colorectal cancer liver metastases because these surgeons can contribute to safe and potentially effective oncologic care.

Patient Selection

Patient selection involves perioperative risk assessment, determining the tech-nical feasibility and resectability of the liver metastases, and evaluation of predictive prognostic criteria for long-term disease-free survival.

Operative Risk Assessment

Patients undergoing a major surgical procedure ideally are free of co-mor-bid disease that threatens intraoperative and postoperative survival. In reality, many patients have one or more medical problems in addition to their colorectal cancer liver metastases. Patients with associated conditions that limit life expectancy more than the liver metastases are not candidates for liver resection. Operative risk assessment is similar to that for other major abdominal procedures, but patients being considered for liver resection must also undergo an evaluation of functional hepatic reserve to reduce the occurrence of postoperative hepatic failure.

Most patients with liver metastases from colorectal cancer do not have cirrhosis. Questions about chronic liver disease, such as hepatitis B or C virus infection or chronic ethanol abuse, are asked during conversations with the patient and family members. If the presence of cirrhosis is suspected from the history or from laboratory and radiographic studies, confirmation can be obtained by a preoperative percutaneous core needle biopsy. In the absence of cirrhosis, at least 20% of the normal hepatic parenchyma must remain following resection. Ensuring that an adequate amount of normal, functional liver remains is accomplished by preoperative and intraoperative assessment of the volume of normal liver parenchyma to be resected and thus the volume that will remain. Most patients tolerate a right or left hepatic lobectomy, but difficulty may occur when a trisegmentectomy is contemplated or if the patient has underlying chronic liver disease. In patients with cirrhosis or other chronic liver disease, the safety of liver resection must be carefully assessed because some patients tolerate little more than segmental or wedge resections.

Technical Feasibility

Certain technical limitations contraindicate exploration for resection. Obvious tumor involvement of the portal vein bifurcation, hepatic vein confluence, or the inferior vena cava as determined on preoperative radiographic studies are examples. Resections involving the portal vein bifurcation and hepatic vein confluence are avoided as they impair vascular integrity to the remaining liver. It is technically possible to resect segment I, the caudate lobe, when involved by colorectal metastasis. However, I have not yet encountered a patient in whom this operation was indicated for a liver metastasis. Likewise, inferior vena cava resection is technically feasible but probably not indicated for most patients with liver metastases because adequate tumor-free resection margins cannot be obtained.

Prognostic Criteria

Assessment of operative risk and technical feasibility is often more straightforward than determining the probability of long-term disease-free survival. When considering prognostic variables, one is attempting to predict the biologic behavior of a malignancy and to determine if intervention is occurring at the correct time in its natural history. Survival without hepatic resection or other treatment for colorectal metastases is usually easy to predict; essentially all untreated patients are dead within 5 years of diagnosis. Because prospective data regarding the efficacy of surgical resection for colorectal liver metastases are scarce, we are forced to compare natural history data with the results of retrospective surgical series to determine the survival benefit associated with liver resection. When analyzed from this perspective, surgical resection of colorectal liver metastases improves 5-year survival from almost zero to 30–50%.[1,3–8] Controversy exists when a therapy for malignant disease is applied without randomized prospective data. However, resolution of any conflict regarding resection of colorectal liver metastases may be impossible, as most physicians do not allow their patients to be randomized between a potentially curative treatment versus observation. Therefore it is necessary for the surgeon to individualize each situation, adhering to absolute indications for operation and assigning the appropriate value to the relative contraindications to resection to determine a treatment strategy.

Series on the natural history of untreated patients have demonstrated that the progression of liver metastases is often slow and dependent on a number of factors, including the extent of disease (both intra- and extrahepatic), patient performance status, and primary tumor differentiation and stage.[3,5,8] The most important of these factors is tumor burden, specifically hepatic replacement by tumor and the presence of extrahepatic disease. Untreated patients with any extrahepatic metastasis or with liver-only disease replacing more than 50% of the normal liver volume rarely survive more than 2 years. Wagner and colleagues reviewed the Mayo Clinic data on survival in patients with untreated colorectal liver metastases and demonstrated the importance of the extent of hepatic involvement as a predictor of survival.[3] Patients with a solitary unilobar metastasis had a median survival of 21 months compared to 15 months for patients with multiple liver lesions. In fact, more than 20% of the patients with a solitary metastasis survived at least 3 years with no treatment. The findings of Goslin et al. were similar: Patients with four or more liver metastases had a median survival of 10 months compared to 24 months for patients with three or fewer metastases.[8] Extrahepatic tumor recurrence, diagnosed at the same time as the hepatic metastases, is another indicator of poor prognosis, with a reduction in median survival from 18 months for liver-only disease to 9 months. Poorly differentiated primary tumors and the presence of nodal metastases at the time of primary tumor resection also seem to affect survival adversely, but they appear to be factors only when the liver tumor burden is low.[5]

Multiple surgical series have examined the merit of resection of colorectal liver metastases. Most are single-institution retrospective reviews, and some are multicenter studies; only one is a prospective evaluation. None is a randomized prospective clinical trials. One of the first significant evaluations of the effectiveness of hepatic resection of colorectal metastases was a multicenter retrospective study of 859 patients from 24 institutions.[1] This study also helped define selection criteria for patients not likely to benefit (regarding long-term survival) from a resection. Factors that were deemed to be absolute contraindications to hepatic resection because of no long-term survival benefit were portal lymph node metastases, coexistent extrahepatic recurrence, and the presence of four or more liver metastases. Relatively poor prognostic variables, but not contraindications to resection, were the presence of mesenteric nodal metastases in the primary colorectal cancer resection specimen and a disease-free interval of less than 12 months. Distribution of metastases (i.e., unilobar versus bilobar) and the size of the lesions proved to have no adverse effect on survival. The 33% five-year actuarial overall survival rate and 21% five-year disease-free survival rate reinforced the previously perceived benefit of liver resection in properly selected patients.

Coexistent extrahepatic disease, other than the primary tumor, is a contraindication for liver resection, even if the extrahepatic disease is resectable. Altogether twenty-four patients in The Hepatic Tumor Registry had portal or celiac lymph node metastases (or both), and none survived 5 years.[1] Patients with coexistent recurrence at sites other than lymph nodes had a median survival of less than 18 months, and there were no 5-year disease-free survivors.

Patients with more than three intrahepatic metastases had a 5-year disease-free survival of 7% versus 25% for patients with three or fewer metastases, a difference that was statistically significant. The number of metastases that can be effectively resected resulting in long-term survival benefit may be debated given the improvements in diagnostic imaging and resection techniques. The study reported by Hughes et al. covered 37 years from 1948 to 1985.[1] The accuracy of pre- and intraoperative liver imaging has improved markedly, as most of the patients in that series were treated before the development of modern imaging techniques. Furhman et al. reported that as many as four lesions can be resected with a 44% five-year actuarial survival rate when there is no evidence of extrahepatic tumor and resection margins are tumor-free.[6] Thus in the future, resection of more than four hepatic colorectal metastases may be an accepted treatment, but this protocol must await further study to provide definitive proof.

The importance of the disease-free interval between resection of the primary colorectal cancer and the diagnosis of liver metastases remains a controversial issue. The retrospective study by Hughes et al. suggested better survival for patients presenting more than 12 months after treatment of the primary tumor compared to less than 12 months[1] (42% vs. 24% five-year survival rates), but strong arguments can be made against using this measure an absolute contraindication to resection. Steele and Ravikumar effectively argued that waiting to determine biologic favorability of liver metastases diagnosed within 12 months of the primary cancer causes undue patient anxiety, may convert a resectable tumor to an unresectable tumor, and tests the hypothesis that metastases can metastasize.[5] Therefore a short disease-free interval should be used as only a relative contraindication to liver resection for management of these patients because some experience a significant long-term survival benefit.

The only prospective evaluation of partial hepatectomy for colorectal metastases was conducted by the Gastrointestinal Tumor Study Group and reported by Steele et al. in 1991.[7] Patients were divided into three groups depending on the immediate operative outcome. The curative group underwent excision of all measurable hepatic tumor with negative margins. Patients who underwent noncurative resection (tumor involving the resection margins or extrahepatic disease) comprised the second group, and patients with anatomically unresectable liver disease were the final group. Median survival for the curative group was 37 months compared to 21 months and 16.5 months for the noncurative resection and unresectable groups, respectively. There was no significant increase in survival advantage in the group of patients undergoing a noncurative resection. This study also emphasized the safety of modern liver resection for colorectal metastases as performed by multiple surgeons at various institutions with low operative mortality (2.7%) and morbidity (13.0%) rates.

Adequate tumor-free surgical margins are imperative for successful surgical treatment of colorectal cancer liver metastases. This statement is supported by results from the Hepatic Tumor Registry, the Gastrointestinal Tumor Study Group, and single-institution reviews.[1,4,7] Cady et al. reported a 60% five-year survival rate for patients with tumor-free liver resection margins larger than 1 cm, a 30% rate if margins were negative but less than 1 cm from the liver metastases, and no 5-year survivors when margins were positive.[4] As expected, the liver-only and the total liver recurrences were higher among patients with close and positive margins when compared to patients with at least a 1-cm tumor-free margin.

In summary, patient selection for resection of colorectal cancer liver metastases involves assessment of operative risk, technical feasibility, and potential for long-term survival (Table 8.1). To give the patient a reasonable chance for long-term survival, the metastatic liver tumor(s) must be confined to the liver, number four or fewer lesions, and be resectable with a 1-cm or larger tumor-free margin, all while leaving an adequate volume of functional hepatic parenchyma. The primary tumor stage and the length of the disease-free interval are viewed as no more than relative contraindications to resection depending on the specific situation.

TABLE 8.1. Contraindications to resection of colorectal cancer liver metastases

Absolute contraindications
Extrahepatic recurrence
More than four liver metastases
Main portal vein bifurcation involvement by tumor
Hepatic vein confluence/inferior vena cava involvement by tumor
Inability to obtain at least a 1-cm tumor-free margin
Inability to preserve an adequate volume of functional hepatic parenchyma
Relative contraindications
Lymph node positive primary colorectal cancer
Disease-free interval of less than 1 year

Resection

Successful hepatic resection can be viewed as a series of steps that begins before the operation, continues through the procedure, and culminates with postoperative care and recovery. Each step is equally important, as each must be completed to proceed safely to the next. Thorough preoperative planning facilitates proper patient selection with its attendant advantages. Proper preparation by the surgeon reduces operative risk and contributes to a better long-term prognosis.

Preoperative Preparation

The primary objective of preoperative patient selection is to exclude patients who will not benefit from resection and those who may be harmed or not survive the physiologic stress of the surgery. As noted previously, I consider extrahepatic recurrence of colorectal cancer and more than four liver metastases to be absolute contraindications to resection. Therefore the primary focus of preoperative evaluation is to identify these patients and avoid an unnecessary abdominal operation. CT generally offers the best imaging preoperatively to evaluate the number and extent of liver metastases and to identify extrahepatic metastases in the lungs, lymph nodes, or peritoneal cavity. The optimal CT technique for defining the extent of intrahepatic disease is debatable and has continued to change with improvements in equipment and software. Some advocate CT portography as the most sensitive method for visualizing small lesions in the liver.[9] In my practice, dynamic bolus intravenous contrast CT has proved to be equally effective for evaluating the number and location of liver metastases.

Thoracic evaluation is usually accomplished with standard posteroanterior and lateral chest radiographs. Questionable lesions on these radiographs are evaluated further with chest CT or biopsy as indicated. One must remember that patients with benign conditions such as sarcoidosis and other inflammatory disorders may present with radiographic findings that mimic metastatic disease.

Presacral changes identified on CT scans after low anterior and abdominoperineal resections for primary colorectal cancer are a radiologic challenge to distinguish between benign postoperative changes and recurrent disease. Excluding a pelvic recurrence of cancer may require monoclonal antibody scans, magnetic resonance imaging (MRI), or biopsy in addition to CT. Colonoscopy should be considered to detect any evidence of an anastomotic recurrence, and it is indicated to exclude a new primary colorectal tumor should the disease-free interval be more than 2 years or if the entire colon was never completely evaluated before the primary colorectal cancer operation.

Most patients with metastatic colorectal liver metastases do not have underlying cirrhosis, in contrast to patients with hepatocellular carcinoma; therefore the issue of sufficient functional hepatic reserve depends on the volume of liver to be resected. Preoperative serum liver function tests that suggest concomitant chronic liver disease should lead to further evaluation. A percutaneous liver biopsy indicating severe hepatitis or cirrhosis can prevent needless exploration and postoperative hepatic failure. For most patients undergoing partial hepatectomy for colorectal metastases, the goal of assessing hepatic reserve is to estimate the volume of liver that will remain after-resection. Fatal postoperative liver failure is rare if at least 20–30% of normal (noncirrhotic), vascularized liver volume is preserved. Some patients develop mild jaundice after such an extensive liver resection, but in most cases it is transient and the serum bilirubin returns to normal.

Intraoperative ultrasonography (IOUS) is used to clarify marginal cases for resection by identifying small tumors not detected on preoperative CT scans or by demonstrating involvement of key vascular structures precluding a margin-negative resection. This point is especially important in my practice, as I use hepatic artery infusion pump chemotherapy for patients with liver-only disease found intraoperatively to be unresectable because of the number or location of the hepatic tumors. During these times of cost containment, many third-party payers do not cover the cost of additional imaging studies if similar tests have already been performed. Because most patients do not have the liver metastases diagnosed with CT portography, the role of IOUS becomes more important.

The liver is a highly vascular organ that receives approximately 20% of the cardiac output. The inability to control hemorrhage during elective liver surgery initially thwarted efforts to resect hepatic neoplasms. Uneventful hepatic resection requires that the surgeon be familiar with the myriad potential vascular variations and apply the basic principle of vascular surgery; inflow and outflow control. Failure in either of these areas may result in uncontrollable intraoperative bleeding or excessive transfusion requirements.

Hepatic arterial anatomy is variable. These variations can usually be identified intraoperatively and managed so there is little impact on successful completion of the liver resection. Preoperative angiography is thus not required for anatomic definition unless placement of a hepatic arterial infusion pump is considered. Portal venous anatomy is more predictable, with the most common hazard being the posterior branch of the right portal vein. This branch often exits within 1 cm of the main portal vein bifurcation and courses almost directly posteriorly. Brisk hemorrhage occurs during isolation of the main right portal vein branch if the posterior branch is entered inadvertently.

The hepatic veins are the source of most of the intraoperative blood loss during hepatic resection. The portal triad inflow vasculature is relatively easy to control prior to parenchymal transection, but the hepatic veins cannot always be controlled extrahepatically. Thus the relevant hepatic veins must be ligated during parenchymal transection, failure to do so results in excessive back-bleeding. Variations in the pattern of hepatic venous drainage are often present, primarily of the right lobe, which have been well described by

Nakamura and Tsuzuki.[10] A thorough review of their manuscript is mandatory for surgeons involved in liver surgery. IOUS of the liver is also helpful for identifying the intrahepatic course of the hepatic veins.

Resection Technique

I view the surgical procedure of liver resection as having three components: determination of resectability, inflow and outflow vascular control, and parenchymal dissection. Failure to perform the first two steps leads to a lack of success with the last. Impatience during the parenchymal dissection may result in tumor-involved margins, excessive blood loss, or postoperative complications with resultant prolonged hospitalization.

Liver resection for colorectal metastases requires excellent exposure of both the upper abdomen and pelvis because the surgeon must search for other sites of recurrence and have adequate exposure of the liver and suprahepatic vena cava. A variety of incisions can be utilized, but I prefer a bilateral subcostal incision, with a superior midline extension (if needed) to enhance exposure of the inferior vena cava and hepatic veins. This incision also provides exposure to the remainder of the abdomen and pelvis for a thorough evaluation to exclude coexistent extrahepatic tumor recurrence. I usually begin with only a right subcostal incision. The porta hepatis and celiac regions can be palpated through this incision, as can a large area of the abdomen and pelvis. Suspicious lymph nodes (> 1 cm in diameter or firm) or peritoneal implants are biopsied for frozen section pathologic analysis. Both lobes of the liver can be adequately palpated and initial IOUS accomplished. Should an unresectable lesion be encountered, the smaller incision is less morbid for the patient. If there are no findings that preclude a liver resection, the incision is extended to a bilateral subcostal incision.

After completing the manual and visual exploration of the abdomen, pelvis, liver, and lymph node bearing areas, the liver is completely mobilized by dividing the "ligaments" for a more thorough hepatic evaluation. IOUS is used again at this point to exclude any previously undetected liver metastases and to assess the proximity of the metastases to vascular and ductal structures. Findings during this more thorough IOUS examination may alter the extent of the hepatic resection. Currently, I use IOUS selectively to determine the feasibility of nonanatomic segmental resection versus formal lobectomy and to clarify indeterminate lesions identified on preoperative CT. Until one has personally evaluated the quality and accuracy of CT at their own institution, I urge routine use of IOUS in all patients undergoing liver resection. It allows an internal audit of the quality and accuracy of the local CT equipment and increases the surgeon's proficiency with IOUS as an intraoperative diagnostic tool.

Once satisfied that the liver resection can proceed, the next step is to obtain vascular control. The extent of the hepatic resection correlates with the amount of portal dissection. A segmental or wedge resection of the liver can be safely accomplished with total portal inflow occlusion. I prefer to occlude all portal structures with a vascular clamp, with the jaws tightened only enough to occlude arterial flow. A clamp occlusion with greater pressure may result in injury to the bile duct or hepatic artery. The duration of hepatic inflow occlusion and warm ischemia that is safe is controversial, but I have found that limiting occlusion to 15-minute intervals with 2–3 minutes of flow in between is well tolerated. The purpose of releasing inflow occlusion briefly is to provide blood flow to the hepatic parenchyma and to allow venous decompression of the gastrointestinal viscera.

For a formal right or left hepatic lobe resection, I prefer individual ligation of the appropriate hepatic arterial and portal venous branches in the porta hepatis. This technique causes vascular demarcation of the hepatic parenchyma which helps to guide the line of resection and permits blood flow to be maintained to the remaining lobe. Control of the left lobe vasculature is usually straightforward because the extrahepatic portions of these vessels are relatively long. The right hepatic artery is also easy to identify, but the right portal vein may provide more of a technical challenge. The right portal vein bifurcates into anterior and posterior branches, which may occur extrahepatically or intrahepatically, with the posterior branch coursing directly posteriorly. The short segment of the posterior branch of the right portal vein may be difficult to visualize and expose. I often place a small vascular clamp across the upper portion of the main portal vein to occlude right portal venous flow. The intrahepatic portion of the right portal vein can then be securely ligated within the hepatic parenchyma during the parenchymal dissection. This method prevents unintended entry into the right portal vein and still maintains extrahepatic inflow occlusion. During a right trisegmentectomy resection, I clamp the entire porta hepatis inflow, as the parenchymal dissection occurs through the medial aspect of the left lobe. Individual vascular control of vessels in the porta hepatis is more time-consuming during this extended resection and adds little to blood loss reduction.

The amount of posterior liver mobilization and inferior vena cava (IVC) exposure depends on the planned resection. Anterior wedge resections require only enough mobilization to allow satisfactory exposure of the tumor and resulting resection bed. A posterior liver tumor requires complete mobilization of the liver and exposure of the IVC. For left lobe resections, enough IVC is exposed to allow control of the middle and left hepatic veins safely. For right lobe resections, the retrohepatic inferior vena cava should be exposed fully to allow access to the right hepatic vein. Numerous smaller accessory hepatic veins usually exist and drain directly from the liver into the IVC. Ligation of these accessory veins prior to transecting the liver reduces blood loss and facilitates a safe posterior parenchymal dissection. These small accessory veins may be controlled with vascular clips; however, I often find these clips do not remain securely in place throughout the procedure, and dislodgment of a clip leads to aggravating bleeding. Therefore I ligate these vessels with silk ties or suture ligatures. I approach the IVC from its superior and lateral aspect by retracting the liver in an inferior and medial direction, which elevates the liver. After the right adrenal gland is visualized, dissection from an inferior to superior direction along the anterior surface of the IVC enables mobilization and ligature control of the small accessory hepatic veins. With adequate mobilization, it is possible to determine if extrahepatic division and suture ligation of the right hepatic vein is possible, or if it would be safer to control this vessel within the hepatic parenchyma.

Complete suprahepatic and infrahepatic IVC control is required with some posterior tumors. It enables complete vascular occlusion of the liver but may also stress cardiac activity significantly by reducing venous return. If this situation is required, I encircle the IVC immediately above the renal veins with an umbilical tape, which can be subsequently used for IVC occlusion. The suprahepatic cava is exposed but not encircled so long as a straight or slightly angled vascular clamp can be placed, if needed, immediately under the diaphragm to complete IVC occlusion. These steps are also warranted if the posterior dissection of the liver is expected to be difficult owing to anatomic exposure constraints related to patient body habitus or tumor encroachment near the IVC or hepatic veins.

The liver parenchyma can be divided by a variety of methods. I prefer to proceed so that the intrahepatic vascular and bilary structures are visualized prior to being transected, thereby reducing blood loss and preventing postoperative bilary leakage. For limited hepatic resections, the electrocautery device on the maximum coagulation setting is sufficient. For more complicated nonanatomic, segmental, and formal lobe resections I prefer the ultrasonic scalpel which gently dissects and removes the liver tissue and exposes the vascular and bilary structures within the parenchyma. The vascular and bilary structures can be clipped or ligated and then divided. When possible, I maintain a 2 cm margin of nonaffected liver parenchyma over the metastasis. Care must be taken to avoid dissecting too near the tumor; at least a 1cm tumor-free margin is the goal of every liver resection.

The ultrasonic scalpel is merely a technologic advancement when compared to the finger fracture, pool-tip-sucker, or Kelley clamp methods of parenchymal fracture in which major vascular and bilary structures are unharmed and exposed for precise identification and ligation. The advantage of the ultrasonic dissecting instrument is the precision it allows when exposing not only large vascular structures but also the many small tributaries and branches. These small vessels can be cauterized, clipped, or ligated under direct vision, which reduces blood loss, improves visualization, and reduces stress to the patient, surgeon, and anesthesiologist. The slight increase in operative time associated with parenchymal dissection using the ultrasonic scalpel is compensated by a reduction in the need for blood transfusions, replacement fluids, and hemostatic efforts.

The final aspect of the resection involves ensuring hemostasis and preventing bile leakage from the cut edge of the liver. All obvious vascular and bilary structures should be ligated. The cut edge of the liver parenchyma is extensively coagulated, and a portion of the greater omentum is mobilized and secured over its surface. Closed suction drains are placed in a dependent area around the operative site to evacuate any residual blood or bile that may accumulate for the first few days. I also resuspend the liver with sutures along the falciform ligament following right lobe and trisegmental resections. This maneuver is intended to prevent angulation and obstruction of the hepatic or common bile duct that can occur when the remaining left lobe settles into the large open space left by the resection.

Postoperative Care

Postoperative care focuses primarily on intravascular volume management and prevention of pulmonary complications. Fluid requirements decrease after the first 24 hours, and judicial diuretic administration can hasten recovery by reducing edema and ascites. When the closed abdominal suction catheter drainage becomes serous and the volume increases, it signals the onset of fluid mobilization and the need to reduce intravenous fluid infusion rates. Postoperative ileus is usually of short duration, which allows resumption of enteral medications, fluids, and nutrition within 48 hours of surgery. Drains are removed 48–72 hours pafteroperation in the absence of evidence of a biliary leak. A significant percentage of patients develop a sympathetic pleural effusion, but only rarely does it become symptomatic, requiring drainage.

Results

In 1963 the operative mortality rate for major hepatic resection was 50%. Modern series report operative mortality rates of less than 5%.[2] This dramatic improvement is the result of lessons learned from military conflicts, application of principles of vascular surgery, better understanding of intrahepatic anatomy, and the use of natural history data to select appropriate candidates for liver resection. Tsao et al. reported a mortality rate of 1.2%, a morbidity rate of 36%, and a median hospital stay of 9 days following hepatic resection for malignant tumors.[2] Furhman et al. reported a similar operative mortality rate (2.8%) and an average hospitalization of 8 days.[6] My own unpublished results for liver resection are similar, with a 30-day mortality rate of 2.8%, a morbidity rate of 30.0%, and a median hospital stay of 6.5 days. The current emphasis on efforts to reduce blood loss are reflected by the finding that 42% of patients reported by Tsao et al. required blood transfusion during the operation or within the first 48 hours postoperatively compared to 23% of the patients in my series.

Furhman and colleagues have also demonstrated a significant improvement in 5-year survival rates with application of a few basic principles for patient selection and operative technique.[6] They stressed preoperative selection by excluding from exploration the patients with extrahepatic metastases or more than four intrahepatic lesions, and they advocated careful intraoperative exploration to exclude patients with coexistent lymph node or peritoneal metastases not detected on preoperative radiographic evaluation. Lastly, confirmation of the number of intrahepatic metastases and their proximity to major vascular and biliary structures using IOUS can help to ensure that the tumor is completely extirpated with a more than 1-cm tumor negative margin. Using the criteria, these authors reported a 5-year survival rate of 44%.

Conclusions

Many issues wait to be resolved concerning hepatic resection for colorectal cancer liver metastases. Such issues include the role of adjuvant therapy following resection, further refinement of patient selection, and determination of the true survival benefit associated with liver resection. The latter issue may not be fully addressed owing to the difficulty of conducting a randomized clinical trial that includes a no-treatment arm. The other questions will be answered in time with a continued review of surgical results, selection criteria, and the use of prospective evaluation of adjuvant therapy.

Hepatic resection is not the perfect treatment for colorectal carcinoma liver metastases. Even a 44% five-year survival rate means that 56% of patients die, most from recurrent disease. The development of intra- and extrahepatic recurrences after liver resection for colorectal metastases indicates that postmetastectomy adjuvant therapy programs must address both the liver and extrahepatic sites. The efficacy of adjuvant chemotherapy is not yet determined, but trials evaluating both regional and systemic chemotherapy are under way.

References

1. Registry of Hepatic Metastases. Resection of the liver for colorectal carcinoma metastases: a multi-institution study of indications for resection. Surgery 103:278, 1988
2. Tsao J, Loftus J, Nagorney D, et al. Trends in morbidity and mortality of hepatic resection for malignancy. Ann Surg 220:199, 1994
3. Wagner J, Adson M, Van Heerden J, Adson M, Ilstrup D. The natural history of hepatic metastases from colorectal cancer: a comparison with resective treatment. Ann Surg 199:502, 1984
4. Cady B, Stone M, McDermott W, et al. Technical and biologic factors in disease-free survival after resection for colorectal cancer metastases. Arch Surg 127:561, 1992
5. Steele G, Ravikumar T. Resection of hepatic metastases from colorectal cancer: biologic perspectives. Ann Surg 210:127, 1989
6. Furhman G, Curley S, Hohn D, Roh M. Improved survival after resection of colorectal liver metastases. Ann Surg Oncol 2:537, 1995

7. Steele G, Bleday R, Mayer R, et al. A prospective evaluation of hepatic resection for colorectal carcinoma metastases to the liver: gastrointestinal Study Group Protocol 6584. J Clin Oncol 9:1105, 1991

8. Goslin R, Steele G, Zamcheck N, Mayer R, MacIntyre J. Factors influencing survival in patients with hepatic metastases from adenocarcinoma of the colon or rectum. Dis Colon Rectum 25:749, 1982

9. Heiken J, Weyman P, Lee J, et al. Detection of focal hepatic metastases: prospective evaluation with CT, delayed CT, DT during arterial portography, and MR imaging. Radiology 171:47, 1989

10. Nakamura S, Tsuzuki T. Surgical anatomy of the hepatic veins and the inferior vena cava. Surg Gynecol Obstet 152:43, 1981

9

Hepatic Arterial Infusion Chemotherapy for Colorectal Cancer Metastasis to the Liver

Lee M. Ellis, Judy Chase, Yehuda Patt, and Steven A. Curley

The liver is the most common site of distant organ metastasis in patients with colorectal carcinoma. Of the 160,000 patients who develop colorectal carcinoma each year in the United States, half develop a recurrence at some point in their lifetimes, with the liver being the most common site (70%).[1] Although we have developed a better understanding of the molecular determinants that lead to colorectal cancer progression and metastasis, little progress has been made in therapy for metastatic disease. Fewer than 10% of patients who develop liver metastasis can undergo potentially curative resection.[2] Despite advances in surgical technology and imaging techniques, at least half of the patients who undergo liver resection for metastatic colorectal cancer suffer a recurrence. Systemic chemotherapy for liver metastasis from colorectal cancer results in only one-third of patients obtaining a partial response, with complete responses being anecdotal.[3,4]

The concept of hepatic regional perfusion of chemotherapy [hepatic arterial infusion (HAI)] was first investigated more than 40 years ago. HAI is based on the principle of improving the therapeutic index by increasing drug delivery directly to the site of tumor while decreasing systemic drug exposure and toxicity. This treatment initially required monthly percutaneous hepatic artery catheterizations with the patient remaining bedridden for several days each cycle. The development of totally implantable infusion pumps for long-term delivery allowed more widespread application of hepatic regional chemotherapy and fostered an evolution toward the current treatment philosophy. In this chapter we (1) describe the rationale for HAI therapy; (2) outline the surgical techniques utilized for HAI catheter placement; (3) review results of randomized trials comparing HAI therapy to systemic chemotherapy; (4) describe the rationale in the development of various chemotherapeutic regiments; (5) review toxicity/complications of HAI therapy; and (6) review current HAI strategies and indications for HAI therapy at The University of Texas M. D. Anderson Cancer Center.

Rationale for HAI Therapy

The rationale for HAI therapy is based on several principles. First, although liver metastasis from gastrointestinal malignancies are believed to reach the liver by way of the portal vein, once a tumor grows beyond several millimeters in diameter it derives most of its blood supply from the hepatic artery. Ridge et al. studied the relative distribution of blood flow to colorectal cancer liver metastases in 11 patients. This study demonstrated that more than twice as much of the nutrient blood supply to the tumor was delivered via the hepatic artery via the portal vein.[5] In an attempt to determine the role of the site of hepatic infusion of chemotherapy in tumor response, Daly et al. randomized 25 patients with colorectal cancer metastases to the liver to receive floxuridine (FUDR) by portal vein infusion or HAI.[6] Fifty percent of the patients who underwent HAI responded, whereas none of the patients in the portal vein infusion group did so.[6] Thus delivery of chemotherapeutic agents to the tumor-bearing liver is enhanced by HAI and may be more efficacious against hepatic metastases than portal vein infusion or systemic therapy. HAI provides a higher concentration of drug to the tumor, whereas the normal liver tissue is exposed to proportionately less drug owing to its dual blood supply provided by the portal vein and hepatic artery.

Second, depending on the drug utilized, the concentration of drug that can be delivered to the liver far exceeds the dose that can be given systemically due to the fact that certain drugs are extracted by the liver at a high rate (Table 9.1). In the pioneering studies of Ensminger and associates, it was shown that 94–99% of FUDR was extracted during the first pass through the liver.[7] First-pass extraction of 5-fluorouracil (5-FU) was somewhat less at 19–81% (depending on the infusion rate). Hepatic tissue levels of intraarterially administered FUDR and 5-FU are 400 and 100 times higher, respectively, than systemic tissue levels.[8] Thus although higher doses are delivered to the liver [and tumor(s)], the extrahepatic tissues are exposed to relatively lower drug levels with a resultant decrease in systemic toxicity.

TABLE 9.1. Pharmacology of selected drugs when administered via the hepatic artery

Drug	Hepatic/systemic drug level ratio	% Hepatic extraction
Floxuridine	400	95–99
5-Fluorouracil	10–100	19–81
Mitomycin C	3	15–20
Cisplatin	5	10–20
Doxorubicin	~2	20–30

Surgical Techniques for HAI Catheter Placement

Successful implantation of HAI pumps requires the coordinated efforts of the surgeon, invasive radiologist, operating room staff, and nuclear medicine radiologist.[9] Attention to detail is imperative to gain the maximum benefit from the use of HAI therapy.

Preoperative and Intraoperative Evaluation

Transfemoral arteriograms are obtained before surgery in all patients to define celiac and superior mesenteric artery anatomy, identify any accessory branches supplying the stomach and duodenum, and rule out portal venous occlusion. There are two common types of anomalous hepatic arterial supply: accessory vessels and replaced vessels. An accessory vessel is an additional artery supplying a lobe when the normal right and left lobar vessels arising from the celiac artery are present. A replaced hepatic vessel occurs when the right or left hepatic artery does not arise from the common hepatic artery but, instead, arises from another branch of the celiac artery or the superior mesenteric artery.

A right subcostal incision from the midline to the anterior axillary line is used for exploration. A thorough operative assessment is necessary to exclude extrahepatic malignant disease, particularly in porta hepatis lymph nodes. With rare exceptions, if extrahepatic metastases are located and malignancy is confirmed histologically by frozen-section examination, placement of HAI devices is contraindicated.

Hepatic Artery Dissection

We routinely begin the dissection of the porta hepatis by performing a cholecystectomy. This measure ensures that the patient will not suffer from postoperative chemotherapy-related "chemical" cholecystitis.

Dissection of the proper hepatic artery begins immediately medial to the common bile duct. The dissection is carried out proximally along the artery until the gastroduodenal artery is located. Only the first 0.5 cm of the common hepatic artery must be dissected to allow application of a vascular clamp. The gastroduodenal artery and the proper hepatic artery 2–3 cm distal to the gastroduodenal artery are dissected free circumferentially; small arterial branches are clamped, divided, and ligated. The right gastric artery must always be ligated and divided to prevent perfusion of drug to the stomach (misperfusion).

A meticulous dissection of the tissues along the superior border of the stomach and duodenum is performed to ligate and divide all vascular structures from the distal antrum to the common bile duct (Fig. 9.1). In addition, a modified Kocher maneuver is performed to ensure that any aberrant ves-

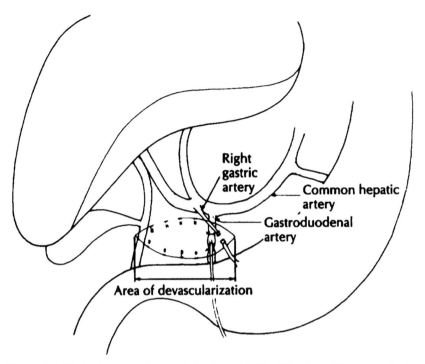

FIGURE 9.1. Gastroduodenal devascularization with distal ligation of the gastroduodenal artery, ligation of the right gastric artery, and division and ligation of the vascular tissues from the distal antrum to the common bile duct. A modified Kocher
maneuver is performed to ensure that any aberrant vessels from the hepatoduodenal
ligament to the duodenum are interrupted.

sels from the hepatoduodenal ligament to the duodenum are interrupted. This
gastroduodenal devascularization is an essential component of the procedure that greatly reduces the risk of drug misperfusion to the stomach and
duodenum.

Variant lobar vessels are exposed and, before ligation, clamped with
noncrushing vascular clamps. When a variant lobar artery is clamped, cy-
anosis of the hepatic lobe supplied by the variant vessel is common. The cy-
anosis is transient in most cases because of intrahepatic collateral arteries.

When a left hepatic artery arising from the left gastric artery is present,
the variant vessel usually can be identified and ligated in the superior
aspect of the gastrohepatic ligament immediately adjacent to the liver.
A right hepatic artery arising from the superior mesenteric artery follows
a retroduodenal course to the porta hepatis; this aberrant vessel can be
identified in the porta hepatis lying within the 90-degree arc beginning
lateral to the common bile duct and extending directly posterior to the
portal vein.

Placement of Pump or Port

A separate right-sided transverse incision is made 5–6 cm inferior to the sub-costal incision for subcutaneous placement of the pump device. A pocket is created in the subcutaneous fat with a thin flap (4–6 mm) overlying the pump. A thick flap makes palpation of the pump access diaphragm difficult or impossible. The pocket should be made entirely caudad to the incision because the pump may migrate upward and the surgeon wants to avoid having any portion of the wound overlying the access ports. The pump should be positioned so the access ports are inferior to the transverse incision, with the bolus access port between the 3 and 6 o'clock positions. Complete hemostasis in the pocket is essential to avoid hematoma formation and to minimize infectious complications.

The pump is placed in the pocket, and the catheter is brought through the fascia and peritoneum of the abdominal wall. The course of the catheter is evaluated as it passes from the pump through the abdominal wall to ensure that there is no acute angulation or kinking of the catheter. The pump is fixed in the pocket with several nonabsorbable sutures placed through the suture loops on the pump.

If an arterial injection port is utilized, the subcutaneous pocket is created superior to the subcostal incision so the port overlies the chest wall (and ribs) just medial to the anterior axillary line. This location offers better stability for the port chamber during injection of chemotherapeutic drugs. We currently do not advocate use of arterial ports because of the high risk of device-related complications (see Device Complications, below).[10,11]

Cannulation Technique

For patients with standard hepatic arterial anatomy (Fig. 9.2), the gastroduodenal artery is ligated 1.5–2.0 cm distal to its origin. An angled vascular clamp, such as a Satinsky clamp, is placed at the junction of the hepatic and gastroduodenal arteries to occlude the gastroduodenal artery while flow is maintained in the hepatic artery. A small arteriotomy is made just proximal to the ligature on the gastroduodenal artery. A beaded catheter is introduced into the gastroduodenal artery and advanced until it abuts the vascular clamp. The catheter tip should lie a the junction of the gastroduodenal and hepatic arteries without extending into the lumen of the hepatic artery (Fig. 9.2). Bidirectional fixation of the catheter is achieved by placing ligatures on either side of the bead. This maneuver is important for preventing subsequent displacement of the catheter either proximally into the hepatic artery or distally into the gastroduodenal artery. The angled vascular clamp is removed after the ligature behind the catheter bead is tied. The proper position of the catheter tip is confirmed before the ligature in front of the bead is tied.

The gastroduodenal artery is also the preferred cannulation site in most patients with variant hepatic arterial anatomy. Although the cannulation tech-

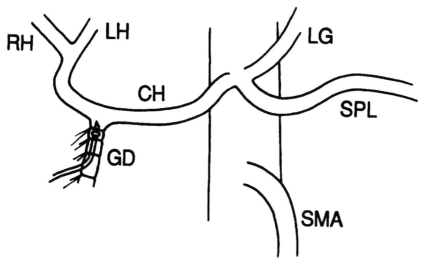

FIGURE 9.2. Standard hepatic arterial anatomy with distal ligation and cannulation of the gastroduodenal artery. GD = gastroduodenal artery; CH = common hepatic artery; RH = right hepatic artery; LH = left hepatic artery; LG = left gastric artery; SPL = splenic artery; SMA = superior mesenteric artery.

nique does not differ for these patients, the variant vessels must be ligated. Figures 9.3–9.8 illustrate our approach for commonly encountered hepatic arterial variations.

Complete or partial stenosis of the entire celiac axis or its branches is encountered occasionally. Preoperative arteriography is essential for identifying such lesions and can frequently show reversal of flow through the gastroduodenal artery. The result may be disastrous if the gastroduodenal artery is ligated and cannulated in such a case. In this situation, we ligate the common hepatic artery proximally and place the catheter into the distal common hepatic artery, with the tip advanced to the junction of the gastroduodenal, common hepatic, and proper hepatic arteries.

When dual catheters are required, a dual catheter pump or two individual pumps must be used to ensure complete hepatic perfusion. The two catheters must never be joined through a Y connector to a single pump because the differential resistance of the catheters may result in incomplete perfusion.

Confirmation of Bilobar Liver Perfusion and Absence of Misperfusion

Total hepatic perfusion and absence of gastroduodenal misperfusion must be exhibited before the operative procedure is concluded. The former is particularly important if variant lobar vessels have been ligated. A 10% fluorescein solution (3 ml) is injected through the pump bolus access port or the

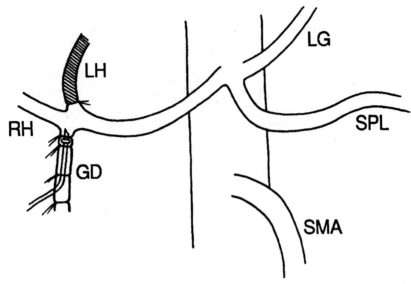

FIGURE 9.3. So-called trifurcation variant of hepatic arterial anatomy with ligation of the left hepatic artery and perfusion of the entire liver through the right hepatic artery via intrahepatic collateral vessels. See Figure 9.2 for abbreviations.

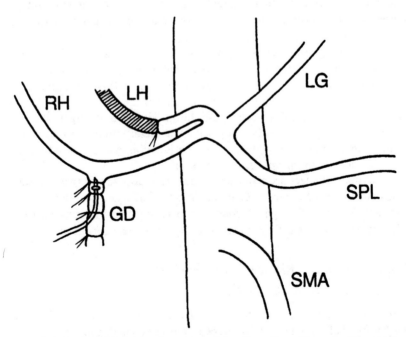

FIGURE 9.4. Replaced left hepatic artery arising from the celiac axis. The replaced left hepatic artery is ligated, with hepatic arterial perfusion through the right hepatic artery. See Figure 9.2 for abbreviations.

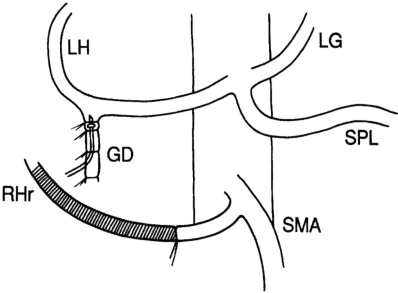

FIGURE 9.5. Replaced right hepatic artery originating from the superior mesenteric artery. The replaced right hepatic artery is ligated, with perfusion of the liver through the left hepatic artery. It should be noted that a replaced right hepatic artery such as this one is located lateral and usually posterior to the common bile duct. Caution must therefore be taken during the porta hepatis dissection to avoid injury to this vessel as it courses lateral to the common bile duct. This vessel can also be injured during cholecystectomy. See Figure 9.2 for abbreviations.

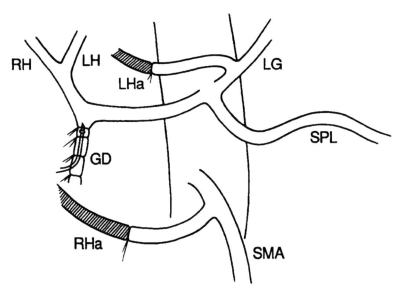

FIGURE 9.6. Accessory left hepatic or right hepatic arteries or both may be encountered. In such situations the accessory vessels can be ligated with standard placement of the infusion catheter into the gastroduodenal artery. See Figure 9.2 for abbreviations.

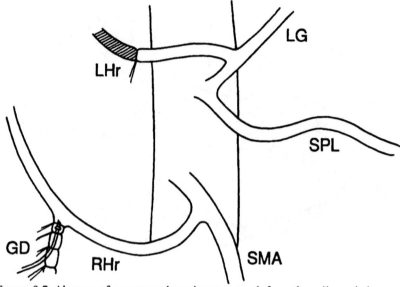

FIGURE 9.7. Absence of a common hepatic artery trunk from the celiac axis is noted. If an adequate side vessel such as a gastroduodenal vessel from the replaced right hepatic artery can be located, the side vessel can be cannulated in a standard fashion, placing the tip at the junction of the side vessel and the replaced hepatic artery. The replaced left hepatic artery is ligated. See Figure 9.2 for abbreviations.

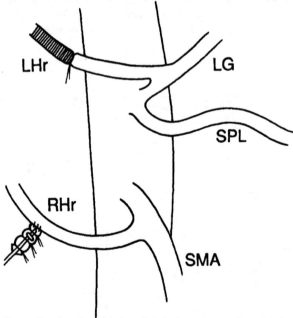

FIGURE 9.8. Example of replaced left and right hepatic arteries with inadequate side branches for cannulation. In this situation a side branch to the replaced right hepatic artery is created surgically, and the left hepatic artery is ligated. See Figure 9.2 for abbreviations.

port chamber; and the liver, stomach, and duodenum are examined with a Wood's light. This step allows identification of any areas of misperfusion into the stomach or duodenum and documents bilobar perfusion of the liver. To verify the absence of extrahepatic perfusion and the adequacy of hepatic perfusion, we obtain scintillation scans on postoperative day 3 or 4. Technetium-99 macroaggregated albumin (0.5 μCi) is diluted in 6 ml normal saline solution and injected slowly though the pump side port for 2–3 minutes; afterward, multiple projections are obtained.

If the infusion of fluorescein during the operation shows perfusion of any part of the stomach or duodenum, a search ensues immediately for the responsible vessel or vessels. After the arterial branches responsible for the misperfusion are identified and ligated, a second intraoperative study is performed to confirm an absence of misperfusion. If more than 40–45 minutes have elapsed, washout of the fluorescein will have occurred, and a repeat injection of fluorescein is needed. When the vessels causing gastroduodenal misperfusion are located quickly, an injection of methylene blue can be used to confirm the absence of blue staining of the stomach and duodenum. After ligation of variant hepatic arteries, it is difficult to confirm cross-perfusion of the liver using methylene blue, so fluorescein is preferred to show bilobar hepatic perfusion.

Impact of Surgical Experience and Variant Arterial Anatomy

A thorough understanding of hepatic arterial anatomy is necessary to ensure proper hepatic infusion with minimal complications. Curley et al. reviewed the histories of 180 patients who underwent placement of implantable hepatic arterial devices at M. D. Anderson Cancer Center to determine the incidence and surgical management of variant hepatic arterial anatomy and the complications associated with surgical placement of these devices.[12] Ligation of variant vessels or nonstandard cannulation was performed in more than one-third of the patients (Table 9.2). Response rates and treatment were no different in this group of patients than in patients with standard hepatic arterial anatomy. Although early operative complications (within 30 days of operation) occurred in only 10 patients (6%) (Table 9.3), late complications

TABLE 9.2. Sixty-eight variant hepatic arterial vessels ligated during operation or occluded at the time of angiography

Variant vessel	Ligation (no.)	Preoperative angiographic occulsion (no.)
Left hepatic (type 1 variant)	16	0
Replaced left hepatic	19	5
Replaced right hepatic	22	1
Accessory left hepatic	3	0
Accessory right hepatic	2	0
Total	62	6

TABLE 9.3. Early complications (within 30 days of operation) in patients undergoing placement of HAI device

Complication	Pump incidence (n = 143)		Port incidence (n = 37)	
Laceration of common				
hepatic artery	1	(0.7%)	0	
Bleeding from gastroduodenal				
artery	1	(0.7%)	0	
Puncture of infusion catheter	1	(0.7%)	0	
Catheter disconnected from				
device	0		1	(2.7%)
Skin necrosis over device	0		1	(2.7%)
Gastric misperfusion:				
missed right gastric artery	1	(0.7%)	0	
Pump pocket hematoma	4	(2.8%)	0	
Total	8	(5.6%)	2	(5.4%)

"Reproduced with permission from Curley SA[12]"

(more than 30 days after operation) or device-related malfunctions developed in 52 patients (29%).

Other studies have demonstrated the impact of surgical experience and variant hepatic arterial anatomy on outcome. Campbell et al. evaluated the role of the surgeon's experience and the presence of variant arterial anatomy on complications associated with HAI chemotherapy in 70 patients who had undergone surgical placement of HAI catheters and pumps.[13] Inexperienced surgeons (< 10 procedures) had a complication rate of 37%, whereas experienced surgeons (≥ 10 procedures) had significantly fewer complications (7%) ($p < 0.01$). Experienced surgeons had no complications when dealing with variant anatomy, in contrast to inexperienced surgeons, for whom the complication rate related to mismanagement of variant arterial anatomy was 42% (8/19). Civelek et al. also demonstrated the effect of anatomic arterial variations on complications with HAI therapy.[14] Despite pre- or intraoperative attempts to correct arterial abnormalities, more than 90% of patients with variant hepatic arterial anatomy had misperfusion, and more than 80% had subsequent clinical complications. This figure was in contrast to the complication rate of less than 10% in the group with normal hepatic arterial anatomy. Thus the importance of a thorough understanding of the appropriate management of variant hepatic arterial anatomy cannot be understated.

HAI Versus Systemic Chemotherapy

Investigators initially evaluated the efficacy and safety of HAI therapy in patients with unresectable liver metastases from colorectal cancer. These early demonstrated that HAI therapy delivered by implantable pumps was feasible, with few complications and response rates ranging from 30% to 80%.[15-17] In most of these early studies, survival was improved compared to that of historical controls. However, at the time of the reports, most of the patients had died, either from progressive hepatic disease or extrahepatic recurrence.

Because of the potential improvement in response with little systemic toxicity, it was necessary to compare the safety and efficacy of HAI therapy to "standard" systemic chemotherapy. Since the late 1980s, six prospective randomized trials have been completed comparing HAI to systemic chemotherapy.[18-23] In all studies, response rates were greater in the HAI arm than in the control arm (Table 9.4). The improved response rates did not always translate into improvements in survival. Nevertheless, it cannot be concluded from these studies that HAI therapy is no better than systemic chemotherapy. Careful analysis of these trials reveals numerous factors that do not allow a direct comparison between the two therapies studied. One controversial factor in these studies is the drug regimens utilized. For example, most current systemic regimens for metastatic colorectal cancer are based on the use of 5-fluorouracil (5-FU),[4] whereas most HAI regimens are based on the use of fluorodeoxyuridine (FUDR).[12,15,17,18,21-26] Many of the prospective randomized studies failed to compare response and survival rates between these two standard regimens. In studies from Memorial Sloan-Kettering Cancer Center (MSKCC), the National Institutes of Health (NIH), and the Northern California Oncology Group (NCOG), systemic therapy consisted of FUDR.[18,21,22] In a study from France, the "control" arm consisted of patients treated according to the standard care of the administering physician, and half of the patients in the control arm did not receive any systemic chemotherapy.[20] More important, two studies (NCOG and MSKCC) included a crossover arm for patients who failed to respond to systemic chemotherapy.[18,21] Thus data concerning survival are uninterpretable. In other studies[19-22] patients with extrahepatic disease were included in the HAI arm; this group of patients is unlikely to benefit from HAI therapy because the extrahepatic disease is not exposed to adequate doses of drug.

In many of the randomized and nonrandomized studies, patients did not receive the intended duration or dose of HAI chemotherapy because of complications secondary to hepatobilary toxicity,[18,20,21] particularly biliary sclerosis related to FUDR. Only recently have less toxic regimens been formulated that provide the same efficacy (response rate of approximately 50%) with less toxicity. Therefore should the studies be repeated today with these more innovative regimens, the intended drug dose would more likely be delivered. The prospects of performing such studies in today's environment are poor for several reasons. First, managed-care providers are less likely to support new studies: despite flaws in study design, previous studies failed to demonstrate a survival benefit, yet the cost of HAI therapy was significantly higher than that of systemic treatment. Second, ethically it would be difficult to design a study in which crossover was not an option offered to patients who failed to respond to the treatment in one arm of the study.

A more recent study by Allen-Mersh et al. examined the issues of quality of life and survival in patients with colorectal cancer metastasis to the liver

TABLE 9.4. Prospective randomized trials of HAI versus systemic therapy for colorectal cancer metastases to the liver

Site/group	Regimen	No. of pts.	Response rate (complete or partial)	Median overall survival (months)	Notes
MSKCC	IA: FUDR 0.3 mg/kg/day	48	50*	17	Crossover
	Systemic: FUDR 0.15 mg/kg/day	51	20	12	
NIH	IA: FUDR 0–0.3 mg/kg/day	21	62*	17	Extrahepatic disease
	Systemic: FUDR 0.125 mg/kg/day	29	17	12	
NCOG	IA: FUDR 0.2–0.3 mg/kg/day	50	42*	17	Crossover and extrahepatic disease
	Systemic: FUDR 0.075 mg/kg/day	65	10	16	
Mayo Clinic	IA: FUDR 0.3 mg/kg/day	33	48*	12.6	Extrahepatic disease
	Systemic: 5-FU 500 mg/m²/day q5wk	36	21	10.5	
France	IA: FUDR 0.3 mg/kg/day	70	43*	15	Extrahepatic disease
	Systemic: 5-FU[a]	41	9	11	
London	IA: FUDR 0.2 mg/kg/day	51	—	13.5*	Variable regimens/no therapy in systemic arm
	Systemic: variable	49	—	7.5	

5-FU = 5-florouracil; FUDR = floxuridine; IA = intraarterial; MSKCC = Memorial Sloan-Kettering Cancer Center; NIH = National Institutes of Health; NCOG = Northern California Oncology Group.

[a]See text for explanation of no dose being listed.

*Significantly different ($p \leq 0.05$).

"Reproduced with permission from Curley SA[12]"

treated with HAI.[23] Altogether 100 patients were randomized to receive either "conventional therapy" (palliation or systemic chemotherapy or both: control group) or 14-day cycles of HAI therapy with FUDR (0.2 mg/kg/day) alternating with 14 days of "rest." Survival was significantly longer in the HAI group than in the control group (median 405 days vs. 226 days) ($p = 0.03$). Overall, the quality of life was similar in the two groups. HAI therapy altered the cause of death in that only 31% of HAI patients died of liver disease, whereas 78% of patients died of liver disease in the control arm.

Two meta-analyses of the prospective randomized studies have been done to evaluate the response to HAI therapy compared to that after systemic chemotherapy or no antitumor treatment. In both studies only a marginal increase in survival was noted in the HAI groups compared to the systemic therapy groups. Hence the question of the clinical utility of HAI chemotherapy was raised.[24,25]

Although the flaws in study design previously mentioned do not allow firm conclusions to be drawn regarding any clear-cut survival benefit with HAI therapy, several key points have emerged from these trials. The use of HAI in the treatment of patients with colorectal cancer metastases to the liver requires a dedicated team including a surgeon, pharmacologist, radiologist, and medical oncologist who have knowledge of hepatic arterial anatomy, drug pharmacology, potential toxicity, complications, and alternative therapies. Second, selection of patients for HAI therapy greatly affects the efficacy of therapy. For example, patients with extrahepatic disease (metastasis to portal lymph nodes or distant sites) or extensive hepatic replacement by tumor should not be considered for HAI therapy because there is clearly no survival benefit in this group of patients.

HAI Regimens

Since the advent of HAI therapy, chemotherapeutic regimens have evolved in an effort to maximize response while minimizing toxicity. Initial regimens utilizing FUDR at relatively high doses (0.3 mg/kg/day) were associated with unacceptable hepatobiliary toxicity.[21,26] Therefore numerous regimens have been developed that use lower doses of FUDR combined with other chemotherapeutic agents, shorter durations of FUDR, FUDR combined with agents that inhibit the development of biliary sclerosis, biomodulating agents in an attempt to increase response rates, or 5-FU.

Sugihara reported on 68 patients treated with HAI therapy consisting of 5-FU at a dosage of 360 mg/m^2 for 7 days followed by 180 mg/m^2 for 21 days.[27] This phase was followed by 7 days of no infusion alternating with 7 days of infusion at the lower dose. A 50.9% response rate was obtained in the 53 evaluable patients. The median survival time for all patients was 11 months: 18 months for responders and 7 months for nonresponders. Patients with minimal extrahepatic disease were included in this study. Although there was no hepatobiliary or hematolgoic toxicity, infusion route-related complications occurred in 20 patients treated with percutaneous catheters instead of an implanted pump. Gastrointestinal complications (including severe abdominal pain, bleeding requiring operation, and vomiting) occurred in 18 patients.

To minimize the hepatic toxicity associated with hepatic intraarterial FUDR and the systemic toxicity following HAI of 5-FU, Stagg et al. had previously evaluated a regimen of HAI therapy using FUDR alternating with 5-FU in a phase II trial.[28] Patients with colorectal cancer metastasis to the liver received FUDR 0.1 mg/kg/day by HAI for 7 days followed by a 15 mg/kg HAI bolus of 5-FU on days 15, 22, and 29. The cycle was repeated every 35 days. Of 64 evaluable patients, 33 (51.6%) experienced a complete or partial response, with a median survival in all patients of 22.3 months. Importantly, no patient required termination of treatment owing to toxicity.

In a follow-up study, Davidson and associates from M. D. Anderson Cancer Center treated 57 consecutive patients with HAI therapy with the regimen outlined by Stagg and associates.[29] Cycles were initiated approximately every 35 days in the absence of toxicity. More than half (52.6%) of the patients had received no prior systemic or HAI treatment. Using this regimen, a response rate of 54.4% was obtained (6 complete responses, 25 partial responses). Another 14 patients (24.6) had stable disease. Median survival for the entire group was 18 months; patients who responded or had stable disease had a median survival of 19 months, whereas patients who had progressive disease had a median survival of 13 months. Importantly, 14 patients (24.6%) required cessation of therapy secondary to FUDR treatment owing to an elevated serum alkaline phosphatase or bilirubin level or both. Two of these patients (3.5%) developed biliary sclerosis requiring biliary stenting. Five patients (8.8%) experienced systemic toxicity related to 5-FU that required temporary cessation of therapy and dose reduction. The remaining 38 patients (66.7%) experienced minimal or no toxicity. Overall, 82.4% of patients were able to maintain full-time employment or usual activities during HAI treatment.

In an effort to minimize the incidence to biliary sclerosis associated with HAI of FUDR, Kemeny et al. evaluated the effect of adding dexamethasone to FUDR.[30] Fifty patients were randomized to receive either FUDR (0.3 mg/kg/day for 14 of 28 days) or FUDR plus dexamethasone (20 mg for 14 of 28 days). Overall, patients in the FUDR plus dexamethasone group received higher total doses of FUDR with a decreased incidence of elevated serum bilirubin levels. Complete and partial response rates were greater in patients in the FUDR plus dexamethasone group than in the FUDR-only group (8% and 63% vs. 4% and 36%, respectively). There was also a trend toward increased median survival in the FUDR plus dexamethasone group (23 months vs. 15 months) ($p = 0.06$).

Based on the principle that leucovorin modulates and enhances the anticancer activity of fluoropyrimidines, Kemeny et al. examined the effect of

FUDR and leucovorin on antitumor response and toxicity rates.[26] High-dose FUDR (0.3 mg/kg/day) and leucovorin (30 mg/m²/day) for 14 days afforded a more than 50% response rate, although sclerosing cholangitis developed in two of the first eight patients treated at these doses. The remainder of the 24 patients in this trial were treated with less aggressive regimens, and no hepatobiliary toxicity occurred. The overall response rate in the entire group was 72% with a median survival of longer than 27 months.

In a follow-up study, the same group examined other HAI regimens utilizing various doses and schedules of FUDR and leucovorin in previously untreated patients with unresectable colorectal cancer metastases to the liver.[31] One group received FUDR (0.3 mg/kg/day) and leucovorin (30 mg/m²/day) for 14 days followed by a 4-week rest period; a second group received FUDR (0.25 mg/kg/day) and leucovorin (30 mg/m²/day) for 14 days followed by a 2-week rest period; and a third group received FUDR (0.3 mg/kg/day) with a lower dose of leucovorin (15 mg/m²/day) for 14 days followed by a 2-week rest period. Complete/partial response rates for groups 1, 2, and 3 were 30%, 54%, and 75%, respectively, with biliary sclerosis rates of 17%, 15%, and 6%. The median survival of all patients treated with FUDR and leucovorin in this study was 28.8 months.

Other groups have utilized unique HAI regimens with similar results.[32] A multicenter study sponsored by the National Register of Implantable Systems from Rome, Italy randomized 109 patients with colorectal cancer metastasis to the liver to receive escalating doses of systemic 5-FU (250, 375, or 500 mg/m²/day on days 1–5) with bolus or continuous HAI of cisplatin (24 mg/m²/day on days 1–5). Overall response rates were slightly higher in the bolus infusion arm. The overall combined complete/partial response rate for both groups was 34.6%. Toxicity was similar among groups.

Warren et al. examined the effect of the combination of HAI of 5-FU (1.5 g/m² over 24 hours) with leucovorin (400 mg/m²) infused intravenously during the initial and final 2 hours for treatment of patients with colorectal color cancer metastases to the liver.[33] Weekly treatments were given in cycles of 6 weeks' duration. The combined complete and partial response rate was 48% with a median time to progression of 8 months.

Kerr et al. also used HAI 5-FU and systemic leucovorin and added a pharmacokinetic study.[34] Forty-three patients received the 48-hour regimen every 2 weeks. Leucovorin was given at a dosage of 200 mg/m² over 2 hours followed by a loading dose of 5-FU (400 mg/m²) given by HAI over 15 minutes. This phase was followed by a 22-hour HAI of 5-FU at doses ranging from 0.8 to 1.84 mg/m². The same doses of chemotherapy were given on day 2. Only 7 of 30 patients demonstrated evidence of progressive disease. The authors favored this regimen, stating that the high levels of 5-FU delivered to the liver provided a good response in that organ and were associated with systemic 5-FU levels similar to those with intravenous regimens. The toxicity related to HAI of 5-FU was tolerable.

Treatment of Disease Refractory to Systemic Chemotherapy

Hohenberger et al. used HAI of 5-FU to treat 16 patients with colorectal cancer metastasis to the liver who had progressive disease while receiving systemic chemotherapy.[35] Three patients had a partial response, and five patients had stable disease. Kemeny et al. treated 95 patients with colorectal cancer metastasis to the liver who had previously failed to respond to systemic therapy (given as adjuvant therapy or treatment of metastatic disease).[36] Patients were randomized to receive either FUDR alone or FUDR, mitomycin C, and carmustine. There was no significant difference in response rates between the two groups, but the chemotherapy-related toxicity was significantly greater in the second group. The overall response rate was 39% and the median survival 16.8 months. In patients who had received prior adjuvant therapy, the response rate was 57%, in contrast to 35% in the patients who had received prior systemic therapy for metastatic disease.

See Current M. D. Anderson Strategies and Indications for HAI below.

Toxicity/Complications of HAI Therapy

Chemotherapy-Related Complications

Although early studies of HAI therapy appeared promising because of the high antitumor response rates, the responses were associated with significant toxicity. The nutrient blood supply to the gallbladder is derived from branches just distal to the proper hepatic artery bifurcation, and HAI therapy was initially associated with high rates of chemical cholecystitis. This problem led to the common practice of routine cholecystectomy as an inherent component of the operative procedure for HAI catheter placement.

Other problems with misperfusion of the drug included exposure of the distal stomach and proximal duodenum to the chemotherapeutic agent. Nearly 20% of patients in early HAI studies experienced complications related to gastritis or duodenitis. With improvements in surgical technique (see above), this complication should be avoidable. However, in patients who receive numerous cycles of HAI therapy, we have seen the late development of collateral vessels, which may lead to aberrant perfusion of the stomach or duodenum. In this case, embolization of these newly formed vessels may be achieved by radiographically guided percutaneous intervention.

The most common complication related to HAI therapy with FUDR is chemical hepatitis/biliary sclerosis. Initial studies utilized FUDR delivered at a rate of 0.3 mg/kg/day over 14 days alternating with 14 days of no therapy. Although response rates at this dose were promising, most investigators had to reduce the dose of drug because of an increase in the serum alkaline phosphatase or bilirubin level (or both).[18,21] The chemical hepatitis manifested by increases in hepatic transaminases is almost always reversible. In the early stages biliary sclerosis is also reversible, but if therapy is not discontinued or modified at the first sign of toxicity the biliary sclerosis may be permanent. This complication is diagnosed by endoscopic retrograde cholangiopancreatography (ERCP). Strictures of major biliary radicals necessitate stent placement. If biliary sclerosis is detected early, HAI of dexamethasone alone without chemotherapeutic agents may prevent progression of the biliary sclerosis. Chemical hepatitis is the most common side effect following HAI of 5-FU but is reversible with cessation of therapy.

Device Complications

Vaughty et al. reviewed the literature regarding technical complications associated with HAI pumps.[37] The overall incidences of pump pocket infection and hematoma/seroma were 1.2% and 6.3%, respectively. Hematomas and seromas can easily be drained percutaneously in the clinic. However, most pump infections (except cellulitis) fail to respond to antibiotics and require relocation of the pump to another site on the abdominal wall. Preferably, an uninfected segment of catheter, one that is intraabdominal or tunneled subcutaneously, should be spliced onto a new pump/catheter or one that has been disinfected (soaked in povidone-iodine solution). In he review by Vaughty et al. pump malfunction occurred only 0.7% of the time; a catheter break, misplacement, migration, leak, or kinking occurred in 5.3%, of cases. Although a 5% incidence of arterial thrombosis or aneurysm was noted, it must be considered in light of the protocols utilized. In our experience, patients who respond to HAI therapy and thus receive repeated courses of HAI may develop a fluid collection around the tip of the catheter detectable with CT. The etiology is unknown but is likely related to periarteritis. Most patients with this finding develop pain with continued infusion; the pain is relieved by cessation of HAI of chemotherapeutic agents.

Fordy et al. evaluated 95 patients undergoing a total of 959 HAI treatments by either an implanted pump (64 patients) or a port (31 patients).[11] The use of a port was associated with a significant increase in catheter occlusion and treatment interruption when compared to the use of a pump. Overall, the continuous-infusion pump offered a thru-fold lower incidence of treatment interruption and a 30-fold lower incidence of catheter occlusion. We have also found that ports are associated with a significantly higher incidence of device-related complications compared with pumps.[10]

Current M. D. Anderson Strategies and Indications for HAI

It is necessary to consider several important variables when formulating treatment strategies for HAI therapy. First, the appropriate patient population must be chosen in order to administer therapy to those most likely to benefit. Second, placement of the pump requires that the surgical team be well versed in hepatic arterial anatomy and experienced with the surgical implantation procedure. Third, the drug regimen must be carefully selected to optimize response while minimizing toxicity. Finally, the oncologist must be aware of the potential complications of HAI therapy, be able to recognize toxic effects at an early stage, and know that appropriate interventions.

At present, with rare exception, we reserve the use of HAI therapy for patients who have failed to respond to systemic therapy or have developed intolerable complications secondary to toxicity. Only patients who have no evidence of extrahepatic disease are considered for HAI therapy, and they must be able to have access to a medical oncologist or a surgeon who is well acquainted with the nuances of this treatment modality. Rarely, we treat patients who had a partial response to systemic chemotherapy but had intolerable side effects such as refractory diarrhea, intractable tearing, or severe mucositis.

In general, the HAI chemotherapeutic regimen with which to initiate therapy is controversial. A number of questions regarding HAI therapy are still unanswered, so it is important that patients be entered into clinical HAI trials when available. In the absence of clinical trials, we usually recommend initiating HAI therapy with what we believe is the least toxic regimen but with comparable response rates. Therefore we often initiate HAI therapy with an alternating FUDR (0.1 mg/kg/day, days 1–7 and 5-FU (15 mg/kg, bolus infusion days 15, 22, and 29) regimen.[29] Liver function tests are monitored on days 1, 8, and 22; a complete blood count (CBC) and platelets are monitored on days 15, 22, and 29. In patients with elevated serum carcinoembryonic antigen (CEA) levels, the CEA should be assayed at the start of each cycle. FUDR should be withheld for any increased serum alkaline phosphatase or bilirubin level that does not return to baseline by the next treatment cycle or for any increase greater than 2.5 times baseline. In this setting FUDR should be completely eliminated from the HAI regimen; the 5-FU may be continued on a weekly basis without an increased risk of biliary sclerosis. If uncontrolled diarrhea, mucositis, or any hematologic toxicity develops, the 5-FU should by withheld until all toxicity resolves. HAI therapy can then be reinitiated with the 5-FU dosage decreased to 10 mg/kg. Two or three cycles or therapy are usually completed (10–15 weeks) prior to restaging. In the absence of significant toxicity, treatment is continued until objective evidence of progression is observed at hepatic or extrahepatic sites.

Patients who have hepatic progression on the FUDR/5-FU regimen may be treated with a variety of HAI regimens. If patients have not experienced hepatobiliary toxicity, we often initiate FUDR/leucovorin + mitomycin C (MMC). FUDR 0.2 mg/kg/day + leucovorin 10 mg/m^2/day are co-infused × 7 days, repeated every 28 days. HAI of MMC at a dose of 10 mg/m^2 is administered over 2 hours and repeated every 6–8 weeks. Patients who have experienced hepatobiliary toxicity may be treated with single agent (MMC)

HAI every 6–8 weeks. The most common side effects from MMC HAI include acute nausea, lethargy, fatigue, and delayed hematologic toxicity including neutropenia, anemia, and thrombocytopenia. The CBC and platelets should be monitored at least every 2 weeks during MMC therapy. MMC should be held for a white blood cell count that is less than $3500/min^3$ or a platelet count less than $80,000/min^3$.

Patt et al. completed a phase II trial of HAI 5-FU and recombinant human interferon-α2b (rINFα2b) in patients refractory to systemic 5-FU/leucovorin.[38] Forty-eight patients were given a 6-hour HAI of rINFα2b 5 mu/m² followed by an 18-hour HAI or 5-FU 1500 mg/m² daily for 5 days, repeated every 28–35 days. The partial response rate was 33% and the median survival 15 months. Grade 3–4 treatment-related toxicity included mucositis, neutropenia, and thrombocytopenia. No hepatobiliary toxicity was encountered. This regimen appears to have more systemic toxicity than other HAI regimens, but the lack of hepatobiliary toxicity may permit salvage HAI therapy in patients not able to tolerate FUDR-containing regimens. Reduction of the INFα2b and 5-FU dosage to 4 mu/m² and 1200 mg/m², respectively, or shortening the schedule to 4 days has decreased the incidence of the grade 3–4 toxicity to a more acceptable level and is recommended for off-protocol use.

We have investigated the use of HAI therapy as an adjuvant to resection of hepatic metastases. Twenty patients with colorectal liver metastasis who underwent hepatic resection with curative intent were implanted with HAI ports (with a valved-tip arterial catheter) for administration of adjuvant HAI therapy.[10] Patients were to be treated with weekly 5-FU (15 mg/kg) for 6 months. With a median follow-up of 33 months, 9 of 18 evaluable patients developed recurrent disease. The liver was the only site of recurrence in 3 of 18 (17%) patients. Catheter thrombosis occurred 11 times in eight patients, although 8 of these occlusions were successfully treated with thrombolytic therapy.

Other studies are under way to determine the role of adjuvant HAI therapy following hepatic resection and cryotherapy. Currently, outside of a clinical trial, we do not advocate the use of HAI therapy as an adjunct to resection or cryotherapy.

Conclusions

For treatment of patients with colorectal cancer metastases confined to the liver, HAI therapy provides response rates that exceed those with systemic therapy. Because of study designs, however, it has been difficult to correlate these findings with improved patient survival. Currently, we reserve HAI therapy for patients who have failed to respond to systemic therapy or who have intolerable adverse effects. The role of HAI therapy in the adjuvant setting remains undefined. When HAI therapy is used, it is necessary to have an experienced team manage the care of the patient: The surgeon must have intricate knowledge of hepatic arterial anatomy and its variants and of the natural history of liver metastases; the invasive radiologist must likewise understand hepatic arterial anatomy; the medical oncologist/surgeon must be able to recognize and treat complications promptly; and the pharmacist must know drug administration, pharmacokinetics, and potential complications. Because most patients who undergo HAI treatment have failed to respond to other therapies, it is the oncologist's obligation to evaluate new regional infusion regimens so long as toxicity remains reasonable.

References

1. Pestana C, Reitemeier RJ, Moertel CG, et al. The natural history of carcinoma of the colon and rectum. Am J Surg 108:826, 1964
2. Steele G Jr, Ravikumar TS. What's new in general surgery: resection of hepatic metastases from colorectal cancer: biologic perspectives. Ann Surg 210:127, 1989
3. O'Dwyer PJ, Minnitti CJ. Randomized trials with 5-fluorouracil in the treatment of advanced colorectal cancer. In: Cohen AM, Winawer SJ (eds) Cancer of the Colon, Rectum, and Anus. New York, McGraw-Hill, 1995 pp. 993–947
4. Moertel CG. Chemotherapy for colorectal cancer. N Engl J Med 330:1136, 1994
5. Ridge JA, Bading JR, Gelbard AS, et al. Perfusion of colorectal hepatic metastases: relative distribution of flow from the hepatic artery and portal vein. Cancer 59:1547, 1987
6. Daly JM, Kemeny N, Sigurdson E, Oderman P, Thom A. Regional infusion for colorectal hepatic metastases: a randomized trial comparing the hepatic artery with the portal vein. Arch Surg 122:1273, 1987
7. Ensminger WD, Rosowsky A, Raso V, et al. A clinical-pharmacological evaluation of hepatic arterial infusions of 5-fluoro-2'-deoxyuridine and 5-fluorouracil. Cancer Res 38:3784, 1978
8. Alexander HR, Bartlett DL, Fraker DL, Libutti SK. Regional treatment strategies for unresectable primary or metastatic cancer confined to the liver. In: PPO Updates. Principles & Practice of Oncology, Vol 10. Philadelphia, Lippincott-Raven, 1996 p. 19
9. Curley SA, Hohn DC, Roh MS. Hepatic artery infusion pumps: cannulation techniques and other surgical considerations. Langenbecks Arch Chir 375:119, 1990
10. Curley SA, Roh MS, Chase JL, Hohn DC. Adjuvant hepatic arterial infusion chemotherapy after curative resection of colorectal liver metastases. Am J Surg 166:743, 1993
11. Fordy C, Burke D, Earlam S. Twort P, Allen-Mersh TG. Treatment interruptions and complications with two continuous hepatic artery floxuridine infusion systems in colorectal liver metastases. Br J Cancer 72:1023, 1995
12. Curley SA, Chase JL, Roh MS, Hohn DC. Technical considerations and complications associated with the placement of 180 implantable hepatic arterial infusion devices. Surgery 114:928, 1993

13. Campbell KA, Burns RC, Sitzmann JV, et al. Regional chemotherapy devices: effect of experience and anatomy on complications. J Clin Oncol 11:822, 1993
14. Civelek AC, Sitzmann JV, Chin BB, et al. Misperfusion of the liver during hepatic artery infusion chemotherapy: value of preoperative angiography and postoperative pump scintigraphy. AJR 160:865, 1993
15. Balch CM, Urist MM, Soong SJ, McGregor M. A prospective phase II clinical trial of continuous FUDR regional chemotherapy for colorectal metastases to the liver using a totally implantable drug infusion pump. Ann Surg 198:567, 1983
16. Niederhuber JE, Ensminger W, Gyves J, et al. Regional chemotherapy of colorectal cancer metastatic to the liver. Cancer 53:1336, 1984
17. Sterchi JM, Richards F, White DR, et al. Chemoinfusion of the hepatic artery for metastases to the liver. Surg Gynecol Obstet 168:291 1989
18. Kemeny N, Daly J, Reichman B, et al. Intrahepatic or systemic infusion of fluorodeoxyuridine in patients with liver metastases from colorectal carcinoma: a randomized trial. Ann Intern Med 107:459, 1987
19. Martin JK Jr, O'Connell MJ, Wieand HS, et al. Intra-arterial floxuridine vs systemic fluorouracil for hepatic metastases from colorectal cancer: a randomized trial. Arch Surg 125:1022, 1990
20. Rougier P, Laplanche A, Huguier M, et al. Hepatic arterial infusion of floxuridine in patients with liver metastases from colorectal carcinoma: long-term results of a prospective randomized trial. J Clin Oncol 10:1112, 1992
21. Hohn DC, Stagg RJ, Friedman MA, et al. A randomized trial of continuous intravenous versus hepatic intraarterial floxuridine in patients with colorectal cancer metastatic to the liver: the Northern California Oncology Group trial. J Clin Oncol 7:1646, 1989
22. Chang AE, Schneider PD, Sugarbaker PH, et al. A prospective randomized trial of regional versus systemic continuous 5-fluorodeoxyuridine chemotherapy in the treatment of colorectal liver metastases. Ann Surg 206:685, 1987
23. Allen-Mersh TG, Earlam S, Fordy C, Abrams K, Houghton J. Quality of life and survival with continuous hepatic-artery floxuridine infusion for colorectal liver metastases. Lancet 344:1255, 1994
24. Harmantas A, Rotstein LE, Langer B. Regional versus systemic chemotherapy in the treatment of colorectal carcinoma metastatic to the liver: is there a survival difference? Meta-analysis of the published literature. Cancer 78:1639, 1996
25. Meta-Analysis Group in Cancer. Reappraisal of hepatic arterial infusion in the treatment of nonresectable liver metastases from colorectal cancer. J Natl Cancer Inst 88:252, 1996
26. Kemeny N, Cohen A, Bertino JR, et al. Continuous intrahepatic infusion of floxuridine and leucovorin through an implantable pump for the treatment of hepatic metastases from colorectal carcinoma. Cancer 65:2446, 1989
27. Sugihara K. Continuous hepatic arterial infusion of 5-fluorouracil for unresectable colorectal liver metastases: phase II study. Surgery 117:624, 1995
28. Stagg RJ, Venook AP, Chase JL, et al. Alternating hepatic intra-arterial floxuridine and fluorouracil: a less toxic regimen for treatment of liver metastases from colorectal cancer. J Natl Cancer Inst 83:423, 1991
29. Davidson BS, Izzo F, Chase JL, et al. Alternating floxuridine and 5-fluorouracil hepatic arterial chemotherapy for colorectal liver metastases minimizes biliary toxicity. Am J Surg 172:244, 1996

30. Kemeny N, Seiter K, Niedzwiecki D, et al. A randomized trial of intrahepatic infusion of fluorodeoxyuridine with dexamethasone *versus* fluorodeoxyuridine alone in the treatment of metastatic colorectal cancer. Cancer 69:327, 1992

31. Kemeny N, Seiter K, Conti JA, et al. Hepatic arterial floxuridine and leucovorin for unresectable liver metastases from colorectal carcinoma: new dose schedules and survival update. Cancer 73:1134, 1994

32. Cortesi E, Capussotti L, Di Tora P, et al. Bolus vs. continuous hepatic arterial infusion of cisplatin plus intravenous 5-fluorouracil chemotherapy for unresectable colorectal metastases. Dis Colon Rectum 37:S138, 1994

33. Warren HW, Anderson JH, O'Gorman P, et al. A phase II study of regional 5-fluorouracil infusion with intravenous folinic acid for colorectal liver metastases. Br J Cancer 70:677 1994

34. Kerr DJ, Ledermann JA, McArdle CS, et al. Phase I clinical and pharmacokinetic study of leucovorin and infusional hepatic arterial fluorouracil. J Clin Oncol 13:2968, 1995

35. Hohenberger P, Schlag P, Herrmann R, Räth U. Intrahepatic 5-FU retreatment of liver metastases of colorectal cancer that were progressive under previous systemic chemotherapy. Am J Clin Oncol 12:447, 1989

36. Kemeny N, Cohen A, Seiter K, et al. Randomized trial of hepatic arterial floxuridine, mitomycin, and carmustine versus floxuridine alone in previously treated patients with liver metastases from colorectal cancer. J Clin Oncol 11:330, 1993

37. Vaughty JN, March RDW, Cendan JC, Chu NM, Copeland EM. Arterial therapy of hepatic colorectal metastasis. Br J Surg 83:447, 1996

38. Patt Y, Hoque A, Lozano R, et al. Phase II trial of hepatic arterial infusion of fluorouracil and recombinant human interferon alfa-2b for liver metastases of colorectal cancer refractory to systemic fluorouracil and leucovorin. J Clin Oncol 15:1432, 1997

10

Cryosurgery
for Hepatic Malignancies

Daniel J. Gagné and Mark S. Roh

It was estimated that there would be 131,200 new cases of colon and rectal cancer in 1997 in the United States and 54,900 deaths due to colon and rectal cancer.[1] Ninety percent of patients who die from colorectal cancer have liver metastases.[2] The liver is the most prevalent site of first or only recurrence.[3] Liver metastases occur in 40–75% of patients with colorectal cancer, but only 10–30% have metastatic disease limited to the liver.[4,5] Surgical resection of hepatic metastases remains the treatment of choice when feasible, but only 5–10% of patients are considered candidates for liver resection.[6,7] Patients with limited liver metastases from colorectal cancer who do not undergo hepatic resection rarely survive more than 2 years after diagnosis.[8,9] Five-year survival rates of 25–35% have been reported in patients who have undergone hepatic resection of colorectal metastases.[10,11] Unfortunately, at least 75% of patients with limited liver-only metastases are not candidates for surgical resection.[12] Patients who have multiple metastases involving both the right and left lobes of the liver, metastatic lesions in proximity to major blood vessels or biliary structures where a 1-cm margin of clearance cannot be achieved, or more than three or four liver metastases have usually been considered to have unresectable lesions and do not qualify for standard hepatic surgical resection.[8,10,13,14]

Cryosurgery is a potentially curative treatment modality for patients with unresectable colorectal metastases confined to the liver, and it is a possible treatment for selected patients with primary hepatocellular cancer as well liver metastases from other primary tumors.[15–17] Cryosurgery is the *in situ* destruction of tissue by a freeze-thaw process.[16] The primary advantage of cryosurgery over resection is the preservation of normal hepatic parenchyma, allowing destruction of tumors deep in the liver without major resection.[18] Cryosurgery allows destruction of tumors without significant blood loss, and multiple lesions affecting both lobes of the liver can be treated by combined resection of one lobe with localized tumor cryoablation in another lobe, thereby increasing the total number of tumors that can be treated.[16,19]

Most patients treated with hepatic cryotherapy have multiple colorectal cancer metastases, although hepatomas, a small number of metastatic neuroendocrine tumors, and miscellaneous other tumors metastatic to the liver have also been treated. The objectives of this chapter are to discuss the history of cryosurgery, patient selection, techniques, patient outcomes, and future directions of cryosurgery of the liver.

History of Cryosurgery

James Arnott, and English physician, in 1845 was the first to use the destructive effect of freezing (cryosurgery) to treat cancer.[20] Iced saline solutions (−18° to 22°C) were used to treat advanced carcinomas of the breast and uterine cervix. The benefits described included relief of pain, reduction in the size of the tumor, and amelioration of bleeding and discharge.

It was not until the development of liquefied gases (oxygen, nitrogen, hydrogen) at the end of the 1800s and the turn of the century that liquefied air was used to treat skin diseases. It was also implied then that carcinoma of the skin could be cured by these techniques.[20] For dermatologic malignancies, where target tissues are easily accessible and often small, cryosurgery has become standard treatment.[21] Important experimental studies during the 1950s demonstrated the feasibility of producing focal areas of destruction in the brain, heart, and liver.

Modern cryosurgery received substantial impetus from the development of automated cryosurgical apparatus using liquid nitrogen circulated through an insulated metal sheath in 1961.[22] In 1963, following successful application of cryosurgery to treat Parkinson's disease, Cooper suggested that primary and metastatic liver tumors might be treated by cryosurgery and that freezing might produce an immunizing effect.[23]

During the late 1960s and early 1970s at the Surgery Branch of the National Cancer Institute and other institutions, numerous experiments were performed using application of extreme cold to kill cancer cells. Cryosurgery was done in many animal models, including guinea pigs, rats, dogs, primates, and hamsters and in numerous *in vitro* studies.[24] Gage et al. and Dutta and Gage showed the feasibility of freezing large volumes of liver tissue in dogs with no detrimental sequelae.[25,26] The cryosurgically destroyed tissue underwent total necrosis, which was followed by inflammatory cell migration in the margins of the lesion. The cryolesion was left *in situ* to be gradually reabsorbed by the body, and within 6–8 weeks after the procedure the cryolesion became a fibrotic scar. No incidence of hepatic abscess formation was seen in these studies. Gage et al. also demonstrated that large blood vessels tolerate freezing without rupture of occlusion so long as the vessels are not ligated prior to freezing,[25] leading the way to cryosurgery of lesions close to the inferior vena cava and portal vein. Cryosurgery has since been used for tumors of the skin,[21,27] bronchus,[20] breast,[28] prostate,[25,29] bone,[30] and pharynx.[20]

Early attempts to destroy liver tumors involved direct application of liquid nitrogen to the surface of the liver.[31–33] Early investigators reported success (limited to superficial lesions) with this crude method, but wide clinical acceptance of this modality was limited because of the amount of normal liver tissue that was damaged and the inability to treat deep lesions.[34]

Two technical advances during the 1980s have made hepatic cryosurgery more feasible for general practice: (1) vacuum-insulated probes and (2) intraoperative ultrasonography.[3,34] Vacuum-insulated probes allow controlled freezing of tumors even at great depths within the liver and avoid direct contact of liquid nitrogen with the liver. Liquid nitrogen (−196°C) is circulated through an insulated sheath, producing subzero temperatures within the enclosed tip of the probe and freezing the surrounding tumor with destruction of only a rim of normal tissue around each lesion.[35,36] By avoiding direct contact of liquid nitrogen with the liver, the use of the probe avoids the risk of nitrogen gas embolus, which can occur with open probes.[37]

The development of intraoperative ultrasound techniques allowed further applications for cryosurgery.[16,36,38-40] A major difficulty of utilizing cryosurgery for hepatic malignant disease was determining the exact volume of frozen tissue during treatment. The zone of freezing and the extent of damaged tissue in relation to the margins of the tumor must be accurately known to ensure total tissue destruction.[41] Initially, cryosurgery was monitored via thermocouples or electrodes (sensitive to changes in tissue impedance). This technique proved to be inadequate for hepatic cryosurgery, as placement of the thermocouples was largely guided by palpation.[32] Lesions with deep margins or irregular contours are difficult to assess by palpation, so thermocouple probe placement was inaccurate.[42] Lesions that are not visible or palpable could not be monitored or treated using visual guidance or thermocouple monitoring.[42]

Onik et al. described the following ultrasonic characteristics of frozen liver.[41] During freezing the cryolesion has a hypoechoic center and a hyperechoic margin, and it shows marked acoustic shadowing. During thawing the hyperechoic rim gradually recedes, and the diameter of the lesion visualized becomes smaller. After complete thawing, the cryolesion becomes less echogenic than before freezing and is therefore easily distinguishable from the surrounding normal hepatic parenchyma by ultrasonography.[35,42] Nonfrozen tissue must be used as an acoustic window to visualize the cryolesion adequately, and it is necessary to scan the liver in several areas for complete visualization of the frozen tissue.[41,42] Intraoperative ultrasonography can define the margins of the tumor and the extent of freezing in relation to the tumor margin.[41] The cryosurgical margin is particularly easy to discern because the tumor, whose echogenicity does not change after freezing, stands out against the lower echogenicity background of the frozen normal liver.[42] Postsurgical pathologic examination has shown excellent correlation between the lesion size and its ultrasonic image.[41,43]

The use of real-time intraoperative ultrasonic monitoring of the cryosurgery process was demonstrated experimentally in dogs.[35] Gilbert et al.[35] and Onik et al.[41] demonstrated *in vitro* and in animals that the entire freezing and thawing cycle can be monitored easily using real-time intraoperative ultrasonography; this capability was later demonstrated in a few small series of human patients.[26,38,42] Cryoprobes utilizing circulating liquid nitrogen, which produced a spherical iceball around each metastasis and which were controlled by operative ultrasonography were developed during the late 1980s. They were demonstrated to provide a technically feasible, effective method of tumor ablation.[36,38,39]

Mechanism of Action of Cryosurgery

Cryotherapy involves direct freezing of lesions *in situ,* which then undergo coagulation necrosis, in time leaving only a contracted fibrotic mass.[44] At temperatures below −20°C, most cells die as a direct consequence of internal freezing, secondary vascular thrombosis, or exposure to concentrated electrolytes during thawing.[39,45]; however, experimental and clinical reports have shown that temperatures in the −40° to −50°C range must be produced to be certain of cell death,[30,46] as intracellular freezing occurs in almost all cells by −40°C.[27] Cryosurgery destroys tumors in a non-tissue-selective manner in that normal and tumor tissue are sensitive to destruction,[47] but the work of Bischof et al. with human liver tissue indicated that cancerous cells may be more resistant to freezing than normal tissue.[48]

Cryosurgery causes tissue destruction and cell death by several mechanisms, both directly and indirectly[30,39,47] The direct cellular damage is a result of the physiochemical effects of (1) intracellular ice formation, (2) extracellular ice formation, and (3) solute–solvent shifts, causing cell dehydration and rupture.[49] The indirect cell damage results from a loss of structural integrity as well as vascular channel and small-vessel obliteration with resulting hypoxemia.

Damage from freezing is caused principally by the formation of ice crystals.[33] The rate of freezing determines in which compartment ice crystals develop and, as a consequence, the mechanism of cell death. A slow rate of cooling results in ice formation in the extracellular space first.[48] Ice crystal formation in the extracellular space creates an extremely hyperosmolar environment as ice forms as pure solid water, excluding all electrolytes and organics.[47] The cells are killed by a mechanism known as the "solution" effect,[49] which is an osmotic gradient that draws water from the cell and results in cell and tissue shrinkage, damage to the membrane, and protein denaturation. The resulting high intracellular ionic concentration leads to cell death.

In contrast, shrinkage is less important during rapid freezing, which produces intracellular ice crystals that have a direct mechanical effect on the cell membrane.[33] Intracellular freezing occurs in almost all cells by −40°C [27]. At high rates of cooling, water cannot leave the cells fast enough to maintain osmotic equilibrium across the cell membrane as with extracellular ice crystal formation. Equilibrium is therefore achieved by ice forming within the cells.[49] As one cell freezes, communication channels between cells provide preferred routes of ice propagation to the other cells.[47] Cell destruction is greater with intracellular ice formation.[49]

Upon thawing, solutes and a large uptake of water into the cells cause them to rupture.[49] During early warming, small ice crystals grow together with larger crystals; this recrystallization is a destructive process and destroys tissue because of the grinding action of ice.[47] For maximal tissue damage during the thawing process, the warming should be slow and passive.[47,49]

Change in the microcirculation are also noted with the freeze–thaw cycle.[33] During freezing, ice forms and propagates along the vascular system, resulting in continuous ice crystals in the vascular space; at low cooling rates the cells surrounding the smaller blood vessels dehydrate, and the water leaving the cells freezes in the adjacent blood vessels. These blood vessels, in turn, expand in diameter as much as twofold. During cryosurgery the expansion of blood vessels occurs at regions of slow freezing, including the outer edge of the frozen lesion. This expansion probably destroys the structural integrity of the vascular system, thereby depriving surviving cells of their blood supply.[50] Immediately on thawing, blood flow increases for up to 1 hour. Increasing damage to the walls of small vessels leads to the deposition of platelet–fibrin thrombi, with reduction and ultimately cessation of blood flow.[51] The resulting ischemia contributes to cell death.

Bischof et al.[48] described the pattern of cell damage around a cryoprobe and how it may affect the destruction of the tumor.[49] During cryosurgery three main areas of freezing occur: (1) an area near the cryoprobe where the freezing is rapid; (2) an area in the middle of the cryosurgical iceball where the tissue experiences intermediate cooling rates; and (3) an area at the periphery of the cryosurgical iceball where slow rates of cooling occur. In area (1), near the probe, where the cooling rate is rapid, extensive intracellular ice forms that is considered lethal to the cells. Far from the probe, in area (3), the tissue experiences the slowest rate of cooling, which leads to extensive cellular dehydration and consequent overdistention and thrombosis of the vasculature. The final region of freezing is an intermediate cooling zone, area (2), where a distribution of intracellular and extracellular ice occurs. The tumor, by resisting dehydration, may effectively increase the intermediate zone, area (2), to such an extent that the vascular thrombosis typical of area (3) is never achieved, and therefore some of the tumor tissue survives. The highest cytotoxicity is achieved nearest the cryoprobe during a rapid freeze following intracellular ice crystallization; and cells at the edge of the ice ball may survive.[49,52]

The temperature within the tumor is not uniform and is proportional to the distance from the probe tip.[30,33] In the human liver, the temperature gradient is about 10°C/mm, which limits use of the single-probe technique to tumors less than 5 cm in diameter, as liquid nitrogen (−196°C) is the agent most commonly used.[53] The advancing edge of the freezing tissue, which appears on the ultrasonic image as a hyperechoic border, is about 0°C.[30] The inner edge of the rim, which is 3–4 mm inside of the leading edge, has been stated to be about −20°C. The location of the −40°C isotherm is critical for effective therapy.[30] A rapid cooling rate moves the isotherm toward the periphery. Tests with high-efficiency modern probes cooled to −195°C places the critically important −40°C isotherm 5–6 mm inside the border of the frozen zone in frozen volumes 6–7 cm in diameter.[30] Although ultrasonography accurately identifies the edge of the iceball, the latter does not always correlate exactly with the eventual area of necrosis[54]; and adoption of a 1-cm ultrasonographic margin ignores the great differences in temperature gradient across iceballs of varying diameter.[54]

Lam et al.[43] confirmed the accuracy of ultrasound scans for depicting the size of the frozen solid hepatic tissue by comparing the ultrasonic cryolesion and the visceral cryolesion. The temperature of frozen liver closest to the cryoprobe was −180°C and that of frozen tissue at the periphery of a cryolesion was −25°C, with a gradient of temperatures in between. Tissue necrosis was complete within the entire volume of tissue encompassed by the ultrasonic cryolesion. Additional but varying necrosis around the frozen tissue occurs by microcirculatory failure.[50]

Other experimental evidence indicates that other factors affecting the diameter of the iceball include probe diameter and interruption of hepatic vascular inflow by clamping the hepatic artery and portal vein (Pringle maneuver).[55-57] Obstruction of portal inflow may be of value when large lesions are treated.[55] A large probe tip surface area results in a large area of maximum cell destruction; multiple probes can increase the effective surface area.[33,46,55]

The histology of acute resected cryosurgical lesions has been described.[38,42,47] Microscopically, the frozen normal liver shows coagulative and hemorrhagic necrosis of individual hepatocytes with small, shrunken, pyknotic nuclei and loss of all of the nuclear details. The cytoplasm is fuzzy and granular with indistinct borders. The sinusoids are moderately congested and hemorrhagic, a finding that could be seen clearly under low power alone.[35] Tumor tissue similarly underwent coagulative necrosis with loss of nuclear detail and cytoplasmic shrinkage in the frozen area. Histologic changes after freezing are much more striking in tumor tissue than in the normal liver, with definite cytologic changes consistent with necrosis even after only one freeze-thaw cycle. An abnormal amount of extracellular fluid is also present in the thawed cryolesion.[35] The edema and hemorrhage are probably responsible for the acoustic changes (reduced echogenicity) observed in the cryolesion. Cryolesions resected at 1 week reveal complete destruction of hepatic architecture and extensive eosinophilic infiltration.[47] An intense inflammatory reaction is seen at the junction of the necrotic and viable regions, with proliferation of hepatocytes peripheral to this zone.

Biliary ducts do not withstand cryosurgery as well as large blood vessels. Gage et al. first demonstrated and reported in animal experiments the necrosis of bile ducts secondary to cryosurgery.[25] This result has also been demonstrated clinically in numerous reports of biliary fistulas.[13,16,56,58,59]

These biliary fistulas can usually be treated succesfully by percutaneous drainage.[4,16]

Freeze-Thaw Cycles

Numerous experimental models have compared the tissue destruction of a single freeze-thaw cycle to that seen with double or triple freeze-thaw cycles. Most report that repeated freezing is more damaging than a single freeze-thaw cycle. Neel et al.[46] reported that repeated freeze-thaw cycles in primate livers achieved more uniform cell death and a larger volume of necrosis than a single cycle. Many reports show an improvement in the rate of growth of the iceball and in its final size after repeated cycles of tissue freezing, and a reduction in thawing rate after repeated freezes has been demonstrated.[49] Hepatic cryosurgery in sheep achieved a significantly higher percentage of destruction of a given iceball diameter following a twin freeze-thaw cycle.[56] It may be due to an increase in thermal conductivity during the initial freeze that makes subsequent cycles more effective or the rapid enlargement of intracellular crystals by freezing water newly taken into the cell during warming.[27,33] Ravikumar et al.[40,47] demonstrated in a experimental model using chemically induced rate colon carcinoma subcutaneous isografts that two or three freeze-thaw cycles were equally effective for controlling tumor growth completely; and that a single freeze-thaw cycle resulted in a 10% failure rate for controlling the local tumor growth. The tumor cubes were immersed in liquid nitrogen and were completely thawed at room temperature before the next freeze cycle was started and then isografted subcutaneously into the rat thigh. The microcirculatory shutdown and indirect destructive mechanism of cryosurgery was probably not a factor in these experiments, as these isografts were subcutaneous. The liver seems to be particularly sensitive to the effects of cryotherapy because of its vascular nature and therefore probably does not require a double freeze-thaw cycle for adequate necrosis.[56]

Morris and colleagues compared single and "double" edge-only freeze-thaw cycles and found that double cycles achieved greater destruction, as measured by serum liver cell enzymes.[54,60] In the double-freeze group, the original iceball was not allowed to thaw completely; only approximately a 0.5- to 1.0 -cm rim of iceball was allowed to thaw before refreezing. Patients undergoing hepatic cryotherapy with a double-freeze cycle clearly had considerably higher aspartate aminotransferase (AST) values than the single-freeze group. Edge-only double freeze-thaw cycles also result in a more marked thrombocytopenia than that seen after a single freeze-thaw cycle.[61] To avoid the significant morbidity and mortality that can be associated with cryoshock and because of the thrombocytopenia that develops after a complete twin freeze-thaw cycle, many groups now uses this edge-only refreeze technique.[57,61] Morris et al. strongly cautioned against allowing a complete thaw prior to the second freeze to avoid the possible complications of severe coagulopathy and respiratory and renal failure.[57,61]

The number and method of freeze-thaw cycles used for cryosurgery of hepatic malignancies has evolved over the years, but most groups now use the double freeze-thaw cycle. It consists of (1) a single rapid freeze, (2) a slow thaw of the outer 1-cm edge of the iceball, (3) an edge-only refreeze, and then (4) a complete thaw and termination of the cryosurgical procedure.

Extrahepatic Effects of Cryosurgery

Extrahepatic effects of cryosurgery, such as an immunizing agent or autovaccine released from the freeze-thaw process, that would be effective against further cancer growth had been suggested by Cooper.[23] It has been demonstrated in both rabbit and humans that antigens are released by cell lysis following freezing.[27] Cryosurgery is known to release fixed tumor-tissue antigens that may provoke an immunologically favorable reaction, leading to enhancement of the specific immune response to the tumor.[62] Reports have noted regression of untreated tumors after cryosurgery, possibly indicating that an immunologic response to the cryosurgery is responsible.[35] An autoantibody response, regional lymph node reactivity, and enhanced tumor resorption have been documented following experimental cryotherapy. Natural killer cell cytotoxicity was found to be enhanced following cryosurgery of normal liver and liver sarcoma tumor in a rat model of cryosurgery.[63] Jacob et al.[53,64] studied the cryodestruction of Walker carcinomas implanted in rat liver and showed significantly increased survival in the rats undergoing cryodestruction of the tumors rather than surgical resection or tumor infarction. Many other experimental studies have demonstrated no immune-mediated regression of remaining untreated tumor and no lengthening of survival.[47,62] The cryoimmune effects seen in some experimental models have yet to be substantiated in humans.[21,40,47]

Patient Selection and Eligibility

Preoperative clinical assessment and performance status of the patient, including the patient's cardiovascular and respiratory status must be adequate to undergo operation. General medical risk factors that are contraindications (e.g., severe chronic obstructive palmonary disease or coronary artery disease) for general anesthesia or intraabdominal surgery are also contraindications for cryosurgery in most centers. Candidate patient criteria and selection for cryosurgery is not the same at all centers, as there is no clear consensus in the literature regarding the number and size of tumors that should be treated by cryosurgery.

Most patients treated with hepatic cryotherapy have multiple colorectal cancer metastases. Surgical resection remains the treatment of choice, but cryosurgery may be appropriate if tumors are considered unresectable or the patient is a poor risk for liver resection. Cryosurgery may also be used to freeze the margin of the resected tumor. Colorectal cancer metastases have usually been considered unresectable if there are more than three or four hepatic metastases, both right and left lobes are involved, or a 1-cm margin of clearance cannot be achieved (i.e., single tumor metastasis close to vital vascular or biliary structures). The presence of extrahepatic malignancy is also considered a contraindication for surgical resection of hepatic metastases and remains a contraindication to cryosurgery at most centers. Ross et al.[14] reported that portal lymph nodes within the perfusion territory of a regional perfusion catheter may be an exception, but most believe that the presence of metastatic lymph nodes in the porta hepatis is invariably associated with recurrence and death despite resection of hepatic metastases and so is a contraindication to major hepatic resection.[65]

Candidates for cryosurgery are considered when they meet the following conditions.[13,16,66]

1. There is a biopsy-proved hepatic lesion or the combination of a rising level of serum carcinoembryonic antigen (CEA)— or α-fetoprotein (AFP) in hepatocellular carcinoma—and the appearance of a lesion on ultrasonography, computed tomography (CT) scan, or magnetic resonance imaging (MRI) of the liver. A negative biopsy of a suspicious lesion is not proof of benignity, and percutaneous liver biopsy is not recommended.[48]
2. There is no evidence of residual disease at their primary resection site.
3. There is no evidence of extrahepatic disease (occasional exceptions are seen with cases of colorectal cancer, provided complete excision can be performed subsequently, i.e., lung metastases).[67]
4. Hepatic disease is considered unresectable due to technical considerations (its location next to vascular or biliary structures, its bilobar nature, or its size) or to underlying cirrhosis.
5. All liver lesions determined by preoperative imaging can potentially be destroyed by cryosurgery alone or in combination with surgical resection; palliation is not a goal.

Pulmonary CT scanning is performed to exclude extrahepatic disease. CT during arterial portography is done to define accurately the number and position of hepatic lesions.[4,47,57] CT during arterial portography (CTAP) is the most sensitive preoperative imaging technique for detecting hepatic metastases from colorectal cancers[67] and is the procedure of choice for the preoperative selection of suitable candidates for hepatic resection.[68] This technique involves the administration of contrast material through the superior mesenteric artery or the splenic artery. This technique results in selective enhancement of the liver parenchyma through the portal vein; the intrahepatic vascular structures are well demonstrated. Hepatic tumors, with their predominant arterial supply, are shown as hypodense perfusion defects.[68] CTAP has a sensitivity in the range of 85–95% when preoperative scans were compared with the histologic resection specimen.[68–70] Some of the few metastases that have been missed by CTAP have been located at the hepatic dome.[67] This lack of sensitivity for the detection of metastases at this location is well known and is probably due to respiratory movements.[67]

The abdominal CT scan may detect intraabdominal extrahepatic disease. CT, ultrasonography (US), and MRI are ineffective for detecting lymph node metastases and differentiating hyperplastic nodes from those invaded by tumor.[71] These modalities are also insensitive for detecting peritoneal studding and metastases to the surface of the liver. Preoperative staging is disappointingly inaccurate, as up to 50% of the patients have unsuspected disease in the liver or in extrahepatic locations, obviating any further attempt at liver metastasis resection.[4,72]

As mentioned earlier, there is no clear consensus in the literature regarding the size and number of tumors that should be treated by cryosurgery. Most investigators believe that tumor larger than 5–6 cm is a contraindication to cryosurgery. Tumors this size are not easily treated by cryosurgery because the size of the iceball needed to ablate the tumor is limited.[4,17] Two or more probes can be used together, but the large amount of necrotic tumor can have adverse consequences on the kidneys, lungs, and coagulation systems.[4,13,14,19,73] Another relative contraindication for cryosurgery in some centers includes the presence of more than five metastases.[14,17] Candy et al. do not perform resection in those patients who have five or more nodules in the liver but still attempt resection with or without cryotherapy if they have only three or four metastases.[65] As the presence of more than four hepatic metastases does not always portend a grim prognosis,[9] some groups are more aggressive in their inclusion criteria and believe that more than 10 lesions is a relative contraindication for cryosurgery.[4] The total amount of liver volume involved by hepatic metastases and subsequent iceball lesions must also be taken into account, as some think that only 35–40% of the liver can be frozen safely,[74] whereas others state that less than 50% liver involvement is a possible indication for cryosurgery.[4]

The only absolute contraindication to resection is extrahepatic disease or the inability to remove the entire tumor.[11,75,76] Medically fit patients without extrahepatic disease should be considered for resection of hepatic metastases from colorectal cancer, regardless of the distribution of the tumors, preoperative CEA level, or disease-free interval.[11]

Preoperative Preparation

After a patient is deemed a candidate for liver resection and possible cryosurgery, further preoperative investigations should include laboratory tests [electrolytes, blood urea nitrogen (BUN), creatinine, glucose, complete blood count (CBC), platelet count, blood coagulation studies, liver function tests, carcinoembryonic antigen (CEA) level to monitor response and follow-up], chest radiography, and electrocardiography (ECG). Preoperative preparation includes the use of a single-dose intravenous prophylactic antibiotic.

Operative Technique

The operative technique is relatively consistent from group to group and has been described in a number of references.[13,14,16,19,47,57] Briefly, the patient is placed in the supine position on the operating table. Large-caliber central venous lines for rapid intravenous access and pulmonary artery catheter monitoring are placed. The use of compressors and Foley urine catheter is routine. The patient' upper or lower extremities (or both) are covered with forced-air heating blankets (Bair Hugger)[77] to avoid clinically significant hypothermia, which can occur as a result of the open abdomen and the intense freezing of a high-blood-flow organ with cryotherapy[13,19,45]; heated intravenous fluids are also used to avoid hypothermia. The patient's core temperature is monitored carefully throughout the procedure.

Although some centers perform diagnostic laparoscopy first to exclude extrahepatic disease, most patients undergo a right subcostal incision first, dividing the oblique muscles and rectus abdominis, thereby avoiding midline adhesions from the patient's previous colonic resection. Adhesions are dissected to allow full access to the liver, gallbladder, and hepaticoduodenal ligament. The abdominal cavity is then explored to exclude the presence of extrahepatic disease, such as local recurrence (primary resection site) or more commonly peritoneal or lymphatic (colonic mesentery and hilus) spread, which would exclude the patient from liver resection or cryotherapy. A thorough search is undertaken for nodal deposits in the porta and periaortic area. Peritoneal implants may be subtle and are often better detected by touch than by sight. They are perceived as roughened areas or raised seed-like projections.[78] When the decision is made to proceed, the incision is extended by adding a left subcostal incision to gain further access. The ligamentum teres is divided and ligated, and the falciform ligament is divided. A sternal lifting retractor or costal margin retractor and frame is placed to elevate the lower end of the chest and sternum for better hepatic exposure. The operating table is than tilted in a head-up (15–20 degrees) position. The liver is than mobilized for full assessment (manually, visually, and by intraoperative US) of the hepatic disease and to allow access in the event of major hemorrhage. Some groups place a tape around the portal inflow to provide the ability to occlude inflow.[57] Complete mobilization also aids in placement of the cryosurgery probes and monitoring the formation of the iceball. Superficial liver metastases, which cannot be seen, are best detected by feeling with the fingertips.[78] They often lie 1–2 mm below the surface of the liver and feel like grains of rice. Bimanual palpation is important and is a means of feeling deeper lesions, although deep, small lesions are likely to be missed.[8]

The liver is surveyed by US using 5.0- and 7.5-MHz (T-probe) intraoperative ultrasound (IOUS) transducers. The depth of sound penetration penetration with 7.5-MHz transducers is approximately 6–8 cm, which is usually sufficient during IOUS examination.[79] Deeper penetration requires that a 5.0-MHz transducer be used, although it has slightly decreased resolution.[42]

High-frequency, high-resolution US can detect 3- to 4-mm tumors. A flat T-shaped side-viewing probe is essential for examining the liver under the abdominal wall or the diaphragm. A pencil-like cylinder front-viewing probe with sector images is suitable for scanning structures deep in the operative field, such as the extrahepatic bile duct or blood vessels. It is important to perform IOUS in a systematic manner so as not to miss an occult lesion. When lesions are identified, they are imaged in both the transverse and longitudinal planes so the precise relations of the lesion to relevant surrounding structures (i.e., hepatic and portal veins) are evaluated.[79] The number of lesions with their relations to the major biliary and vascular structures are determined and mapped. The feasibility of surgical resection is determined; a safe route for the cryoprobes is planned to avoid the major vascular and biliary structures and to freeze a 1-cm margin of normal tissue.

The decision on whether to resect only, use cryosurgery only, or use a combination of the two is made at laparotomy. Cryosurgery is not a substitute for resection. Conventional liver resection is used where possible, and cryosurgical ablation is used when conventional surgical resection is not possible.

The probes to use and their ideal positioning to achieve adequate freezing is then planned. Using a sterotaxic US-guided technique, an echogenic 18-gauge hollow needle is placed in the tumor. Using the Seldinger technique, a J-tip guidewire is then passed through the needle for placement of a dilator and sheath introducer cannula. The guidewire and dilator are then withdrawn, and the cryoprobe is placed through the cannula into the tumor. Laparotomy pads are placed to protect adjacent structures from freezing injury. The CMS accuprobe System (Cryomedical Sciences, Rockville, MD) uses vacuum insulated cryoprobes that utilize supercooled liquid nitrogen and has a capacity for five stimultaneous probes. The use of multiple probes permits overlapping of frozen areas during treatment of large cancers. The new apparatus features the use of disposable probes, a choice of design that ensures consistent, high quality probe performance, whereas reusable probes are subject to sporadic performance and slow deterioration of freezing capacity as time passes.[30] A wide variety of probe diameters, lengths, and shapes are currently available for endoscopic, laparoscopic, and percutaneous placement. Two of the cryoprobes available through this system are the 3 mm diameter blunted probe, which can create a freeze zone of up to 4 cm, and the 8 mm diameter trocar point probe, which can create a freeze zone of up to 6 cm. A flat surface probe can be used for surface lesions or to freeze an inadequate resection margin. Multiple probes can be used to create an overlapping iceball to freeze large lesions or multiple lesions. One or more probes are inserted into the target lesion(s) and cooled in sequence; then maximum cooling power is applied so freezing occurs as rapidly as possible. The maximal freeze cycle is initiated by circulating liquid nitrogen at −196°C through the cryoprobe, and US is used to monitor the freezing. The cryolesion and freeze margin are easily seen on US an hyperechoic rim with posterior acoustic shadowing slowly developing from the center of the lesion.[41,42] The edge of the iceball is monitored by US until the entire tumor is enveloped with a 1 cm margin of normal liver parenchyma.

Just before the initial freeze cycle, patients are given mannitol, low-dose dopamine, and sodium bicarbonate to induce a high urine output and alkalinize the urine to prevent acute renal failure from the myoglobinemia and myoglobinuria that results from cryosurgery.[4] High urine output and alka-linization of the urine are continued into the postoperative period.

Each lesion is frozen for 15 minutes, followed by a 10-minute natural thaw period without active rewarming and a second 15-minute freeze.[4,57] For groups that are inflow occlusion, occlusion is removed after the first freeze, and the edge of the lesion is allowed to thaw for 1 cm.[57] When a second freezing cycle is used, only partial ("edge only") thawing is allowed to occur until the iceball has receded, as demonstrated on US by approximately 5–10 mm, and again a 1 cm frozen margin around each tumor is obtained.[13,57]

For large lesions, the efficacy of cryotherapy can be increased by occluding the hepatic vascular inflow by placing a vascular clamp across the hepaticoduodenal ligament and clamping the hepatic artery and portal vein (Pringle's maneuver).[14] Vascular inflow is occluded prior to commencement of the freeze cycle.[80,81] Hepatic inflow occlusion has been shown to increase the zone of necrosis within the area of iceball formation.[6,56] The duration of clamping should not exceed 1 hour but may be reapplied after a 15-minute recovery period. Hepatic inflow occlusion is not used by all groups performing cryosurgery.[66] Cirrhotic livers, as seen with hepatocellular cancer in particular, are probably more vulnerable to ischemic injury than normal livers; and the Pringle manuever should probably be avoided in such situations.[82]

After the second freezing cycle is completed, the probe is actively rewarmed and withdrawn from the liver. The still-frozen tract made by the cryoprobe is packed with oxidized cellulose Gelfoam or Surgicel to control bleeding through the probe tract. Bleeding areas at the periphery are coagulated with electrocautery or an argon beam coagulator. Iceball cracks are common when the iceball involves the surface of the liver.[57] Considerable hemorrhage can occur from these cracks.

Some centers performing cryosurgery now routinely place a hepatic artery infusion catheter via the gastroduodenal artery and subcutaneous reservoir for postoperative chemotherapy in all patients undergoing cryosurgery for colorectal metastases.[14,47,54,57] Cholecystectomy and ligation of the right gastric artery is routinely performed to prevent cytotoxic cholecystitis and peptic ulceration.[45] At the end of the cryosurgery and thawing, hemostasis is checked and the abdominal wound is closed. Some centers routinely place a suction drain above and below the liver.[14]

Postoperative Care

Patients undergoing hepatic cryosurgery are routinely admitted to an intensive care unit (ICU) for 1–2 days postoperatively. Warming devices continue to be used to prevent hypothermia during the immediate postoperative period. Postoperative laboratory evaluation consists of a CBC, platelet count, coagulation profile, electrolytes, glucose, BUN, and serum creatinine level. Abnormal coagulation and blood studies are treated with fresh frozen plasma (FFP), platelets, packed red blood cells (pRBCs), and cryoprecipitate as necessary. The postoperative laboratory profile and the serum myoglobin level are checked every morning for the first few postoperative days. A maintenance intravenous infusion of 5% dextrose in water (D_5W) with 20 mEq KCl and HCO_3 and a renal-dose dopamine infusion is continued to maintain adequate urine output. The patient's urine is checked every 6 hours to maintain the pH above 7 and each morning to monitor the myoglobin level. The intravenous sodium bicarbonate and renal-dose dopamine are discontinued once the urine is free of myoglobin, which is usually within 3 days.[4,13,16]

Complications of Hepatic Cryosurgery

A number of complications have been associated with hepatic cryosurgery.

Death: Mortality rates is most of the cryosurgery series range from 0% to 4%, with more complications occurring in patients with extensive disease and aggressive treatment. These patients usually develop severe coagulopathies that cannot be controlled and eventually lead to multisystem organ failure and death.[4,16,25] Liver failure[13,62,81] and myocardial infarction[13,66] have also been reported as causes of perioperative death.

Hypothermia: Mild hypothermia occurs to some degree in most cryosurgery patients. The duration of tissue freeze and the operating time do not appear to have any direct bearing on the degree of hypothermia.[45] Mild hypothermia has been found to reduce platelet function and decreases activation of the coagulation cascade, increasing the risk of blood loss and the incidence of ventricular tachycardia and morbid cardiac events.[83] Significant arrhythmias may occur during cryotherapy, possibly due to a cold stream of blood returning to the heart, direct myocardial cooling, or a sudden potassium load from cell lysis.[14,45] Most groups routinely use a warming device (i.e., Bair Hugger[77]) and warm intravenous fluid.

Biliary fistulas: Bile duct injury that resulted in either a bile leak or biliary cutaneous fistula occurred in 5 or 47 patients in one series,[4] and seven bile leaks developed in 20 patients in whom cryosurgery was used to freeze an inadequate resection margin.[84] It is best managed by radiographically placed percutaneous transhepatic catheters.[4,16,58,59]

Bleeding: The mean blood loss during cryosurgery is approximately 750 ml in reported series[14,70]; about one-third of patients require blood transfusion.[54] Lesions at the liver surface have a greater tendency to bleed than those deep in the liver parenchyma. More than 2000 ml of blood loss is unusual, but significant blood loss may occur with "cracking" of the iceball during thawing (see below).

Thrombocytopenia: Thrombocytopenia and platelet consumption are common after hepatic cryosurgery and have been reported in many series.[4,14,45,58,66,74] Thrombocytopenia is usually worst on postoperative day 3, usually self-limiting, and rarely requires platelet transfusion.[14] If extreme, it may contribute to a bleeding diathesis. Thrombocytopenia has been found to be related to the day 1 AST value, and an AST value of more than 1000 U/L indicates a high risk of impending thrombocytopenia.[14,57,61] Conversely, a low AST level is likely to mean that the patients will not have a large fall in platelet count during the subsequent few days. The double edge-only freeze-thaw cycle results in a more marked fall in platelet count, which may be responsible for the coagulopathy seen in some of these patients.[61] A complete double freeze-thaw would probably only exacerbates the problem by causing greater hepatocellular injury.[61]

Liver surface cracking-fracture: Surface cracking in the iceball lesion during thawing is an iatrogenic form of liver trauma that can result in significant hemorrhage; it has been reported in many series.[13,16,45,57,58,62] First described by Onik et al.,[16] this cracking is secondary to the thermal stresses that occur during the rapid freezing and thawing process and is likened to the cracks that occur in an ice cube when it is placed in warm water. Ross and Morris[84] and Morris et al.[54] reported that significant cracking that required liver suturing occurred in 25% (10/40) of their patients who had hepatic cryotherapy not combined with resection of the primary tumor or other metastatic disease. The average blood loss was 740 ml (range < 100–1800 ml), and the patients were transfused with a mean 2.4 units of blood (range 0–226 units). Liver cracking can usually be managed by packing.

Consumptive coagulopathy: A mild consumptive coagulopathy develops to some extent in every cryosurgery patient and is easily treated with fresh frozen plasma.[25] A marked consumption coagulopathy can result in significant intraperitoneal bleeding at sites other than the cryoablated tumor.[74,85]

Prothrombin: Prothrombin times elevated up to 1.5 times normal and uncorrectable with vitamin K were reported in all 47 patients in one series.[4] They have been reported by others as well.[66]

Cryogenic shock: Cryoshock syndrome—thrombocytopenia, disseminated intravascular coagulation, renal failure, hepatic failure, and adult respiratory distress syndrome—secondary to massive systemic release of necrotic tissue has been reported.[13,57,73] Ross et al. did not allow cryolesions to thaw completely before refreezing, as this situation may be causally associated with potentially fatal cryoshock syndome.[14]

Iatrogenic cryoprobe injuries: Perforation of the opposite lobe liver capsule[66] and freezing injury to adjacent tissue (right hemidiaphragm, lung right lower lobe, and skin[74]) have been reported.

Electrolyte disturbances: One episode of ventricular tachycarida has been reported during thawing of a pericaval lesion. It was possibly due to hyperkalemia, based on the theoretic possibility of an acute increase in potassium from intracellular stores as cells lyse when thawing.[14,59]

Nitrogen embolism: Nitrogen embolism was reported with the use of an open-contact probe where liquid nitrogen directly contacted the liver and the tumor being frozen.[37] Nitrogen gas is 500 times the volume of an equivalent amount of liquid nitrogen, so even small amounts of liquid nitrogen entering the hepatic veins can produce a significant nitrogen embolus as it expands to a gas.

Abscess (intrahepatic): Intrahepatic abscesses are relatively rare though postoperative CT scans often show gas bubbies in cryolesions. An intrahepatic abscess developed in 1 of 18 patients in one series[16] and in 1 of 11 patients in another series.[58] Both resolved on percutaneous drainage.

Abscess (subphrenic): Only one subphrenic abscess has been reported, and it was in a patient who underwent right hepatic lobectomy and cryoablation of a left-lobe metastasis.[39,86] The abscess was related to the resection and was drained under CT guidance.

Pleural effusions and atelectasis: Pleural effusions and atelectasis have been reported in many series[4,16,45,54,57,62,77,85,87] and occur in nearly all patients. Probably secondary to the irritative process underneath the diaphragm, they occur most commonly on the right side, are usually asymptomatic, and rarely have to be drained.

Acute renal failure, acute tubular necrosis: Acute renal failure is rare if intraoperative blood pressure, hydration, fluid resuscitation, and urine output are maintained.[14] Diuresis with diuretics or mannitol is used if urine output is low or pink discoloration of the urine is noted. Many groups routinely induce diuresis to avoid renal failure induced by myoglobinuria (see below). Acute tubular necrosis developed in 3 of 86 patients in one series, none of whom required dialysis.[13] Morris and Ross[57] reported acute renal failure in 2 of 149 patients due to postoperative bleeding and intraoperative anaphylaxis; both patients recovered.

Myoglobinuria: Onik et al.[16] first reported myoglobinuria in 7 of 18 patients; the remainder of the patients were not tested, as the surgeons became aware of this complication only late in their series of patients. Myoglobin can be detected intraoperatively immediately after the iceball thaws, and it usually resolves in 1–3 days.[16] Just before the initial freeze cycle, patients are given mannitol, low-dose dopamine, and sodium bicarbonate to induce a high urine output and alkalinize the urine to mitigate the effects of the myoglobinuria.[4] Myoglobinuria can be demonstrated to some degree in virtually all patients.[13] Because this phenomenon appears to be related to the volume of tissue frozen, Onik et al. became aware of the complication only late in their experience, when tissue freezing became more extensive. The mechanism of myoglobinuria from hepatic freezing can only be speculation; the problem consistently appeared in patients who had multiple lesions or large lesions frozen, and it appeared subclinically in all other patients once it was recognized as a possible problem.[13] No patient has needed dialysis in their series.

Transient elevation of liver enzymes: Many series report a rise in AST postoperatively.[39,45,66,74,85] Such a rise has been shown to correlate with the destruction of hepatic tissue and release of this intracellular enzyme and with postoperative thrombocytopenia.[45,57,61] Hyperbilirubinemia has been reported,[45,62] as has hypoalbuminemia.[45]

Leukocytosis: A transient leukocytosis is common during the postoperative period.[39,47]

Pyrexia: Postoperative pyrexia is a common finding.[45,47,58] Patients may have temperatures as high as 39°C for 3–4 days after surgery, with negative cultures for any signs of systemic sepsis.[86] The cryonecrotized liver may well be responsible.[14] Radiographic imaging may fail to demonstrate an abscess; and routine cultures of urine, sputum, blood, and drainage fluid reveal no focus of infection.

Hypoglycemia: Goodie et al.[45] reported one episode of asymptomatic hypoglycemia recorded postoperatively in a patient who had undergone previous hepatic resection; in this case a significantly reduced hepatic mass probably led to impaired glucose homeostasis.

Postoperative Follow-up After Cryosurgery

Standard follow-up of patients who have undergone cryosurgery includes serial clinical examinations, CT scans, chest radiographs, serial liver function tests, and CEA levels.[4,47] Tumor markers (CEA) and CT scans are used to evaluate the response.

CT Scan

Computed tomography with intravenous contrast is used to follow cryosurgery of liver tumors. CT arterioportography is of little value after cryosurgery, as it rarely distinguishes a cryolesion from a malignant tumor.[88] A baseline CT scan is usually obtained during the first week after cryosurgery. Follow-up scans are usually performed every 4 months for the first year, every 6 months over the next 2 years, and then annually the next 2 years.

A baseline CT scan as early as 5–7 days after cryoablation normally shows a well demarcated region of frozen tissue that is of lower attenuation than normal liver.[88,89] The cryolesions may show evidence of necrosis, and sometimes small foci of central immobile gas bubbles are present in the lesions, mimicking hepatic abscesses.[5,88,89] This picture may add confusion if a patient remains febrile after surgery. These bubbles usually disappear after several weeks. An increase in the number or size of gas bubbles in the cryolesion suggests development of a cryolesion abscess.[88] Right- and left-sided pleural effusions and lung atelectasis are seen in almost all patients.[89] The tracks from the recently inserted cryoprobes may be visible on CT.[88] High-attenuation foci compatible with hemorrhage also may be present in the cryolesions on the baseline postoperative CT scan.[89]

Many cryolesions have a wedge-shaped appearance similar to that typically associated with hepatic infarction.[89] Dilation of the bile ducts can occur if a main duct is frozen; edema of the wall then causes partial luminal occlusion with resultant stenosis and dilation.[88]

Usually after 6 weeks the area of necrosis decreases in size.[36] After a period of 6 months or more, complete resolution of the treated area is demonstrable in about 10% of patients; but in 80% of the patients the scar remains at the site of the treated lesion, persisting as low-attenuation foci without reabsorption of the dead tissue, often for several years.[47] Local recurrence occurs in the remaining 10% of patients, perhaps indicative of incomplete cryoablation at the margin of the lesion.[47] Tumor recurrence should be suspected if a lesion persists or shows increasing attenuation or size.[88] Occasionally, these locally recurrent lesions could again undergo cryoablation in 6–9 months' time.[4,47,74] Histologic proof of complete response could be documented by biopsy of treated lesions.[40] A spherical area of yellowish green fibrous tissue is seen in animals and in patients who have been reoperated after cryotherapy.[6,54]

Carcinoembryonic Antigen

Serical serum carcinoembryonic antigen levels can be used to monitor the effect of hepatic cryotherapy.[90] The therapeutic response is measured by monitoring tumor markers measured at monthly or quarterly intervals. After cryosurgery the CEA levels fall in almost all CEA secretors.[14] The kinetics of fall in the tumor markers after cryosurgery is slower than after liver resection.[56,86] Characteristically, the tumor markers after do not normalize until about 6–8 weeks after surgery. A subsequent rise in CEA level has always been predictive of local or systemic relapse. After investigation to assess the extent of the disease, further cryotherapy or regional chemotherapy may be considered in the absence of extrahepatic disease.

Results of Cryosurgery

Candidate patient criteria and selection for cryosurgery differ among centers, so it is difficult to assess and compare the results of the groups performing the procedure. Most patients treated with hepatic cryosurgery in the United States have metastatic colorectal cancer. As mentioned earlier, 5-year survival rates of 25–35% have been reported in patients who have undergone hepatic resection of colorectal metastases.[10,11] Lesions undergoing cryosurgery are usually considered unresectable, but the patients can now be treated for a disease with a less than 2-year life expectancy.

Steele and Ravikumar et al.[7,86] stated that in properly selected patients, when freeze margins are well defined by US to be 2–3 cm, the results are the same as in patients who have undergone successful wedge, segmental, or lobar resection of isolated metastases but with no mortality among the more than 250 patients and the hospital stay averaging only 5–7 days. Ravikumar et al.[86] reported a 28% disease-free survival after a median follow-up of 2 years with a 72% overall 2-year survival. In another of their series of similar patients Ravikumar reported a 52% disease-free survival after a median follow-up of 18 months and a 73% overall survival.[47]

Morris's group[91] reported a 21% two-year survival in patients treated with cryosurgery and hepatic artery infusion. They also reported[47] a 3-year survival rate of 5% for all patients with colorectal metastases treated with cryosurgery. In 27 of the 52 patients who had a fall in CEA level postoperatively, the CEA returned to the normal range; the median survival of this group exceeded 1000 days, indicating that some patients with unresectable disease can now be offered a survival similar, with at least approximately 3 years follow-up, to that of patients with resectable lesions.

Onik et al.[29] reported a 22% disease-free survival after a mean of 28.8 months and later reported[13] a disease-free survival (based on a normal CT scan and CEA level) of 27% with a mean follow-up of 21 months. Weaver et al.[4] reported an 11% disease-free survival with a median follow-up of 30 months and a 62% overall survival with a mean follow-up of 24 months in a series of patients followed for at least 2 years. Weaver et al. later reported[85] a series of 180 patients with a median survival of 22 months (range 1–85 months); patients followed more than 2 years had a median survival of 26 months (range 4–85 months). Of 70 patients still alive the median survival was 27 months; and of the 166 patients with more than 5-year follow-up the median survival was 40 months (range 9–85 months).

Ravikumar et al., analyzing the recurrence pattern after cryosurgery found a 10% failure rate at the treated site in clinical series[46,56,86] and experimental studies.[40] About 50% of patients who fail experience both hepatic and extrahepatic recurrence; 15% have recurrence only at the extrahepatic sites (lung, peritoneum, bone); and the remaining 35% have failure primarily in the remaining liver, including the 10% with local recurrences. This pattern of recurrence is similar to that in other series.[4,16,57] In an attempt to address the patients with disease recurring in the liver only, placement of hepatic arterial infusion pumps has been added as an adjunct to cryosurgery in selected patient.[47,57]

Cryosurgery for Treatment of Primary Liver Cancer

Liver resection is the best treatment of malignant liver tumors and the sole therapy to offer a chance of cure. However, cure is achieved in only 3–30% of patients, with a 5-year -survival of 12–50% of patients with hepatocellular carcinoma (HCC).[92,93] Cryosurgery is preferred by some for primary hepatoma, as major resections are difficult in the cirrhotic liver, and resection of too much liver results in liver failure.[19,94]

The worldwide experience with cryosurgery for HCC is limited, although the first large studies of hepatic cryosurgery were of patients with HCC.[31,32] In 1979

Zhou et al.[31] reported freezing HCCs in 35 patients who had tumors that were unresectable by traditional surgical means. Cryosurgery, using flat surface probes, was monitored via thermocouple needles blindly placed into the margins of the tumor and seen visually from the hepatic surface. There were no surgical deaths and no complications such as bleeding, tumor rupture, bile leakage, or infection. Survival rates were 55.5% for 1 year, 24.3% for 2 years, and 10% for 3 years. By comparison, patients with similar-stage disease who received chemotherapy had survival rates of 13% for 1 year and 0% for 2 years. The 5-year survival rate of patients with tumors smaller than 5 cm was 12.5%.

This group from Shanghai has since reported on 167 patients with primary liver cancer treated from November 1973 to March 1995 with cryosurgery and hepatic artery ligation, perfusion, or cryosurgery with resection.[94,95] The 1-, 3-, and 5-year survival rates were 73.5%, 47.7%, and 31.7%, respectively. The 1-, 3, and 5-year survival rates were 59.8%, 36.3%, and 23.3%, respectively, for the 76 patients with primary liver cancer treated by cryosurgery only.[94]

Cryosurgery of Neuroendocrine Hepatic Metastases

Cryotherapy of patients with hepatic metastases from neuroendocrine tumors have been reported in several series.[25,36,39,57,58,74,85,86,96] Malignant neuroendocrine tumors metastatic to the liver are relatively rare but can be associated with considerable morbidity due to syndromes of hormonal excess.[96] The neuroendocrine tumors that have been treated include (1) carcinoid tumors; (2) iselet cell tumors of the pancreas such as gastrinoma, VIPoma, and ACTH-producing tumor; and (3) metastatic retroperitoneal paraganglioma. Significant palliation of functioning metastases from various endocrine tumors may be possible by cryoablation, even if there is extrahepatic disease. In one series[96] all patients have radiologic evidence of complete response and excellent reduction of tumor markers, although one patient has had a subsequent recurrence.[57] The four patients with symptoms became asymptomatic with follow-up of 3–7 years. Although not always curative, cryotherapy of liver metastases remains rewarding for this indication as many patients experience total relief and palliation of their hormone-related symptoms.

Cryosurgery of Metastatic Noncolorectal, Nonendocrine Tumors

Patients with untreated metastatic noncolorectal, nonendocrine primary tumors have a dismal prognosis, with a median survival of 2–8 months.[75] Cryosurgery has been performed for a number of these anecdotal cases, but there are no large series and few follow-up survival data. Some of the metastatic noncolorectal, nonendocrine tumors treated are melanoma[57,62]; sarcoma[58,85]; breast,[25,85] renal,[85] ovarian,[25,57,85] cervical,[25] and unknown primary cancers[39,85,86]; cloacogenic cancer from the anal canal[86]; gastric,[62,74] adrenocortical,[19] and pancreatic[19] cancer; desmoid tumor[57]; cholangiocarcinoma[19,62]; hemangiopericytoma (meningeal primary)[81]; and gallbladder cancer.[57]

Future Trends, Directions, and Role of Cryosurgery

Cryoassisted Surgical Resection

The cryoprobe can be used as a physical aid in hepatic resection, serving as a "handle" for resecting the liver tumor by placing the probe within the tumor and freezing the lesion into a sold mass.[97] Welling and Lamping first reported this novel use of the cryoprobe in surgical resections in 10 patients with no complications, morbidity, or mortality associated with the use of the probe handle.[97] This handle allows the surgeon to obtain leverage and provided a taut surface for transection and for better visualization of the hepatic ducts and blood vessels. Another use of this technique is in cases of "close" margins, where the tumor abuts anatomic resection lines. Freezing the tumor along with a margin of surrounding tissue may allow more precise delineation of resection planes and avoid fracturing the liver along the fragile tumor–liver interface.

Polk et al[81] described the following technique of cryoassisted resection: Dissection is performed directly on the iceball or at a slight distance from it. Traction is held on the cryoprobe and iceball complex to provide useful exposure in the line of parenchymal transection. As vessels are encountered, they are controlled individually. The specimen is left attached to the cryoprobe and is allowed to thaw, at which time it is removed and sectioned to ensure adequate resection margins. Should there be doubt as to the adequacy of the margins, a flat cryoprobe may be inserted into the cavity and further freezing of the relevant margin undertaken.

Chemotherapy: Systemic and Hepatic Artery Infusion

Many of the patients in the major cryosurgery series have been treated with preoperative systemic chemotherapy. There is support for treating patients with resection and adjunct cryosurgery before initiating chemotherapy, which result in an even greater survival benefit because the total tumor mass would be reduced. Moreover, such chemotherapy might have a greater effect on micrometastases.[4] Of the patients who fail and whose lesions recur after cryosurgery, approximately 30–35% have failure in the liver only. In an attempt to address the patients with disease recurring in the live only, hepatic arterial infusion pumps have been placed as an adjunct to cryosurgery in selected patients.[47,57] Tumor debulking by cryoablation may work synergistically with hepatic artery infusion (HAI).

Morris's group[91,98] first reported the use of hepatic artery chemotherapy (HAC) in addition to cryotherapy for hepatic metastases from colorectal carcinoma and was first to demonstrate that the use of HAC in this situation is associated with increased survival. Their retrospective study[91] demonstrated an increase in estimated median survival for patients treated with cryotherapy plus HAC versus cryotherapy along (570 days vs. 245 days).

Ravikumar's group offers cryoablation for one or two lesions that are otherwise unresectable and cryoablation plus HAI for three or more lesions.[47] HAI is administered through an Infusaid pump (Infusaid, Norwood, MA) for a period of 1 year, using a regimen of 5-fluorouracil (5-FU) and fluorodeoxyuridine (FUDR). Morris's group routinely place a subcutaneous resevoir an catheter to perfuse the liver in all patients undergoing cyrosurgery.[57]

Laparoscopic and laparoscopy Assisted Cryotherapy for Liver Tumors

Intraoperative ultransonography of the liver can be done via laparoscopy.[50,71] Laparoscopic US has been introduced for evaluating the liver during exploratory laparoscopy, helping to determine the stage and resectability of malignant tumors.[50,79,99] Several groups have not reported laparoscopic and laparoscopy assisted approaches during cryosurgery of the liver.[19,47,62] The use of video-mixer and split-screen features allows simultaneous visualization of the laparoscopic and US images. For this technique the tumors should be easily approachable by the cryosurgical probe. Generally, the tumors treated should be close to the surface of the liver and should not be in the most posterior area of the right lobe.[19] Technical difficulties with laparoscopic US include the inability to delineate the entire circumference of the iceball and to ensure that the cryoablation extends beyond the limits of the lesion, especially in large and posteriorly situated tumors.[62]

The cryoprobes are placed through the midline subxiphoid port or the left subcostal port. The US transducer and laparoscopic camera are placed through the umbilical port or right subcostal port interchangeably. The cryoprobes are placed through the anterior surface of the liver, and the transducers are positioned on the inferior surface of the liver to monitor cryoablation.[19,47]

This approach is generally challenging because of the limited ability to maneuver the probes independently through the fixed trocar sites compared to the easy maneuverability of the probes and liver with the open approach. Maintaining orientation of the tumors and the cryoprobe requires constant monitoring of the area in question through multiple oblique US windows.[19]

Adjunct to Resection

Many groups now routinely complement surgical hepatic resection with cryosurgery. Cryosurgery allows surgical resections now previously possible by allowing "sterilization" of the remaining surgical margin using a wide, flat cryoprobe.[13] Grossly positive or inadequate (< 1 cm) margins following surgical resection can be frozen.

Morris et al.[57,59] reported the use of cryotherapy as an adjunct to liver resection in more than 30 patients. The therapy was either to treat disease in the contralateral lobe after concurrent lobectomy or to freeze an inadequate (< 1 cm) or grossly involved resection margin. There were no operative or 30-day deaths, but bile leaks were more common than after resection alone. Whereas an involved or less than 1 cm margin results in almost certain recurrence at 1 year, their experience at 11 months' median follow-up in the 12 "edge freeze" patients was that only two resection margin recurrences were seen, although four other patients developed tumor elsewhere in the liver. Of eight patients with contralobe lesions, four were tumor-free at 11 months.

Conclusions

Cryosurgery allows many patients who would not otherwise be candidates for surgical resection to be treated for tumors of the liver. It is usually reserved for patients with unresectable tumors, as the prognosis of these patients is worse than for those with resectable disease. Cryotherapy enables combinations of surgery and cryosurgical ablation to be used in patients who previously would never have gotten to the operating room because of a multiplicity of lesions; it offers them the possibility of cure.[25] For patients with metastases confined to the liver, cryosurgery increases the number of patients who can be made potentially disease-free or at least who have no evidence of disease.[4]

References

1. Parker SL, Tong T, Bolden S, et al. Cancer statistics, 1997. CA Cancer J Clin 47:5, 1997
2. Taylor I. Liver metastases from colorectal cancer: lessons from past and present clinical studies. Br J Surg 83:456, 1996
3. Steele G Jr. Cryoablation in hepatic surgery. Semin Liver Dis 14:120, 1994
4. Weaver ML, Atkinson D, Zemel R. Hepatic cryosurgery in treating colorectal metastases. Cancer 76:210, 1995
5. Bismuth H, Adam R, Navarro F, et al. Re-resection for colorectal liver metastasis. Surg Oncol Clin North Am 5:353, 1996
6. Fortner JG, Silva JS, Golbey RB, et al. Multivariate analysis of a personal series of 247 consecutive patients with liver metastases from colorectal cancer. I. Treatment by hepatic resection. Ann Surg 199:306, 1984

7. Steele G Jr, Ravikumar TS. Resection of hepatic metastases from colorectal cancer. Ann Surg 210:127, 1989
8. Adson MA, Van Heerden JA, Adson MH, et al. Resection of hepatic metastases from colorectal cancer. Arch Surg 119:647, 1984
9. Adson MA. Resection of liver metastases—when is it worthwhile. World J Surg 11:511, 1987
10. Hughes KS, Simon R, Songhorabadi S, et al. Resection of the liver for colorectal carcinoma metastases: a multiinstitutional study of indications for resection. Surgery 103:278, 1988
11. Fong Y, Cohen AM, Fortner JG, et al. Liver resection for colorectal metastases. J Clin Oncol 15:938, 1997
12. Blumgart LH, Fong Y. Surgical options in the treatment of hepatic metastasis from colorectal cancer. Curr Probl Surg 32:333, 1995
13. Onik GM, Atkinson D, Zemel R, et al. Cryosurgery of liver cancer. Semin Surg Oncol 9:309, 1993
14. Ross WB, Horton M, Bertolino P, et al. Cryotherapy of live tumours: a practical guide. HPB Surg 8:167, 1995
15. Ravikumar TS, Kane R, Cady B, et al. Hepatic cryosurgery with intraoperative ultrasound monitoring for metastatic colon carcinoma. Arch Surg 122:403, 1987
16. Onik G, Rubinsky B, Zemel R, et al. Ultrasound-guided hepatic cryosurgery in the treatment of metastatic colon carcinoma. Cancer 67:901, 1991
17. McMasters KM, Edwards MJ. Liver cryosurgery: a potentially curative treatment option for patients with unresectable disease. Ky Med Assoc 94:222, 1996
18. Guillen JG, Paty PB, Cohen AM. Surgical treatment of colorectal cancer. CA Cancer J Clin 47:113, 1997
19. Quebbeman EJ, Wallace JR. Cryosurgery for hepatic metastases. In: Condon RE (ed) Current Techniques in General Surgery. Mosby, New York 1997 pp. 1–75
20. Gage AA. Cryosurgery in the treatment of cancer. Surg Gynecol Obstet 174:73, 1992
21. Zacarian SA, Adham MI. Cryotherapy of cutaneous malignancy. Cryobiology 2:212, 1966
22. Cooper IS, Lee A. Cryostatic congelation: a system for producing a limited, controlled region of cooling or freezing of biologic tissues. J Nerv Ment Dis 133:259, 1961
23. Cooper IS. Cryogenic surgery: a new method of destruction or extirpation of benign or malignant tissues. N Engl J Med 268:743, 1963
24. Ramming KP. Cryosurgery: the coming of the surgical ice age? J Surg Oncol 58:147, 1995
25. Gage AA, Fazekas G, Riley EE Jr. Freezing injury to large blood vessels in dogs. Surgery 61:748, 1967
26. Dutta MM, Gage AA. Large volume freezing in experimental hepatic cryosurgery. Cryobiology 16:50, 1979
27. Farrant J, Walter CA. The cryobiological basis for cryosurgery. J Dermatol Surg Oncol 3:403, 1977
28. Staren ED, Sabel MS, Gianakakis LM, et al. Cryosurgery of breast cancer. Arch Surg 132:28, 1997
29. Onik GM, Cohen JK, Reyes GD, et al. Transrectal ultrasound-guided percutaneous radical cryosurgical ablation of the prostate. Cancer 72:1291, 1993

30. Baust J, Gage AA, Ma H, et al. Minimally invasive cryosurgery: technological advances. Cryobiology 34:373, 1997
31. Zhou XD, Tang ZY, Yu YQ. Cryosurgery for liver cancer: experimental and clinical study. Chin J Surg 17:480, 1979
32. Zhou XD, Tang ZY, Yu YQ, et al. Clinical evaluation of cryosurgery in the treatment of primary liver cancer: report of 60 cases. Cancer 61:1889, 1988
33. Bayjoo P, Jacob G. Hepatic cryosurgery: biological and clinical considerations. J R Coll Surg Edinb 37:369, 1992
34. Fong Y. Hepatic cryosurgery. In: Blumgart LH (ed). Surgery of the Liver and Biliary tract, 2nd ed. New York, Churchchill Livingstone, 1994, pp. 1535–1537
35. Gilbert JC, Onik GM, Hoddick WK, et al. Real time monitoring of hepatic cryosurgery. Cryobiology 22:319, 1985
36. Charnley RM, Doran J, Morris DL. Cryotherapy for liver metastases: a new approach. Br J Surg 76:1040, 1989
37. Schlinkert RT, Chapman TP. Nitrogen embolus as a complication of hepatic cryosurgery. Arch Surg 125:1214, 1990
38. Ravikumar TS, Kane R, Cady B, et al. Hepatic cryosurgery with intraoperative ultrasound monitoring for metastatic colon carcinoma. Arch Surg 122:403, 1987
39. Ravikumar TS, Steele GD Jr. Hepatic cryosurgery. Surg Clin North Am 69:433, 1989
40. Ravikumar TS, Steele GS Jr. Kane R. Kane R. Experimental and clinical observations on hepatic cryosurgery for colorectal metastases. Cancer Res 51:6323, 1991
41. Onik G, Cooper C, Goldberg HI, et al. Ultrasonic characteristics of frozen liver. Cryobiology 21:321, 1984
42. Onik G, Kane R, Steele G, et al. Monitoring hepatic cryosurgery with sonography. AJR 147:665, 1986
43. Lam CM, Shimi SM, Cuschieri A. Ultrasonic characterization of hepatic cryolesions. Arch Surg 130:1068, 1995
44. Gage AM, Montes M, Gage AA. Destruction of hepatic and splenic tissue by freezing and heating. Cryobiology 19:172, 1982
45. Goodie DB, Horton MDA, Morris RW, et al. Anaesthetic experience with cryotherapy for treatment of hepatic malignancy. Anaesth Intensive Care 20:491, 1992
46. Neel BH, Ketcham AS, Hammond WG. Requisites for successful cryogenic surgery of cancer. Arch Surg 102:4, 1971
47. Ravikumar TS. Interstitial therapies for liver tumors. Surg Oncol Clin North Am 5:365, 1996
48. Bischof J, Christov K, Rubinsky B. A morphological study of cooling rate response in normal and neoplastic human liver tissue: cryosurgical implications. Cryobiology 30:482, 1993
49. Orpwood RD. Biophysical and engineering aspects of cryosurgery. Phys Med Biol 266:555, 1981
50. Rubinsky B, Lee CY, Bastacky J, et al. The process of freezing and the mechanism of damage during hepatic cryosurgery. Cryobiology 27:85, 1990
51. Whittaker DK. Mechanisms of tissue destruction following cyrosurgery. Ann R Coll Surg Engl 66:313, 1984
52. Homasson JP, Thiery JP, Angebault M, et al. The operation and efficacy of cryosurgical, nitrous-oxide driven cryoprobe. Cryobiology 31:290, 1994
53. Jacob G, Li A, Hobbs K. A comparison of cryodestruction with excision or infarction of an implanted tumor in rat liver. Cryobiology 21:148, 1984

54. Morris DL, Horton MD, Dilley AV, et al. Treatment of hepatic metastases by cryotherapy and regional cytotoxic perfusion. Gut 34:1156, 1993
55. Dilley AV, Warlters A, Gillies A, et al. Hepatic cryosurgery: is portal clamping worth it? Aust NZ J Surg 61:A522, 1991
56. Dilley AV, Dy DY, Warlters A, et al. Laboratory and animal model evaluation of the Cryotech LCS 2000 in hepatic cryotherapy. Cryobiology 30:74, 1993
57. Morris DL, Ross WB. Australian experience of cryoablation of liver tumors. Surg Oncol Clin North Am 52:391, 1996
58. McKinnon G, Temple WJ, Wiseman DA, et al. Cryosurgery for malignant tumours of the liver. Can J Surg 39:401, 1996
59. McCall JL, Ross WB, Morris DL. Cryotherapy with liver resection for the treatment of liver tumours. Gut 35(suppl 2):S15, 1994
60. Stewart GJ, Preketes A, Horton M, et al. Hepatic cryotherapy: double-freeze cycles achieve greater hepatocellular injury in man. Cryobiology 32:215, 1995
61. Cozzi PJ, Stewart GJ, Morris DL. Thrombocytopenia after cryotherapy for colorectal metastases: correlates with hepatocellular injury. World J Surg 18:774, 1994
62. Cuschieri A, Crosthwaite G, Shimi S, et al. Hepatic cryotherapy for liver tumors. Surg Endosc 9:483, 1995
63. Bayjoo P, Rees RC, Goepel JR, et al. Natural killer cell activity following cryosurgery of normal and tumour bearing liver in an animal model. J Clin Lab Immunol 35:129, 1991
64. Jacob G, Kurzer MN, Fuller BJ. An assessment of tumour cell viability after in vitro freezing. Cryobiology 22:417, 1985
65 .Cady B, Stone MD, McDermott WV, et al. Technical and biological factors in disease-free survival after hepatic resection for colorectal cancer metastases. Arch Surg 127:561, 1992
66. Adam R, Akpinar E, Johann M, et al. Place of cryosurgery in the treatment of malignant liver tumors. Ann Surg 225:39, 1997
67. Soyer P, Levesque M, Elias D, et al. Detection of liver metastases from colorectal cancer: comparison of intraoperative US and CT during arterial portography. Radiology 183:541, 1992
68. Moran BJ, O'Rourke N, Plant GR, et al. Computed tomographic portography in preoperative imaging of hepatic neoplasms. Br J Surg 82:669, 1995
69. Ravikumar TS, Buenaventura S, Salem RR, et al. Intraoperative ultrasonography of liver: detection of occult liver tumors and treatment by cryosurgery. Cancer Detect Prevent 18:131, 1994
70. Saini S. Imaging of the hepatobiliary tract. N Engl J Med 336:1889, 1997
71. Kruskal JB, Kane RA. Imaging of primary and metastatic liver tumors. Surg Oncol Clin North Am 5:231, 1996
72. Steele G Jr. Advances in the treatment of early- to late-stage colorectal cancer: 20 years of progress. Ann Surg Oncol 2:77, 1995
73. Nagorny DM. Newer techniques in liver surgery. In: Cameron JL (ed) Current Surgical Therapy, 5th ed. St. Louis, Mosby, 1992, pp. 258–260
74. Shafir M, Shapiro R, Sung M. Cryoablation of unresectable malignant liver tumors. Am J Surg 171:27, 1996
75. Kavolius J, Fong Y, Blumgart LH. Surgical resection of metastatic liver tumors. Surg Oncol Clin North Am 5:337, 1996

76. Fong Y, Blumgart LH, Cohen AM. Surgical treatment of colorectal metastases to the liver. CA Cancer J Clin 45:50, 1995

77. Onik GM, Chambers N, Chernus ST, et al. Hepatic cryosurgery with and without the bair hugger. J Surg Oncol 52:185, 1993

78. Strasberg SM, Callery MP. Treatment of hepatic metastases of colorectal tumors by liver resection and cryotherapy, Probl Gen Surg 12:106, 1996

79. Machi J, Sigel B. Operative ultrasound in general surgery. Am J Surg 172:15, 1996

80. Millikan KW, Staren ED, Doolas A. Invasive therapy of metastatic colorectal cancer to the liver. Surg Clin North Am 77:27, 1997

81. Polk W, Fong Y, Karpeh M, et al. A technique for the use of cryosurgery to assist hepatic resection. J Am Coll Surg 180:171, 1995

82. Fan ST. Technique of hepatectomy. Br J Surg 83:1490, 1996

83. Sessler DI. Mild perioperative hypothermia. N Engl J Med 336:1730, 1996

84. Ross WB, Morris DL. Hepatic cryosurgery: biological and clinical considerations [letter] J R Coll Surg Edinb 38:266, 1993

85. Weaver ML, Atkinson DP, Zemel R. The treatment of unresectable hepatic metastases with cryosurgery. Presented at the Annual Meeting of the Society of Surgical Oncology, Atlanta, March 1996

86. Ravikumar TS, Kane R, Cady B, et al. A 5-year study of cryosurgery in the treatment of liver tumors. Arch Surg 126:1520, 1991

87. Tierney J, Carlin B, Lupetin A, et al. Pleural effusion and atelectasis associated with cryosurgical ablation of hepatic metastases. Am Rev Respir Dis 147:A83, 1993

88. McLoughlin RF, Saliken JF, McKinnon G, et al. CT of the liver after cryotherapy of hepatic metastases: imaging findings. AJR 165:107, 1995

89. Kuszyk BS, Choti MA, Urban BA, et al. Hepatic tumors treated by cryosurgery: normal CT appearance. AJR 166:363, 1996

90. Charnley RM, Thomas M, Morris DL. Effect of hepatic cryotherapy on serum CEA concentration in patients with multiple inoperable hepatic metastases from colorectal cancer. Aust NZ J Surg 61:55, 1991

91. Preketes AP, Caplehorn JRM, King J, et al. Effect of hepatic artery chemotherapy on survival of patients with hepatic metastases from colorectal carcinoma treated with cryotherapy. World J Surg 19:768, 1995

92. Farmer DG, Rososve MH, Shaked A. Current treatment modalities for hepatocellular carcinoma. Ann Surg 219:236, 1994

93. Nagashima I, Hamada C, Naruse K, et al. Surgical resection for small hepatocelluar carcinoma. Surgery 119:40, 1996

94. Zhou XD, Tang ZY, Yu YQ. Ablative approach for primary liver cancer: Shanghai experience. Surg Oncol Clin North Am 5:379, 1996

95. Zhou XD, Tang ZY, Yu YQ, et al. The role of cryosurgery in the treatment of hepatic cancer: a report of 113 cases. J Cancer Res Clin Oncol 120:100, 1993

96. Cozzi PJ, Englund R, Morris DL. Cryotherapy treatment of patients with hepatic metastases from neuroendocrine tumors. Cancer 76:501, 1995

97. Welling RE, Lamping K. Cryoprobe as a "handle" for resection of metastatic liver tumors. J Surg Oncol 45:227, 1990

98. Horton MD, Walters A, Dilley AV, et al. Hepatic artery cytotoxic perfusion therapy after cryotherapy: a single patient control trial? Med J Aust 155:849, 1991

99. John TG, Greig JD, Crosbie JL, et al. Superior staging of liver tumors with laparoscopy and laparoscopic ultrasound. Ann Surg 220:711, 1994

11

Hepatectomy for Noncolorectal Liver Metastases

Todd M. Tuttle

Hepatic resection is the treatment of choice for patients with isolated metastases from colorectal primary tumors. Systemic chemotherapy provides responses in only a few patients and results in a median survival of approximately 12 months.[1-3] By comparison, median survival after hepatic resection of colorectal metastases is approximately 25–35 months with a 5-year survival rate of 25–33%.[4-6] With appropriate patient selection, advances in surgical intensive care, and improved methods for parenchymal dissection to minimize blood loss, the operative mortality rate of hepatectomy is now 5% or less at most major centers.[7,8] Several published reports have identified specific determinants of survival for patients undergoing liver resection for colorectal metastases. Although agreement is not universal for every clinical variable, the importance of tumor-free margins of resection, disease-free interval before development of metastases, stage of the primary colorectal tumor, and the number of metastases is well documented.[6,8,9]

The role of hepatic resection for metastases from malignancies other than colorectal cancer is not as clearly defined. Autopsy data indicate that approximately 40–50% of cancer patients have liver metastases at the time of death (Table 11.1).[10,11] Adenocarcinomas from gastrointestinal sites such as the pancreas, gallbladder, and stomach frequently metastasize to the liver. Ocular melanoma is a rare tumor with a high incidence of hepatic metastases. Conversely, the liver is an infrequent site of involvement in the natural history of metastatic prostate carcinoma. Despite the high incidence of hepatic metastases at death, fewer than 5% of cancer patients have disease confined to the liver. Until recently, few published reports were available to physicians who must decide which patients, if any, should undergo hepatic resection for noncolorectal (NCR) metastases. Some authors have suggested that patients with NCR hepatic metastases fare worse after resection than those with colorectal metastases, whereas others have suggested that an NCR primary tumor is a relative contraindication for hepatectomy.[12-14] Early studies were limited by small numbers of patients, combining survival data of noncolorectal metastases with colorectal metastases, and the lack of assessing specific prognostic factors.[13,14,19]

TABLE 11.1. Incidence of liver metastases at autopsy

Primary tumor	Incidence (%)	
	Edmondson[11]	Pickren[10]
Bronchogenic	42	43
Pancreas	56	52
Breast	53	61
Stomach	64	49
Ovary	48	49
Prostate	13	16
Cervix	32	29
Melanoma—cutaneous	50	36
Melanoma—ocular	—	78
Bladder/ureter	38	29
Esophagus	30	21
Testis	44	55
Endometrial	32	—
Thyroid	17	—
Endocrine	—	25
Oral cavity/pharynx	—	14

Survival After Hepatectomy

In an effort to determine the survival of patients with NCR liver metastases, we performed a retrospective study on all patients undergoing hepatic resection at The University of Texas M. D. Anderson Cancer. From 1985 to 1995, altogether 45 patients underwent potentially curative hepatic resection for NCR metastases. Palliative procedures and en bloc resections of primary tumors with direct hepatic extension were excluded from review. Patients with liver metastases were evaluated by history and physical examination, chest radiography, and computed tomography (CT) of the abdomen, pelvis, and chest. Patients with more than four lesions on preoperative diagnostic imaging studies were considered ineligible for resection. Evidence of tumor abutment to portal or hepatic veins responsible for the blood supply or drainage of the hepatic parenchyma not intended for resection excluded some patients from operation because a tumor-free margin of resection would be impossible. Intraoperative hepatic ultrasonography was used to identify any additional lesions not palpated or visualized on preoperative imaging. In general, patients with extrahepatic disease did not undergo resection, although a few selected patients with extrahepatic disease that could be completely removed underwent liver resection. Surgery was considered curative in intent only if all gross disease was completely removed. Selected patients with NCR liver metastases were treated with two or three cycles of preoperative chemotherapy prior to hepatic resection.

A tumor-free margin was obtained in 44 of the 45 patients in this series. At the time of liver resection, 12 patients had documented extrahepatic disease that was completely removed, rendering the patient free of gross malignant disease. The 5-year actuarial overall survival after hepatic resection for NCR metastases was 44% with a median survival of 54.2 months (Fig. 11.1A). The 5-year disease-free survival was 22% with a median disease-free survival of 15 months (Fig. 11.1B). Eight patients survived more than 5 years after hepatic resection. These survival data are comparable to those from another large series of patients with NCR hepatic metastases treated at Memorial Sloan Kettering Cancer Center.[20] Harrison et al. reported a 5-year survival of 37% (median 32 months) among 96 patients undergoing hepatic resection with 12 five-year survivors.[20]

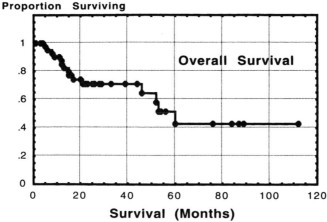

FIGURE 11.1-A.

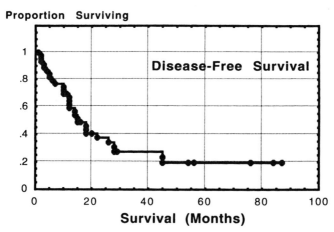

FIGURE 11.1-B.

FIGURE 11.1. Actuarial 5-year overall (A) and disease-free (B) survival following hepatic resection of noncolorectal metastases.

The survival rate following hepatic resection of carefully staged and selected patients with NCR liver metastases is comparable to the survival data following resection of colorectal liver metastases. The same group of surgeons from M. D. Anderson reported a similar 5-year survival following hepatic resection of metastatic colorectal tumors during the same period.[21] Moreover, these data corroborate the findings of other series comparing survival of colorectal versus noncolorectal hepatic metastases following resection.[20,22,23]

Predictors of Survival

Previous studies have identified clinical variables that correlate with improved survival after hepatic resection of colorectal metastases.[5,6] In the series from M. D. Anderson, potential prognostic variables were analyzed in an attempt to determine predictors of survival following hepatic resection of NCR metastases. The number and size of metastases, patient age, and disease-free interval between diagnosis of primary tumor and subsequent hepatic metastases were not significant determinants of overall or disease-free survival. The site of the primary tumor, including an assessment of gastrointestinal versus nongastrointestinal origin, was not a significant prognostic variable in this study. Extrahepatic disease, even though completely resected, was a significant predictor of worse disease-free survival, a finding consistent with survival data from patients with colorectal liver metastases.[6] In fact, only 1 of 12 patients with extrahepatic disease in this series has survived more than 18 months without cancer recurrence.

Investigators from Memorial Sloan Kettering also analyzed various factors predictive of outcome.[20] Disease-free interval, intent of resection (palliative versus curative), and primary tumor type were identified as significant predictors of overall survival. The best outcome was noted for patients with genitourinary or gynecologic tumors. Patients with soft tissue primary tumors exhibited an intermediate survival, and those with metastastic nonsarcomatous gastrointestinal tumors had the worst outcome. It should be noted that the authors of that report arranged tumor types into groups based on anatomic location instead of biologic behavior. For instance, adrenal carcinomas and cervical cancers were included in the same group, and breast cancers and sarcomas were grouped together. Thus the importance of the primary tumor type should not be overemphasized as a prognostic factor.

Survival and Primary Tumor Type

In a review of the published literature and unpublished personal communications, Schwartz analyzed survival following hepatic resection of NCR metastases according to specific tumor type.[14] The prognosis after hepatic resection of metastatic Wilms' tumors was favorable, and several long-term survivors have been identified.[24,25] Resection of metastatic renal cell carcinoma has also provided long-term survival to a number of patients, including one man from our series who has survived 8 years following liver resection.[16,24–26] Similarly, patients with metastastic testicular tumors may experience long-term survival after liver resection.[20] Our series included one patient with previously treated testicular teratoma who developed two separate hepatic metastases 1 year after orchiectomy. He underwent hepatic resection and has not developed tumor recurrence during the 5-years since then. Long-term survival has been reported in a small number of patients with metastatic adrenal tumors, although no 5-year survivors were identified from our series.[20,27]

Hepatic resection of metastatic gynecologic malignancies may provide long-term survival in rare patients. We reported three 3-year survivors after hepatic resection of ovarian metastases. One notable patient from our series developed a 20 cm hepatic metastasis 9 years after total abdominal hysterectomy and bilateral oophorectomy for papillary serous carcinoma of the ovary. An extended right hepatectomy was performed and the patient is alive without disease 10 years after hepatic resection. Another study of 21 patients with hepatic metastases from breast cancer reported a 5-year survival rate of only 9% after liver resection.[28] Anecdotal long-term survivors following liver resection of breast cancer metastases have been observed.[20,29] Our series included a patient who survived tumor-free for 62 months following hepatectomy for metastatic breast cancer before developing recurrent disease.

Soft tissue and gastrointestinal sarcomas frequently metastasize to the liver. Jacques et al. recently reported no 5-year survivors among 14 patients undergoing hepatic resection for sarcoma metastases.[30] In the series from M. D. Anderson, three patients who underwent hepatic resection for metastatic sarcomas have survived more than 3 years. Isolated hepatic metastases from cutaneous melanoma are unusual, and only a few long-term survivors following hepatic resection have been reported in the literature.[20,24] Likewise, long-term survival following resection of metastatic lung, pancreas, stomach, and head and neck cancers is anecdotal only. Certainly, the type of primary tumor may have an impact on the survival of patients with NCR liver metastases. The primary tumor type should not be a sole contraindication for resection of an isolated liver metastasis.

Preoperative Chemotherapy

The most important determinant of outcome from our series of patients treated at M. D. Anderson was response to preoperative chemotherapy. Patients with metastatic hepatic lesions that demonstrated more than 50% reduction in tumor volume in response to preoperative chemotherapy had a significantly improved disease-free survival compared to nonresponders (Fig. 11.2). Importantly, in the group of nonresponders, there are no patients who have survived without cancer recurrence longer than 12 months after hepatic resection. One patient from our series was treated with systemic chemotherapy prior to hepatic resection for metastatic testicular cancer. On histologic examination of the hepatic metastasis, significant tumor necrosis was noted with no viable tumor cells. The patient has survived 7 years without tumor recurrence. Response to preoperative chemotherapy has also been found to be a significant determinant of survival in patients with other malignancies.[31,32] In addition to providing important prognostic information, a short course of preoperative chemotherapy allows time for extrahepatic micrometastases to become clinically detectable, thus potentially sparing a patient a nonbeneficial surgical procedure. Moreover, postoperative adjuvant chemotherapy may be considered in patients with tumors proved to be responsive to preoperative chemotherapy. Finally, preoperative chemotherapy is recommended to reduce tumor volume in an effort to improve the likelihood of obtaining a tumor-free margin of resection.

Tumor Recurrence Following Hepatectomy

Nearly two-thirds of patients develop tumor recurrence following hepatic resection of NCR metastases. In our study 43% of recurrences were intrahepatic only, 27% were extrahepatic only, and 30% were intra-plus extrahepatic. This pattern of tumor recurrence is not dissimilar to the reported results after hepatic resection of metastases from colorectal primary tumors.[33] Clearly, more effective systemic and regional therapies are needed to improve the survival of these patients.

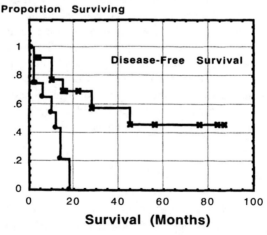

FIGURE 11.2. Actuarial 5-year disease-free survival following hepatic resection of noncolorectal tumors responsive (x) and nonresponsive (o) to preoperative chemotherapy.

Although the results of recent studies are encouraging, one cannot conclude definitively that hepatic resection provides an improved survival compared to nonresection. An alternate explanation for these data is that this group of highly selected patients with NCR liver metastases may have experienced long-term survival without surgical treatment. Only a prospective randomized trial comparing resection with nonresection would address this issue. To date, no such study has been completed on patients with either colorectal or NCR hepatic metastases. Nevertheless, hepatic resection is considered the treatment of choice for patients with isolated colorectal metastases. The survival of patients with unresected hepatic metastases from other solid tumors is well established.[34,35] Most patients die within 12 months of diagnosis, and the 5-year survival is less than 5%. Because the 5-year survival of 37–44% following hepatic resection of NCR metastases is nearly identical to the outcome following resection of metastases from colorectal cancer, it seems unacceptable to deny hepatic resection to appropriately selected patients with isolated NCR metastases. In addition, studies are now reporting increasing numbers of patients surviving more than 5 years without tumor recurrence following hepatic resection of NCR metastases.

Neuroendocrine Hepatic Metastases

It is useful to distinguish neuroendocrine from nonneuroendocrine liver metastases based on differences in tumor biology. Neuroendocrine malignancies are often slow-growing, and patients may survive many years despite advanced metastatic disease. Patients with these tumors comprise the largest group of long-term survivors after resection of NCR liver metastases, even though these malignancies are relatively rare.[36-45] Que et al. reported the results of 74 patients with metastatic neuroendocrine tumors undergoing hepatic resection at the Mayo Clinic from 1984 to 1992.[46] The primary tumors included metastatic carcinoid ($n = 50$), glucagonoma ($n = 8$), multihormonal islet cell carcinoma ($n = 7$), nonfunctioning islet cell carcinoma ($n = 5$), gastrinoma ($n = 2$), insulinoma ($n = 1$), and atypical neuroendocrine tumors ($n = 1$). Of the 74 patients, 28 underwent potentially curative hepatic resection with removal of all gross disease. The overall survival at 4 years was 73% for all patients. Survival among patients who had resection with curative intent versus those with palliative intent did not differ significantly. Patients with hepatic metastases typically develop symptoms from increasing liver size or ectopic hormone production. Importantly, symptomatic relief was obtained in 90% of patients following resection at the Mayo Clinic. Therefore, in contrast to other NCR metastases, noncurative resection may prolong survival and provide effective palliation in selected patients with metastatic neuroendocrine tumors.

Orthotopic liver transplantation has been employed as an alternative to resection for selected patients with metastatic neuroendocrine malignancy.[47-55]

For most patients with primary and metastatic hepatic malignancies, the results of liver transplantation have been disappointing because most of the patients develop early tumor recurrence.[53-56] The unacceptably high recurrence rate has not justified the utilitization of the few available donor organs. Neuroendocrine tumors are generally more indolent, and liver transplantation here may provide improved disease-free survival and significant palliation. Early reports have been limited to small patient numbers and short follow-up.[47-49,52] More recently, Lang et al. reported the results of liver transplantation for neuroendocrine primary tumors from a single institution.[57] Twelve patients underwent transplantation with a median survival of 55 months. Seven of the twelve patients have recurrent or persistent tumor. Le Treut et al. have reported the results of a retrospective, multicenter review of patients undergoing liver transplantation for metastatic neuroendocrine tumors.[58] Thirty-one patients were treated with orthotopic liver transplantation in 11 centers across France from 1989 to 1994. The actuarial overall and disease-free 5-year survival rates were 36% and 17%, respectively. In general, hepatic transplantation for metastatic neuroendocrine tumors should be reserved for patients without extrahepatic disease and in whom other treatments are ineffective.

Recommendations

Although the survival rates following hepatic resection of noncolorectal metastases are promising, most patients develop recurrent tumor. The most important factor in improving chances for survival following hepatic surgery is appropriate patient selection. A standardized approach for managing patients with NCR liver metastases should be adopted. Patients with hepatic metastases require a staging evaluation that includes CT of the chest, abdomen, and pelvis. A regimen of two or three cycles of preoperative tumor-specific chemotherapy is suggested. Restaging is performed with repeat CT after completing neoadjuvant therapy. Hepatic resection is considered for patients who are medically fit, have no extrahepatic disease, and have four or fewer metastatic lesions on CT that can be potentially resected with tumor-free margins. Intraoperative hepatic ultrasonography is necessary to identify lesions not palpated or visualized on preoperative imaging. Patients with extrahepatic disease discovered at operation should not undergo liver resection. Postoperative adjuvant chemotherapy is considered for patients with tumors responsive to preoperative chemotherapy.

References

1. Gastrointestinal Tumor Study Group. Adjuvant therapy of colon cancer: results of a prospectively randomized trial. N Engl J Med 310:737, 1984

2. Arbuck S. Overview of clinical trials using 5-fluorouracil and leucovorin for the treatment of colorectal cancer. Cancer 63:1036, 1989

3. Kemeny N, Younes A, Seiter K, et al. Interferon alpha-2a and 5-flurouracil for advanced colorectal carcinoma. Cancer 66:2470, 1990

4. Fortner J, Silva J, Golbey R, et al. Multivariant analysis of a personal series of 247 consecutive patients with liver metastases from colorectal cancer. Ann Surg 199:306, 1984

5. Scheele J, Stangl R, Altendorf-Hofmann A, et al. Indicators of prognosis after hepatic resection for colorectal secondaries. Surgery 110:13, 1991

6. Hughes K, Simons R, Songhorabodi S, et al. Resection of the liver for colorectal carcinoma metastases: a multi-institutional study of indications for resection. Surgery 103:278, 1988

7. Rosen C, Nagorney D, Taswell H, et al. Perioperative blood transfusion and determinants of survival after liver resection for metastatic colorectal carcinoma. Ann Surg 216:492, 1992

8. Doci R, Gennari L, Bignami P, et al. One hundred patients with hepatic metastases from colorectal cancer treated by resection: analysis of prognostic determinants. Br J Surg 78:797, 1991

9. Cady B, Stone M, McDermott W, et al. Technical and biological factors in disease-free survival after hepatic resection for colorectal cancer metastases. Arch Surg 127:561, 1992

10. Pickren J, Tsukada Y, Lane W: Liver metastasis: analysis of autopsy data. In Weiss L, Gilbert HA (eds) *Liver Metastases*. Boston, GK Hall, 1982, pp. 2–18

11. Edmonson H, Peters R. Neoplasms of the liver. In Schiff L, Schiff E (eds) Diseases of the Liver, 5th ed. Philadelphia, Lippincott-Raven, 1982, pp. 1101–1157

12. Steele G, Ravikumar TS. Resection of hepatic metastases from colorectal cancer: biological perspectives. Ann Surg 210:127, 1989

13. Wolf R, Goodnight J, Krag D. Results of resection and proposed guidelines for patient selection in instances of noncolorectal hepatic metastases. Surg Gynecol Obstet 173:454, 1991

14. Schwartz S. Hepatic resection for noncolorectal nonneuroendocrine metastases. World J Surg 19:72, 1995

15. Pommier R, Woltering E, Campbell J, et al. Hepatic resection for primary and secondary neoplasms of the liver. Am J Surg 153:428, 1987

16. Tomas de la Vega J, Donahue E, Doolas A, et al. A ten year experience with hepatic resection. Surg Gynecol Obstet 159:223, 1984

17. Cobourn C, Makowka L, Langer B, et al. Examination of patient selection and outcome for hepatic resection for metastatic disease. Surg Gynecol Obstet 165:239, 1987

18. Sesto M, Vogt D, Hermann R. Hepatic resection in 128 patients: a 24-year experience. Surgery 102:846, 1987

19. Thompson J, Tompkins R, Longmire W. Major hepatic resection: a 25-year experience. Ann Surg 197:375, 1983

20. Harrison L, Brennan M, Newman E, et al. Hepatic resection for noncolorectal nonneuroendocrine metastases: a fifteen-year experience with ninety-six patients. Surgery 121:625, 1997

21. Fuhrman G, Curley S, Hohn D, et al. Improved survival after resection of colorectal liver metastases. Ann Surg Oncol 2:537, 1995

22. Iwatsuki S, Starzl T. Personal experience with 411 hepatic resections. Ann Surg 208:421, 1988
23. Fong Y, Blumgart L, Fortner J, et al. pancreatic or liver resection for malignancy is safe and effective for the elderly. Ann Surg 222:426, 1995
24. Foster J, Lundy J. Pathlogy of liver metastasis. Curr Probl Surg 18:157, 1981
25. Morrow C, Grage T, Sutherland D, et al. Hepatic resection for secondary neoplasms. Surgery 92:610, 1983
26. Strauss F, Scanlon E. Five-year survival after hepatic lobectomy for metastatic hypernephroma. Arch Surg 72:328, 1956
27. Iwatsuki S, Shaw B, Starzl T, et al. Experience with 150 liver resections. Ann Surg 197:247, 1983
28. Elias D, Lasser P, Montrucolli D, et al. Hepatectomy for liver metastases from breast cancer. Eur J Surg Oncol 21:510, 1995
29. Stehlin J, de Ipoyli P, Greeff P, et al. Treatment of cancer of the liver: twenty years' experience with infusion and resection in 414 patients. Ann Surg 208:23, 1988
30. Jaques D, Coit D, Casper E, et al. Hepatic metastases from soft-tissue sarcoma. Ann Surg 221:392, 1994
31. Thoms W, McNeese M, Fletcher G, et al. Multimodality treatment for inflammatory breast cancer. Int J Radiat Oncol Biol Phys 17:739, 1989
32. Gerner R, Moore G, Pickman J. Soft tissue sarcomas. Ann Surg 181:803, 1975
33. Hughes K, Simon R, Songhoraboi S, et al. Resection of the liver for colorectal carcinoma metastases: a multi-institutional study of patterns of recurrence. Surgery 100:278, 1986
34. Bengmark S, Jonsson P, Surgical treatment of liver metastases in: Weiss L, Gilbert H (eds) *Liver Metastases*. Boston, GK Hall, 1982, pp. 294–297
35. Zinser J, Hortobagi G, Buacar A, et al. Clinical course of breast cancer patients with liver metastases. J Clin Oncol 5:773, 1987
36. Stephen J, Grahame-Smith D. Treatment of the carcinoid syndrome by local removal of hepatic metastases. Proc R Soc Med 65:444, 1972
37. Strodel W, Talpos G, Eckhauser F, et al. Surgical therapy for small-bowel carcinoid tumors. Arch Surg 118:391, 1983
38. Norton J, Sugarbaker P, Doppman J, et al. Aggressive resection of metastatic disease in selected patients with malignant gastrinoma. Ann Surg 203:352, 1986
39. McEntee G, Nagorney D, Kvols L, et al. Cytoreductive hepatic surgery for neuroendocrine tumors. Surgery 108:1091, 1990
40. Makridis C, Oberg K, Juhlin C, et al. Surgical treatment of midgut carcinoid tumors. World J Surg 14:377, 1990
41. Soreide O, Berstad T, Bakka A, et al. Surgical treatment as a principle in patients with advanced abdominal carcinoid tumors. Surgery 111:48, 1992
42. Gramma E, Eriksson B, Martensson H, et al. Clinical characteristic, treatment and survival in patients with pancreatic tumors causing hormonal syndromes. World J Surg 16:632, 1992
43. Ahlman H, Wangberg B, Jansson S, et al. Management of disseminated midgut carcinoid tumours. Digestion 49:78, 1991
44. Goto H, Yamaji Y, Konno T, et al. A glucagon-secreting alpha cell carcinoma of the pancreas. World J Surg 6:107, 1982
45. Nagorney D, Bloom S, Polak J, et al. Resolution of recurrent Verner-Morrison syndrome by resection of metastatic VIPoma. Surgery 93:348, 1983

46. Que F, Nagorney D, Batts K, et al. Hepatic resection for metastatic neuroendocrine carcinomas. Am J Surg 169:36, 1995
47. Makowka L, Tzakis A, Mazzaferro V, et al. Transplantation of the liver for metastatic endocrine tumors of the intestine and pancreas. Surg Gynecol Obstet 168:107, 1989
48. Arnold J, O'Grady J, Bird G, et al. Liver transplantation for primary and secondary hepatic apudomas. Br J Surg 76:248, 1989
49. Alsina A, Bartus S, Hull D, et al. Liver transplantation for metastatic neuroendocrine tumor. J Clin Gastroenterol 12:533, 1990
50. Lobe T, Vera S, Bowman L, et al. Hepaticopancreaticogastroduodenectomy with transplantation for metastatic islet cell carcinoma in childhood. J Pediatr Surg 27:227, 1992
51. Gulanikar A, Kotylak G, Bitter-Suermann H. Does immunosuppression alter the growth of metastatic liver carcinoid after orthotopic liver transplantation? Transplant Proc 23:2197, 1992
52. Farmer D, Shaked A, Colonna J, et al. Radical resection combined with liver transplantation for foregut tumors. Am J Surg 59:806, 1993
53. Iwatsuki S, Gordon R, Shaw B, et al. Role of liver transplantation in cancer therapy. Ann Surg 202:401, 1985
54. O'Grady J, Polson R, Rolles K, et al. Liver transplantation for malignant disease: results in 93 consecutive patients. Ann Surg 207:373, 1988
55. Ringe B, Wittekind C, Bechstein W, et al. The role of liver transplantation in hepatobiliary malignancy: a retrospective analysis of 95 patients with particular regard to tumor stage and recurrence. Ann Surg 209:88, 1989
56. Penn I. Hepatic transplantation in primary and metastatic cancer of the liver. Surgery 110:726, 1991
57. Lang H, Oldhafer K, Weimann A, et al. Liver transplantation for metastatic neuroendocrine tumors. Ann Surg 225:347, 1997
58. Le Treut Y, Delpera J, Dousset B, et al. Results of liver transplantation in the treatment of metastatic neuroendocrine tumors. Ann Surg 225:355, 1997

12

Biology of Colorectal Cancer Liver Metastasis

CHUL HO CHO AND ROBERT RADINSKY

Metastasis—the spread of malignant tumor cells from a primary neoplasm to distant parts of the body where they multiply to form new growths—is a major cause of death from cancer. The treatment of metastatic cancer poses a major problem to clinical oncologists because the presence of multiple metastases makes complete eradication by surgery, irradiation, or drugs nearly impossible. For most tumors, including colorectal carcinoma, the presence of liver metastasis renders the patient essentially incurable. A better understanding of the biology of liver metastases and the molecular events leading to the metastatic phenotype is essential if new and innovative therapeutic approaches are to be developed to treat this disease.

The liver is the site of metastases from cancers of diverse and distant organs, in particular those of the gastrointestinal tract.[1] This phenomenon may be due to the liver's place as the first visceral organ that malignant cells of gastrointestinal origin encounter after release into capillaries, postcapillary venules, and subsequently the portal circulation. However, the interaction or lodgement of circulating tumor cells within an organ is not by itself sufficient for the formation of metastasis. Rather, metastasis is a highly selective process whereby only cells of the necessary genotype and phenotype are capable of completing all steps in the metastatic process. In addition, host organ interactions with the metastatic tumor cell play a crucial role in the survival of cells with metastatic potential and their ability to proliferate to form metastases. Insight into the molecular mechanisms regulating the pathobiology of cancer metastasis and a better understanding of the interaction between the metastatic cell and the organ-specific microenvironment should provide a foundation for the design of new therapeutic approaches. Furthermore, the development of *in vivo* and *in vitro* models that allow isolation and characterization of cells possessing metastatic potential within both primary tumors and metastases will be invaluable in the design of more effective and safe therapeutic modalities.

In this chapter we summarize the biology of colorectal carcinoma liver metastasis with special emphasis on recent reports from our laboratory and others demonstrating that the organ microenvironment can profoundly influence the biologic behavior of metastatic tumor cells including induction of carcinoembryonic antigen (CEA),[2] regulation of the invasive phenotype,[3,4] modulation of multidrug resistance,[5,6] and control of tumor cell survival and proliferation in liver.[7-10] Collectively, these data support the concept that the microenvironment of organs can influence the biologic behavior of tumor cells at different steps of the metastatic process. These findings have obvious implications for the therapy of neoplasms in general and metastases in particular.

Metastatic Cascade

In contrast to our understanding of the development of primary colorectal carcinoma, little is known about the genetic alterations associated with its metastatic ability.[11] Metastasis is a highly selective, nonrandom process favoring the survival of a minor subpopulation of metastatic cells that preexist within the primary tumor mass.[10,11] To produce metastases, tumor cells from this subpopulation must complete a sequence of interrelated steps (Fig 12.1). This process begins with invasion of the surrounding normal stroma by single tumor cells with increased motility or groups of cells from the primary tumor. Once the invading cells penetrate the vascular or lymphatic channels they may grow there, or a single cell or clumps of cells may detach and be transported within the circulatory system. Tumor emboli must survive the host's immune and nonimmune defenses and the turbulence of the circulation, arrest in the capillary bed of compatible organs, extravasate into the organ parenchyma, survive, proliferate, and establish a micrometastasis. Growth of these small tumor lesions requires the development of a vascular supply and continuous evasion of host defense cells. Failure to complete one or more steps of the process (e.g., inability to invade/extravasate, inability to proliferate in a distant organ's parenchyma) eliminates the cells (Fig 12.1). To produce clinically relevant distant metastases, the successful metastatic cell must therefore exhibit a complex phenotype that is regulated by transient or permanent changes at the gene level.[7-11]

There is now wide acceptance that many malignant tumors, including colorectal carcinomas, contain heterogeneous subpopulations of cells. This heterogeneity is exhibited in a wide range of genetic, biochemical, immunologic, and biologic characteristics such as growth rate, antigenic and immunogenic status, cell surface receptors and products, enzymes, karyotypes, cell morphologies, invasiveness, drug resistance, and metastatic potential. It is likely that specific tumor cells or colonies within the larger heterogeneous tumor specimen are the forerunners of distant metastases.[12]

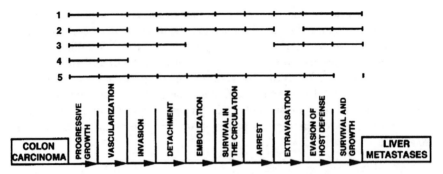

FIGURE 12.1. Sequential linked steps in the pathogenesis of tumor cell metastasis. Tumor cells must complete every step in the process to produce clinically relevant metastases. These steps include the progressive growth and vascularization of the primary neoplasm, tumor cell invasion of the surrounding tissue and detachment from the primary tumor, embolization and survival in the circulation, arrest and extravasation in the target tissue, evasion of host defenses, and finally proliferation at the secondary site of implantation . Failure to complete one or more steps disrupts the linkage and eliminates the cell. 1-metastatic colorectal cancer cell; 2-nonmetastatic tumor cell deficient in invasion and extravasation; 3, 4-nonmetastatic tumor cells due to multiple deficiencies; 5-nonmetastatic tumor cell deficient in the final step of metastasis (i.e., progressive growth ability at the secondary metastatic site). (Adapted from Fidler and Radinsky,[11] with permission).

Biologic Aspects of Colorectal Cancer Liver Metastasis

Cancer of the colon and rectum is the second most prevalent cause of cancer deaths in men and the third most common in women.[13] Most patients with colon cancer present with either Dukes' stage B or C disease. Overall survival for patients undergoing surgical excision of Dukes' stage B or C disease is 60–85% and 40–60%, respectively. Approximately 55% of colorectal cancers recur within 5 years. Despite surgery to remove the primary tumor, half recur regionally, and up to 80% produce distant metastases. The liver is the most common site of these metastases.[14] Surgical treatment of liver metastasis is effective as a curative therapy in only a small number of cases,[15] and chemotherapy and radiation therapy are largely palliative.[16] Once metastases are diagnosed, survival tends to be short, averaging less than 10 months.[17] Therefore diagnosis of patients with colon cancer at an early or premalignant stage and the identification of patients likely to relapse following surgery alone are crucial goals. Given how little is known about the genetic alterations associated with metastasis,[11] an increased understanding of the molecular mechanisms mediating this process is a primary goal of cancer research aimed at improving treatment.

Animal Models

Two criteria must be met when designing an appropriate model for human cancer metastasis. It must use metastatic cells, and these cells must grow in a relevant organ environment. Many investigators have reported on the implantation of human tumor cells into the subcutis of nude mice, but in most cases the growing tumors failed to produce metastases.[10] During the 1980s Fidler's laboratory developed a reproducible model of colorectal carcinoma liver metastasis.[10,18-21] Tumor cells from colorectal cancer surgical specimens were implanted into the spleens of nude mice.[10,18-21] The growth of colorectal cancer in the nude mouse liver directly correlated with the metastatic potential of the cells; that is cells from surgical specimens of primary human colorectal carcinoma (HCC) classified as Dukes' stage D or from liver metastases produced significantly higher numbers of colonies in the livers of nude mice than cells from a Dukes' stage B tumor.[19,20] Importantly, radioactive distribution analyses of colorectal cancer cells demonstrated that shortly after intrasplenic injection the tumor cells reached the liver; hence the production of HCC liver metastasis in nude mice was determined by the ability of the HCC cells to survive and proliferate in the liver parenchyma rather than by the ability of the cells to reach the liver.[21] The initial presence of viable tumor cells in a particular organ does not always predict that the cells will be able to survive and proliferate to produce metastases.[10]

Additional experiments were carried out to select and isolate cells with increasing liver—metastasizing potential directly from heterogeneous primary colon cancers.[19] Briefly, cells derived from a surgical specimen of a Dukes' stage B_2 primary colon carcinoma were established in culture or injected into the subcutis, cecum, and spleen of nude mice. Progressively growing tumors were isolated and established in culture. Implantation of these four culture-adapted cell lines into the cecum or spleen of nude mice produced few liver tumor foci. HCC cells from these few liver metastases were expanded into culture and reinjected into the spleens of nude mice to provide a source for further cycles of selection. Importantly, with each successive *in vivo* selection cycle, the metastatic ability of the isolated and propagated cells increased. Four cycles of selection yielded cell lines with a high metastatic efficiency in nude mice.[19] In parallel studies using a surgical specimen of a Dukes' stage D primary colon cancer, cells from highly metastatic cell lines were isolated, but successive selection cycles for growth in the liver only slightly increased metastatic properties.[19,20] These results demonstrated that highly metastatic cells can be selected from primary colorectal cancers and that orthotopic implantation of these cells in nude mice is a valid model for determining metastatic potential.[10,18-21]

If a human tumor is biologically heterogeneous, some of its cells possess a growth advantage, depending on whether it is transplanted to the skin, cecum, liver, or kidney of nude mice. Data from our laboratory utilizing a genetically tagged HCC cell population validates this statement.[22] Distinct colon carcinoma clones differentially expressing specific mRNA transcripts for metastasis-related genes were the forerunners of the liver metastases.[22] The importance of orthotopic implantation of human neoplasms is also supported by results in other human tumor model systems (for review see Fidler[10]). The correct in vivo model system for human spontaneous metastasis therefore allows interaction of the tumor cells with their relevant organ microenvironment .

Organ-Derived Growth Factors

As early as 1889 Paget proposed that the growth of metastases is due to the specific interaction of particular tumor cells with particular organ environments.[23] This hypothesis, supported both experimentally and clinically, may explain metastatic colonization patterns that cannot be due solely to mechanical lodgement/anatomic considerations.[24] There is considerable evidence that the microenvironment of each organ influences the implantation, invasion, survival, and growth of particular tumor cells, meaning that the outcome of metastasis is influenced by both the intrinsic properties of the tumor cell and host-specific factors.

A mechanism for site-specific tumor growth involves the interaction between receptive metastatic cells and the organ microenvironment, possibly mediated by local growth factors (GFs). These factors are known to mediate the growth of normal and neoplastic cells.[25] Evidence supporting the influence of organ-specific GFs on the metastatic phenotype has been obtained, in part, from experiments on the effects of organ-conditioned medium on the growth of particular neoplastic cells. The presence of stimulatory or inhibitory factors in a particular tissue correlated with the site-specific pattern of metastasis (for reviews see Radinsky[7,9] and Fidler[10]). Collectively, these data suggest a role for organ-derived paracrine growth factors in the regulation of tumor cell proliferation.

Different concentrations of hormones in individual organs, differentially expressed local factors, or paracrine GFs may all influence the survival and growth of malignant cells in particular organs[7] (Fig 12.2). For example, specific peptide GFs are concentrated in distinct tissue environments. One example is insulin-like growth factor-I (IGF-I). IGF-I is synthesized in most mammalian tissue, its highest concentration being in the liver.[26] This GF controls cell cycle progression through G_1.[27] One study demonstrated that carcinoma cells metastatic to the liver were growth-stimulated by hepatocyte-derived IGF-I in direct proportion to IGF-I receptor density on the metastatic versus nonmetastatic tumor cells; the correlation suggests a potential mechanism of selection in the process of liver colonization.[28] Another example is transforming growth factor-β (TGFβ). The principal sources of this peptide are platelets and bone, suggesting that it has roles in healing and bone remodeling processes.[7] Many transformed cells produce increased levels of TGFβ and simultaneously lose their sensitivity to its growth inhibitory effects. Interestingly, moderately or highly metastatic murine fibrosarcoma cells were growth-stimulated by TGFβ_I, whereas nonmetastatic and transformed cells of the identical lineage were growth-inhibited, similar to the nontransformed parental cell lines.[29] Clonal stimulation or inhibition of human colorectal carcinoma cells by TGFβ_I has also been observed and correlated with differential expression of its receptors.[30] These findings indicate that the receptive metastatic cell (compared to its nonmetastatic counterparts) may acquire altered responses to GF signals.[7,10]

Tissue-Specific Repair Factors

Host factors (autocrine or paracrine) that control organ repair or regeneration (or both) may also affect the proliferation of malignant tumor cells. It is interesting to speculate that metastatic cells may therefore proliferate in secondary organs that produce compatible GFs, that is, GFs similar to those involved in the cellular regulation of the normal tissue from which the primary tumor originated (Fig 12.2). For example, colon carcinoma cells utilize and respond to specific GFs that regulate normal colonic epithelium.[31,32] Some of these identical factors also regulate homeostasis and tissue renewal and repair in the liver [e.g., TGFα and hepatocyte growth factor (HGF) (Fig 12.2).[33,34] Do these same factors and receptors participate in the regulation of HCC growth in the liver? There is evidence they do. For instance, after partial (60%) hepatectomy the liver undergoes rapid cell division termed regeneration. We transplanted HCC cells into nude mice that had been subjected to either partial (60%) hepatectomy, nephrectomy, or control abdominal surgery.[35] Those implanted subcutaneously demonstrated accelerated growth in partially hepatectomized mice but not in nephrectomized or control mice. Consistent with these observations is the appearance during liver regeneration of factors in the peripheral blood that stimulate DNA synthesis in grafted hepatic parenchyma concomitant with DNA synthesis by the liver *in situ*.[34] Thus liver regeneration in the nude mouse stimulated the growth of colon carcinoma cells.

Described as a physiologic regulator of liver regeneration, TGFα has been suggested to act by means of an autocrine mechanism.[33] TGFα production by hepatocytes might have a paracrine role as well, stimulating proliferation of adjacent nonparenchymal cells.[33,34] TGFα may also be a component of the paracrine regulatory loop, controlling hepatocyte replication at the later stages of liver regeneration.[33] Therefore when normal tissues such as liver are damaged (possibly by invading tumor cells), GFs are released to stimulate normal organ tissue repair, and these factors may also stimulate the proliferation of receptive malignant tumor cells (see below). Hence tumor cells that originate from or have an affinity for growth in a particular organ can respond to appropriate organ-specific physiologic signals.

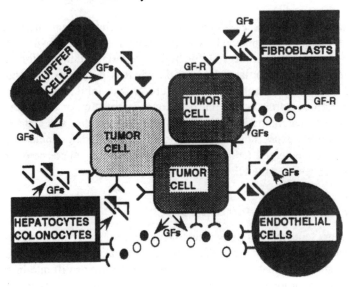

FIGURE 12.2. Model for the paracrine regulation of metastatic colon carcinoma cells in the liver. Paracrine regulation of tumor cells can involve stimulation or inhibition by growth factors in the extracellular environment. Candidate stimulatory ligands include transforming growth factor (TGFα), which is produced by hepatocytes in response to trauma. Experimental evidence indicates that this physiologic regulator of liver regeneration works through an autocrine loop in hepatocytes and through a paracrine mechanism in adjacent nonparenchymal cells through the epidermal growth factor receptor (EGF-R). Another candidate mitogen, hepatocyte growth factor (HGF), is synthesized and secreted from liver endothelial, Kupffer, and Ito cells, which is consistent with its paracrine action in the growth regulation of liver and colonic epithelium.[32-34] Furthermore, after liver damage a rapid increase in HGF production is observed in the Ito and Kupffer cells in parallel with the down-regulation of its receptor, c-Met, in hepatocytes.[34] Hence homeostatic processes such as inflammation and repair that follow damage to an organ facilitate the proliferation of normal cells, and in some cases tumor cells possessing the appropriate receptors. Tumor cells can also release factors that affect the host cells, resulting in a reciprocal relation between the tumor cells and host cells in the tumor microenvironment.[7] GFs-growth factors; GF-R-growth factor receptor. (Adapted from Radinsky,[7] with permission).

Host Tumor–Interactions Regulating Colorectal Cancer Cell Gene Expression During Liver Metastasis

Insight into the molecular mechanisms regulating the different and distinct steps of the metastatic process and a better understanding of the interaction between the metastatic cell and the host microenvironment should provide a foundation for new therapeutic approaches.

Regulation of Carcinoembryonic Antigen Expression by the Organ Microenvironment

An essential step in the formation of liver metastasis is the adherence of tumor cells to the microvasculature of the liver. This process is both active and passive. Tumor cell emboli often circulate as clumps of cells adherent to other tumor cells or platelets. Mechanical trapping of these tumor cells occurs in the hepatic sinusoid, and yet fewer than 1% of these cells survive 5 days, and only a small percentage of them form metastases.[36] The mere trapping of cells in the hepatic circulation does not ensure their survival; cell surface adhesion molecules specific for receptor molecules on the hepatic endothelial cells and extracellular matrix are necessary for attachment and subsequent growth in the liver. Tumor cells expressing specific adhesion molecules on their cell surface may show preferential metastasis to the liver. Interestingly, the tumor marker carcinoembryonic antigen (CEA) may play a role in cell adhesion in liver metastasis from colorectal cancer. Injection of CEA intravenously prior to injecting colon cancer cells in an experimental model of colorectal cancer increased the percentage of mice developing liver metastases.[37] In other studies, transfection and overexpression of CEA increased the metastatic potential of HCC cells.[38]

First described in 1965 by Gold and Freedman,[39] CEA is the most widely used clinical tumor marker for several neoplastic diseases, especially colorectal carcinomas.[40] It serves as a prognostic marker because in most cases an elevated preoperative serum CEA level is associated with a poor prognosis.[41] CEA is a member of the immunoglobulin supergene family functioning as an intercellular adhesion molecule.[37] Cells expressing CEA have been shown to aggregate under in vitro conditions, suggesting that CEA promotes the adhesion of tumor cells to each other (homotypic) or to host cells (heterotypic). Hence tumor cells in circulating aggregates may have an increased capacity to arrest in distant capillary beds, resulting in an increased probability of metastasis.

Although the expression of CEA by HCC cells has been directly correlated with their metastatic potential,[37] its regulation is poorly understood.[41] Previous reports have demonstrated a positive relation between the degree of differentiation of colorectal cancer and CEA production.[37] Several agents that alter the degree of cellular differentiation have also been shown to increase the level of CEA expression in these cell types.[42]

Results from our laboratory indicate that the expression of CEA is regulated by the organ microenvironment.[2] The orthotopic (cecal wall) implantation of colorectal carcinoma cells into nude mice yielded more-differentiated tumors, which then expressed high levels of steady-state CEA mRNA and protein. In contrast, ectopic (subcutis) tumors were less differentiated and produced low levels of steady-state CEA mRNA transcripts and protein. In the cecal wall of nude mice, colorectal cancer cells (isolated from a moderately differentiated adenocarcinoma of the colon from a patient with high preoperative serum CEA levels) produced differentiated lesions with higher levels of CEA mRNA transcripts and protein than lesions produced by colon carcinoma cells (isolated from a poorly differentiated colon adenocarcinoma from a patient with a low preoperative serum CEA level). In culture, however, these different cells produced similar levels of CEA mRNA and protein.

In patients with colorectal carcinomas, an elevated preoperative serum CEA level is associated with poor prognosis.[37,40] The serum CEA level of patients with colorectal carcinoma is influenced by the balance between production of CEA by tumor cells and the ability of the liver to clear CEA from the blood.[40] Thus elevated serum levels of CEA may be due to an increased tumor burden, especially metastatic lesions in the liver [40]. These data do not address this possibility but show that CEA expression is indeed regulated by cell density. When cells enter quiescence, they can exhibit major alterations in cell surface receptors, expression of transcription factors, enzymes, and cellular ultrastructure. The expression of basic fibroblast growth factor (bFGF), *mdr*-1, and type IV collagenases have been shown to be down-regulated in confluent cultures,[43] and colorectal carcinoma cells have been shown to undergo polarization and differentiation when cultured to confluence.[44] We found that dense monolayer cultures or spheroids of the colorectal cancer cell lines produced mucin after reaching confluence and showed increased expression of CEA. Incubation of these cells in serum-free medium decreased cell proliferation and enhanced CEA production. We also treated colorectal cancer cells (high CES production) with mitomycin C and found that growth-arrested cells (under sparse conditions) produced higher CEA levels. This finding suggests that CEA expression is influenced by cell proliferation. Moreover, medium removed from dense cultures increased the expression of CEA in tumor cells growing as sparse monolayers, indicating that CEA expression may be regulated by an autocrine mechanism.

Collectively, these data indicate that the production of CEA by colorectal carcinoma cells can be modulated by specific organ microenvironments, cell density, and autocrine and paracrine factors. Because CEA expression levels and differentiation of tumor cells growing in the cecal wall of nude mice directly correlated with the preoperative serum CEA level and pathologic diagnosis of the original patient surgical specimens, we conclude that the orthotopic implantation of human colorectal carcinoma xenografts provides a relevant model to study the regulation and role of CEA in liver metastasis.

Organ-Specific Modulation of the Invasive Phenotype

As described thus far, the interaction of tumor cells with specific organ environment can modulate tumorigenicity and metastatic behavior. The implantation of HCC cells into the subcutis (ectopic site) or the wall of the cecum (orthotopic site) results in locally growing tumors.[19,20] Metastasis to distant organs, however, is produced only by tumors growing in the wall of the cecum.[19,20] This difference in production of distant metastasis directly correlated with the production of degradative enzymes by the colorectal cancer cells.[3,4]

The ability of tumor cells to degrade connective tissue extracellular matrix (ECM) and basement membrane components is an essential prerequisite for invasion and metastasis.[45,46] Among the enzymes involved in degradation of the ECM are the metalloproteinases, a family of metal-dependent endopeptidases.[45] These proteinases are produced by connective tissue cells as well as many tumor cells and include enzymes with degradative activity for interstitial collagen, types IV and V collagen, gelatin, and proteoglycans. The relative molecular weight (M_r) 72-kDa type IV collagenase is a neutral metalloproteinase capable of degrading type IV collagen within the triple helical domain.[45] Most of the enzyme is secreted into the extracellular milieu in a proenzymatic form.[45]

Expression of 72-kDa collagenase type IV is higher in colon carcinoma cells than in normal colonic mucosa cells,[47] and the metastatic capacity of these tumor cells from orthotopic sites in nude mice directly correlates with the production of this enzyme activity.[3,4,19,20] Intracecal tumors (in nude mice) of metastatic colorectal cancer secreted high levels of 92-kDa and 68-kDa gelatinase activities, whereas tumor cells growing subcutaneously (not metastatic) did not produce or secrete the 68-kDa gelatinase activity.[4,48] Moreover, histologic examination of the colon carcinoma growing in the subcutis or cecum of nude mice revealed that mouse fibroblasts produced a thick pseudocapsule around the subcutaneous tumors but not the cecal tumors.[48] These differences suggest that the organ environment can influence the ability of metastatic cells to produce EC—Mdegradative enzymes.

Other reports have shown that stromal fibroblasts can influence the tumorigenicity and biologic behavior of tumor cells,[49] Fabra et al. investigated whether organ-specific fibroblasts could directly influence the invasive ability of the colorectal cancer cells.[48] Co-culture of fibroblasts from skin, lung, and colon of nude mice with highly invasive and metastatic human colorectal carcinoma cells showed that these cells adhered to and invaded the mouse colon and lung but not skin fibroblasts.[48] Moreover, nude mouse skin fibroblasts, but not colon or lung fibroblasts (orthotopic environments), inhibited the production of 72-kDa type IV collagenases by highly invasive and metastatic colorectal cancer cells. This inhibition was due to the specific interaction between the colorectal carcinoma cells and skin fibroblasts as the skin fibroblasts, did not decrease the production of collagenase or the invasive capacity of control squamous carcinoma cells. These data directly correlated with the studies showing that colon cancer cells can grow in the wall of the cecum and the subcutis of nude mice but are invasive only from the wall of the cecum.[4,20] Moreover, colon carcinoma growing in the subcutis did not produce type IV collagenase.[4] The *in vitro* data directly correlate with the *in vivo* findings and suggest that fibroblasts populating the ectopic and orthotopic organs influence the invasive phenotype of tumor cells.

Regulation of the Multidrug Resistance Phenotype by the Organ Microenvironment

Several intrinsic properties of tumor cells can render them resistant to chemotherapeutic drugs, including increased expression of the multidrug resistance (MDR) genes, leading to overproduction of the transmembrane transport protein P-glycoprotein (P-gp)[50] Increased levels of P-gp can be induced by selecting tumor cells for resistance to natural product amphiphilic anticancer drugs.[50] Numerous reports have also described elevated expression of P-gp simultaneously with the development of the MDR phenotype in solid tumors of the colon, kidney, and liver that had not been exposed to chemotherapy.[51,52] Because the development of MDR in tumor cells is a major barrier to therapy, understanding the mechanisms by which specific mediators affect this process is mandatory if successful treatments are to be designed.

P-glycoproteins are encoded by a small gene family, mdr, which in rodents consists of three highly homologous members (mdr-1, mdr-2, mdr-3).[53] Despite this homology, functional differences exist between the individual mdr genes: mdr-1 and mdr-3, but not mdr-2, are independently overexpressed in MDR cell lines of fibroblastic, lymphoid, and reticuloendothelial origin. Both mdr-1 and mdr-3 confer drug resistance in transfection experiments, and the two encoded proteins appear to have overlapping but distinct substrate specificities.[54] In contrast, overexpression of mdr-2 failed to confer drug resistance.[54]

Expression of mdr gene transcripts in normal tissues is controlled in a tissue-specific manner.[55] Although selection of cells by exposure to various drugs may alter the normal pattern of mdr gene expression, organ-specific factors regulating mdr-1 and mdr-3 expression in normal tissues may determine which gene is overexpressed in an MDR derivative of a particular tissue type.[53]

Clinical observations have suggested that the organ environment influences the response of tumors to chemotherapy. For example, in breast cancer patients, lymph node and skin metastases respond better than lung or bone metastases.[56] Investigations of experimental systems have produced similar results.[56,57] A mouse fibrosarcoma growing subcutaneously in syngeneic mice was sensitive to systemic administration of doxorubicin (DOX), whereas lung metastases were not.[58]

We initiated studies to determine how the organ microenvironment influences the response of tumor cells to chemotherapy. Murine CT-26 colorectal cancer cells growing in the lung (metastases) were relatively resistant to systemic therapy with DOX, whereas those in the subcutis were sensitive.[5,57] CT-26 cancer cells harvested from lung metastases and treated in vitro exhibited more resistance to DOX than cells harvested from subcutaneous tumors or parental cells grown in culture.[5] Resistance was reversible by adding verapamil, and all CT-26 cells demonstrated similar sensitivities to 5-fluorouracil (5-FU). Hence a direct correlation was observed between the increased resistance to DOX (*in vivo* and *in vitro*) of CT-26 cells and expression levels of *mdr*-1 mRNA transcripts and P-gp. The drug resistance and accompanying elevated expression of *mdr*-1 found for cells growing in the lung depended on their interaction with the specific organ environment: Once removed from the lung, the tumor cells reverted to a sensitive phenotype similar to the parental cells, and *mdr*-1 mRNA and P-gp reverted to the baseline levels typical of CT-26 parental cells.

An organ-specific response to DOX is not restricted to CT-26 cells. Previous reports with UV—2237 fibrosarcoma cells[58] and human KM12 colorectal carcinoma cells[57] also demonstrated significant differences in resistance to DOX (but not 5-FU) between subcutaneous tumors (sensitive) and lung or liver metastases (resistant). Similarly, in patients with colorectal carcinoma, high levels of P-gp expression were found on the invasive edge of the primary tumor (growing in the colon[51,52] and in lymph node, lung, and liver metastases.[52] The environmental regulation of the MDR phenotype may explain, in part, the polarized expression of *mdr*-1 in colon carcinomas[58] and the discrepancy between *in vitro* and *in vivo* expression levels of the MDR phenotype.[50,58] The models described here can be used to investigate further the molecular mechanisms that regulate the *in vivo* expression of the *mdr* genes (for reviews see Fidler et al.[6] and kerbel et al.[59]).

Survival and Growth of Colorectal Cancer Cells at Distant Metastatic Sites

A mechanism that would explain the interaction between distinct colon carcinoma cells and the liver environment could involve the proliferation of tumor cells differentially expressing certain GF receptors and their response to liver-derived paracrine GFs. For example, highly metastatic tumor cells from Dukes' stage D colorectal tumors or surgical specimens of liver metastases responded to mitogens associated with liver regeneration induced by hepatectomy in nude mice.[7,10,35] As described above, transforming growth factor-α (TGFα) is a positive regulator of liver regeneration[33,34] and a mediator of the proliferation of normal colonic epithelial cells.[32] TGF-α exerts its effect through interaction with the epidermal growth factor receptor (EGF-R), a plasma membrane glycoprotein that contains a tyrosine-specific protein tyrosine kinase (PTK) in its cytoplasmic domain. The binding of TGFα to the EGF-R stimulates a series of rapid responses, including phosphorylation of tyrosine residues within the EGF-R itself and within many other cellular proteins, hydrolysis of phosphatidylinositol, release of Ca^{2+} from intracellular stores, elevation of cytoplasmic pH, and morphologic changes; after 12 hours in the presence of TGFα, cells synthesize DNA and ultimately divide.[60]

The EGF-Rs are present on many normal and tumor cells.[60] Elevated levels or amplification of the EGF-R has been found in many human tumors and cell lines.[61] These results suggest the physiologic significance of inappropriate expression of the EGF-R tyrosine kinase for abnormal cell growth control.

We examined the expression and function of EGF-R in a series of HCC cell lines whose liver metastatic potential differed. Our results demonstrated that the expression of EGF-R at the mRNA and protein levels directly correlated with the ability of the HCC to grow in the liver parenchyma and hence produce hepatic metastases.[8] The EGF-Rs expressed on metastatic tumor cells were functional based on *in vitro* growth stimulation assays using picogram concentrations of TGFα and were specific, as shown by neutralization with anti-EGF-R or anti-TGFα antibodies. Moreover, EGF-R-associated tyrosine kinase activity paralleled the observed EGF-R levels. Immunohistochemical analysis of the low metastatic parental KM12C colon carcinoma cells demonstrated heterogeneity in the EGF-R-specific staining pattern, with fewer than 10% of the cells in the population staining intensely for EGF-R, whereas the *in vivo* selected highly metastatic KM12SM and KM12L4 cells exhibited uniform, intense staining. Western blotting confirmed the presence of higher EGF-R protein levels in the metastatic KM12L4 and KM12SM cells than in the low metastatic KM12C cells. Finally, isolation of the top and bottom 5% EGF-R-expressing KM12C cells by fluorescence-activated cell sorting confirmed the association between EGF-R levels on the tumor cells and the ability to produce metastatic nodules in the liver.[8,22]

Our analyses indicated a direct correlation between EGF-R levels on cell lines isolated from HCC specimens and the ability to produce liver metastases in nude mice. These findings are more generalized because in our analysis of formalin-fixed paraffin-embedded colon carcinoma surgical specimens for EGF-R transcripts using a rapid colorimetric *in situ* mRNA hybridization (ISH) technique,[62] we found that cell-surface hybridization with EGF-R-antisense hyperbiotinylated oligonucleotide probes in primary and metastatic colon carcinoma specimens directly correlated with immunohistochemistry and Northern blot analyses. Moreover, unlike Northern analyses, ISH showed intratumoral heterogeneity in EGF-R gene expression and identified particular cells expressing high levels of EGF-R in the tissues.[62]

Collectively, these data suggest that EGF-R is involved in tumor progression and dissemination and indicate that this receptor could be used as a target for therapy (for review see Mendelsohn[63]). Anti-EGF-R monoclonal antibodies (mAbs), which block ligand binding, prevent the growth in culture of cells that are stimulated by EGF or TGFα as well as the growth of human tumor xenografts bearing high levels of EGF-R.[63] Studies have also indicated that anti-EGF-R mAbs substantially enhance the cytotoxic effects of doxorubicin or *cis*-diammine/dichloroplatinum on well established xenografts.[64] Furthermore, clinical trials with squamous cell carcinoma have demonstrated the capacity of the anti-EGF-R mAb to localize in such tumors and to achieve saturating concentrations in the blood for more than 3 days without toxicity.[63,64] Other treatments targeting the EGF-R include inhibitors of receptor dimerization,[65] antisense RNA, and EGF-R—specific PTK inhibitors,[66] as well as overexpression of dominant-negative mutant receptors.[67]

Conclusions

A current goal of cancer research is increased understanding of the molecular mechanisms regulating the process of cancer metastasis. Analyses of the interaction of colorectal cancer cells with the microenvironment has increased our understanding of biologic mechanisms mediating organ-specific metastasis. Insight into the mechanisms that mediate the pathobiology of cancer metastasis and better understanding of the interaction between the metastatic cell and the host environment should produce a foundation for new therapeutic approaches. As reviewed here, the liver microenvironment can profoundly influence the pattern of gene expression and the biologic phenotype of metastatic colorectal cancer cells, including induction of CEA, modulation of the invasive phenotype, resistance to chemotherapy, and proliferation of the metastatic cell at the distant metastatic site. Each of these studies indicates that the production of clinically relevant metastases depends, in part, on the interaction of particular tumor cells with specific organ environments. Therefore the successful metastatic cell whose complex phenotype helps make it the decathlon champion must be viewed today as a cell receptive to its environment. The studies presented herein add evidence to support the concept that cancer metastasis is not a random process; it is a regulated process that can be analyzed on the molecular level in the context of the relevant organ environment. This new knowledge should eventually lead to the design and implementation of more effective therapies.

References

1. Pickren JW, Tsukada Y, Lane WW. Liver metastasis: analysis of autopsy data. In: Weiss L, Gilbert H A, (eds). Liver Metastasis, Boston, GK Hall, 1982, pp. 2–18.
2. Kitadai Y, Radinsky R, Bucana CD, et al. Regulation of carcinoembryonic antigen expression in human colon carcinoma cells by the organ environment. *Am J Pathol* 149:1157, 1996
3. Gohji K, Fidler IJ, Tsan R, et al. Human recombinant interferons-beta and -gamma decrease gelatinase production and invasion by human KG-2 renal carcinoma cells. *Int J Cancer* 58:380, 1994
4. Nakajima M, Morikawa K, Fabra A, et al. Influence of organ environment on extracellular matrix degradative activity and metastasis of human colon carcinoma cells. *J Natl Cancer Inst* 82:1890, 1990
5. Dong Z, Radinsky R, Fan D, et al. Organ specific modulation of steady-state mdr gene expression and drug resistance in murine colon cancer cells. *J Natl Cancer Inst* 86:913, 1994

6. Fidler IJ, Wilmanns C, Staroselsky A, et al. Modulation of tumor cell response to chemotherapy by the organ environment. *Cancer Metastasis Rev* 13:209, 1994

7. Radinsky R. Paracrine growth regulation of human colon carcinoma organ-specific metastases. *Cancer Metastasis Rev* 12:345, 1993

8. Radinsky R, Risin S, Fan D, et al. Level and function of epidermal growth factor receptor predict the metastatic potential of human colon carcinoma cells. *Clin Cancer Res* 1:19, 1995

9. Radinsky R. Modulation of tumor cell gene expression and phenotype by the organ—specific metastatic environment. *Cancer Metastasis Rev* 14:323, 1995

10. Fidler IJ. Special lecture: critical factors in the biology of human cancer metastasis: twenty-eighth G. H. A. Clowes Memorial Award Lecture. *Cancer Res* 50:6130, 1990

11. Fidler IJ, Radinsky R. Genetic control of cancer metastasis [editorial]. *J Natl Cancer Inst* 82:166, 1990

12. Kerbel RS. Growth dominance of the metastatic cancer cell: cellular and molecular aspects. *Adv Cancer Res* 55:87, 1990

13. Boring CC, Squires TS, Tong T. *Cancer statistics* 1993. CA Cancer J Clin 41:7, 1993

14. Russell AH, Tong D, Dawson LE, et al. Adenocarcinoma of the proximal colon: sites of initial dissemination and patterns of recurrence following surgery alone. *Cancer* 53:360, 1984

15. Benotti P, Steele G. Patterns of recurrent colorectal cancer and recovery surgery. *Cancer* 70:1409, 1992

16. Buyse M, Zelenuick-Jacquotte A, Chalmers TC. Adjuvant therapy of colorectal cancer: why we still don't know. *JAMA* 259:3571, 1988

17. Pestana C, Reitemeier RJ, Moertel CG, et al. The natural history of carcinoma of the colon and rectum. *Am J Surg* 108:826, 1964

18. Giavazzi R, Campbell DE, Jessup JM, et al. Metastatic behavior of tumor cells isolated from primary and metastatic human colorectal carcinomas implanted into different sites of nude mice. *Cancer Res* 46:1928, 1986

19. Morikawa K, Walker SM, Jessup JM, et al. *In vivo* selection of highly metastatic cells from surgical specimens of different colon carcinomas implanted into nude mice. *Cancer Res* 48:1943, 1988

20. Morikawa K, Walker SM, Nakajima M, et al. Influence of organ environment on the growth, selection, and metastasis of human colon carcinoma cells in nude mice. *Cancer Res* 48:6863, 1988

21. Giavazzi R, Jessup JM, Campbell DE, et al. Experimental nude mouse model of human colorectal cancer liver metastasis. *J Natl Cancer Inst* 77:1303, 1986

22. Singh RK, Tsan R, Radinsky R. Influence of the host microenvironment on the clonal selection of human colon carcinoma cells during primary tumor growth and metastasis. *Clin Exp Metastasis*, 15:140, 1997

23. Paget S. The distribution of secondary growths in cancer of the breast. *Lancet* 1:571, 1889

24. August DA, Ottow RT, Sugarbaker EV. Clinical perspectives of human colorectal cancer metastasis. *Cancer Metastasis Rev* 3:303, 1984

25. Deuel TF. Polypeptide growth factors: roles in normal and abnormal cell growth. *Annu Rev Cell Biol* 3:443, 1987

26. Zarrilli R, Bruni CB, Riccio A. Multiple levels of control of insulin-like growth factor gene expression. *Mol Cell Endocrinol* 101:R1, 1994

27. Stiles CD, Capone GT, Scher CD, et al. Dual control of cell growth by somatomedins and platelet-derived growth factor. *Proc Natl Acad Sci USA* 76:1279, 1979

28. Long L, Nip J, Brodt P. Paracrine growth stimulation by hepatocyte-derived insulin—like growth factor-1: a regulatory mechanism for carcinoma cells metastatic to the liver. *Cancer Res* 54:3732, 1994

29. Schwarz LC, Gingras MC, Goldberg G, et al. Loss of growth factor dependence and conversion of transforming growth factor-β1 inhibition to stimulation in metastatic H—ras-transformed murine fibroblasts. *Cancer Res* 48:6999, 1988

30. Fan D, Chakrabarty S, Seid C, et al. Clonal stimulation or inhibition of human colon carcinomas and human renal carcinoma mediated by transforming growth factor-β1. *Cancer Commun* 1:117, 1989

31. Malden L, Novak U, Burgess A. Expression of transforming growth factor alpha messenger RNA in normal and neoplastic gastrointestinal tract. *Int J Cancer* 43:380, 1989

32. Markowitz SD, Molkentin K, Gerbic C, et al. Growth stimulation by coexpression of transforming growth factor-α and epidermal growth factor receptor in normal an adenomatous human colon epithelium. *J Clin Invest* 86:356, 1990.

33. Mead JE, Fausto N. Transforming growth factor α may be a physiological regulator of liver regeneration by means of an autocrine mechanism. *Proc Natl Acad Sci USA* 86:1558, 1989

34. Michalopoulos GK, DeFrances MC. Liver regeneration. *Science* 276:60, 1997

35. Gutman M, Singh RK, Price JE, et al. Accelerated growth of human colon cancer cells in nude mice undergoing liver regeneration. *Invasion Metastasis* 14:362, 1994–1995

36. Barbera-Guillem E, Smith I, Weiss L. Cancer-cell traffic in the liver. I. Growth kinetics of cancer cells after portal-vein delivery. *Int J Cancer* 52:974, 1992

37. Jessup JM, Thomas P. Carcinoembryonic antigen: function in metastasis by human colorectal carcinoma. *Cancer Metastasis Rev* 8:263, 1989

38. Hashino J, Fukuda Y, Oikawa S, Nakazato H, Nakanishi T. Metastatic potential of human colorectal carcinoma SW1222 cells transfected with cDNA encoding carcinoembryonic antigen. *Clin Exp Metastasis* 12:324, 1994

39. Gold P, Freedman SO. Demonstration of tumor-specific antigen in human colonic carcinoma by immunological tolerance and absorption techniques. *J Exp Med* 121:439, 1965

40. Steele G Jr, Zamcheck N. The use of carcinoembryonic antigen in the clinical management of patients with colorectal cancer. *Cancer Detect Prev* 8:421, 1985

41. Hauck W, Stanners CP. Transcriptional regulation of the carcinoembryonic antigen gene. *J Biol Chem* 270:3602, 1995

42. Toribara NW, Sack TL, Gum JR, et al. Heterogeneity in the induction and expression of carcinoembryonic antigen-related antigens in human colon cancer cell lines. *Cancer Res* 49:3321, 1989

43. Xie B, Bucana CD, Fidler IJ. Density-dependent induction of 92-kd type IV collagenase activity in cultures of A431 human epidermoid carcinoma cells. *Am J Pathol* 144:1058, 1994

44. Pinto M, Robine-Leon S, Appay M-D, et al. Enterocyte-like differentiation and polarization of the human colon carcinoma cell line Caco-2 in culture. *Biol Cell* 47:323, 1983

45. Stetler-Stevenson WG. Type IV collagenases in tumor invasion and metastasis. *Cancer Metastasis Rev* 9:289, 1990

46. Testa JE, Quigley JP. The role of urokinase-type plasminogen activator in aggressive tumor cell behavior. *Cancer Metastasis Rev* 9:353, 1990

47. Levy A, Cioce V, Sobel ME, et al. Increased expression of the 72 kDa type IV collagenase in human colonic adenocarcinoma. *Cancer Res* 51:439, 1991

48. Fabra A, Nakajima M, Bucana CD, Fidler IJ. Modulation of the invasive phenotype of human colon carcinoma cells by fibroblasts from orthotopic or ectopic organs of nude mice. *Differentiation* 52:101, 1992

49. Chung LWK. Fibroblasts are critical determinants in prostatic cancer growth and dissemination. *Cancer Metastasis Rev* 10:263, 1991

50. Chin K-V, Pastan I, Gottesman MM. Function and regulation of the human multidrug resistance gene. *Adv Cancer Res* 60:157, 1993

51. Goldstein LJ, Galski H, Fojo A, et al. Expression of a multidrug resistance gene in human tumors. *J Natl Cancer Inst* 81:116, 1989

52. Weinstein RS, Shriram JM, Dominguez JM, et al. Relationship of the expression of the multidrug resistance gene product (P-glycoprotein) in human colon carcinoma to local tumor aggressiveness and lymph node metastasis. *Cancer Res* 51:2720, 1991

53. Raymond M, Rose E, Housman DE, Gros P. Physical mapping, amplification, and overexpression of the mouse *mdr* gene family in multidrug-resistant cells. *Mol Cell Biol* 10:1642, 1990

54. Devault A, Gros P. Two members of the mouse *mdr* gene family confer multidrug resistance with overlapping but distinct drug specificities. *Mol Cell Biol* 10:1652, 1990

55. Croop JM, Raymond M, Haber D, et al. The three mouse multidrug resistance (*mdr*) genes are expressed in a tissue-specific manner in normal mouse tissues. *Mol Cell Biol* 9:1346, 1989

56. Slack NH, Bross JDJ. The influence of site of metastasis on tumor growth and response to chemotherapy. *Br J Cancer* 32:78, 1975

57. Wilmanns C, Fan D, O'Brian CA, et al. Orthotopic and ectopic organ environments differentially influence the sensitivity of murine colon carcinoma cells to doxorubicin and 5-fluorouracil. *Int J Cancer* 52:98, 1992

58. Staroselsky A, Fan D, O'Brian CA, et al. Site-dependent differences in response of the UV-2237 murine fibrosarcoma to systemic therapy with adriamycin. *Cancer Res* 40:7775, 1990

59. Kerbel RS, Kobayashi H, Graham CH. Intrinsic or acquired drug resistance and metastasis: are they linked phenotypes? *J Cell Biochem* 56:37, 1994

60. Van der Geer P, Hunter T, Lindberg RA. Receptor protein-tyrosine kinases and their signal transduction pathways. *Annu Rev Cell Biol* 10:251, 1994

61. Harris AL, Neal DE. Epidermal growth factor and its receptor in human cancer. In: Sluyser M (ed) Growth Factors and Oncogenes in Breast Cancer. 1987, pp. 60–90

62. Radinsky R, Bucana CD, Ellis LE, et al. A rapid colorimetric *in situ* messenger RNA hybridization technique for analysis of epidermal growth factor receptor in paraffin—embedded surgical specimens of human colon carcinomas. *Cancer Res* 53:937, 1993

63. Mendelsohn J. The epidermal growth factor receptor as a target for therapy with antireceptor monoclonal antibodies. *Semin Cancer Biol* 1:339, 1990

64. Baselga J, Norton L, Masui H, et al. Antitumor effects of doxorubicin in combination with anti-epidermal growth factor receptor monoclonal antibodies. *J Natl Cancer Inst* 85:1327, 1993

65. Lofts FJ, Hurst HC, Sterberg MJE, Gullick WJ. Specific short transmembrane sequences can inhibit transformation by the mutant *neu* growth factor receptor *in vitro* and *in vivo*. *Oncogene* 8:2813, 1993

66. Dinney CPN, Parker C, Dong Z, et al. Therapy of human transitional cell carcinoma of the bladder by oral administration of the epidermal growth factor receptor protein tyrosine kinase inhibitor 4,5-dianilinophthalimide. *Clin Cancer Res* 3:161, 1997

67. Selva E, Raden DL, Davis RJ. Mitogen-activated prsotein kinase stimulationby a tyrosine kinase-negative epidermal growth factor receptor. *J Biol Chem* 268:2250, 1993

13

Gene Therapy
for Hepatocellular Carcinoma

DENNIE V. JONES JR.

Hepatocellular carcinoma (HCC) is one of the most common malignancies in the world, with approximately one million new cases recorded annually.[1] At present, only complete surgical resection has the potential for producing a cure, and then only in a small subset of patients. Other modalities, such as radiotherapy, chemotherapy, or bioimmunotherapy, have produced response in a few patients, but it is clear that most patients derive little or no benefit from the application of such treatments. Virtually all antineoplastic therapies are associated with substantial toxicities due to the often unacceptable adverse effects on normal tissues. As a result, most patients either receive ineffective therapy, or are unable to tolerate therapy that could potentially eradicate their neoplasm. This situation justifies the evaluation of novel modalities.

It has long been recognized that a malignancy is basically a genetic defect, due either to an imbalance in the function of a set of critical genes or the acquisition of new functions by the protein products of mutated genes. For some time, gene therapy has been evaluated as a potential means of treating diseases due to a monogenic defect, such as adenine deaminase deficiency or cystic fibrosis. Many, if not most, of the gene therapy protocols have focused on the therapy of malignant diseases, even though malignancy is the result of multiple genetic lesions. One of the potential goals of genetic therapy is to replace nonfunctional antioncogenes or to increase the level of expression of anti-oncogenes to restore any stoichiometric balance that may exist. As noted by Hug and Sleight,[2] several conditions must exist for successful gene replacement therapy: The normal gene must be produced in ample quantities; appropriate delivery vehicles (vectors) must be utilized that can deliver the nucleic acid to the correct target cells; if stable expression is desired, the DNA must be integrated into the host genome in a stable fashion that does not interfere with the function of other genes; the exogenous DNA should be integrated into either "nonsense" regions of the genome or, under ideal circumstances, undergo homologous recombination with the defective gene; and if replacing a defective gene is the goal, the expression of the exogenous gene should be under the control of its native *cis*-acting sequences.

In addition to attempting to replace single genes thought to be critical in carcinogenesis, genetic therapy has been used in an attempt to augment existing therapies. Much of the work has focused on reversing drug resistance or enhancing immunotherapy. There is much potential here, but clinical studies are only beginning; few patients have been treated with genetic therapies.

The liver has been considered an excellent target organ for genetic modulation; a deficiency of any given specific hepatocyte protein in a metabolic pathway gives rise to many of the metabolic diseases that would be candidates for genetic manipulation. The techniques derived here may be applicable to tumors that arise, or predominantly involve, the liver. Additionally, cells derived from HCC, like the normal hepatocytes from which they are derived, uniquely or preferentially express several proteins; hence it is potentially possible to exploit the genes for these proteins, thereby giving selectivity to the therapy.

In general, genetic therapy of neoplasms may be utilized to protect normal tissues or to target the malignant cells themselves. An example of the former are protocols where drug resistance genes such as *mdr*-1, dihydrofolate reductase, or O-methylguanidine-DNA-methyltransferase are inserted and expressed in autologous hematopoietic stem cells,[3–7] ideally to increase the therapeutic window of greater doses of chemotherapy. Although potentially attractive in concept, this approach is unlikely to prove successful in the therapy of HCC for two reasons. First, many of these enzymes are already constitutively expressed in the normal liver and in most HCCs, which may account, at least in part, for the low degree of tumor responsiveness to the chemotherapeutic agents currently utilized. Thus, whereas normal tissues such as the bone marrow are afforded some degree of protection from the antineoplastic therapy, the tumor is already "protected." Second, notwithstanding the possible exception of hepatic arterial chemotherapy, there is little evidence that dose intensification offers any benefit to the patient with HCC; in fact, most patients have such a degree of underlying hepatic dysfunction that many cannot reasonably be expected to tolerate even "standard doses" of conventional chemotherapy.

A more attractive proposition would be to target the tumor cells themselves and insert into them (i.e., transfect the cells) with active copies of tumor suppressor genes, such as *p53* and *RB1,* oncogene-specific inactivators; genes for enzymes that convert relatively innocuous agents into a cytotoxic species only in or near the malignant cell, or genes that make the tumor cells detectable to the immune system for their subsequent destruction.

Vectors

Of prime consideration is delivery of the genetic material to the tumor bed. *In vivo* it is difficult to inject intravenously or ingest naked DNA and have it reach the malignant cells. Because of the large size and electrical charge of most nucleic acids and the presence of ample serum and tissue nucleases, the introduction of "naked" nucleic acids is usually inefficient.[8] Alternative methods that can be employed to introduce exogenous nucleic acids into eukaryotic cells are calcium phosphate co-precipitation,[9] microinjection,[10,11] and electroporation,[12,13] but none of these methods can be used *in vivo*. Two types of vector that can successfully deliver the nucleic acids are viruses and liposomes.

Viruses

Viruses are essentially replicating (with the assistance of host cell proteins) nucleic acid delivery systems. In theory, any virus could be engineered to carry the gene(s) of interest. Practically speaking, however, few viruses are understood in such detail or meet certain other requirements (e.g., a lack of virulence and the ability to take up limited amounts of foreign DNA) as to render them impractical. Ideally, for liver-directed transduction, a modified hepatitis virus, such as the hepatitis B virus, would be a useful vector, but it is too small to carry sufficient amounts of DNA.[14] The hepatitis A, C, D, and E viruses are nonretroviral RNA viruses and are not usable by present techniques; other hepatitis viruses are insufficiently characterized.

To date, most clinical investigations have centered on retroviruses and adenoviruses. Retroviruses have been the most commonly evaluated viral vector in light of their ability to integrate exogenous DNA into the host cell genome; lack of an apparent required target sequence for integration into the host genome; lack of tissue and species specificity of amphotrophic vectors (those with an ability to infect tissues of different species); and their tendency to integrate their DNA into dividing cells. This last feature is obviously a potential advantage in antitumor therapy, especially for tumors with rapidly dividing cells; however, retroviruses are essentially unable to integrate their vector DNA in nondividing cells.[15]

With the complications associated with large-scale production, retroviral vector titers that can be produced [10^6–10^7 colony forming units (cfu)/ml] are often too low to treat moderate to large tumors; such low titers are due to the limited output of the "packaging" cell lines, and the difficulty retrieving the vectors by ultracentrifugation of large volumes of culture medium. Furthermore, the vector itself may be damaged by the ultracentrifugation process, further reducing its viability. Such low levels of vector titers in the inoculum limit the number of cells that can be successfully transduced, as most vectors replicate poorly *in vivo*. Bowles and colleagues described a low-speed centrifugation process that allows recovery of up to nearly 500 times as much vector from a large volume of tissue culture medium (1 liter).[15]

There may also be an upper limit upon the size of the inoculum that can be infused. When Bowles et al. attempted to administer a β-galactosidase-expressing retroviral vector to male rats via portal vein infusion (24 hours after partial hepatectomy to stimulate hepatocyte division), animals that had received more than 2×10^8 cfu died of hemorrhage during the infusion or developed disseminated intravascular coagulopathy or portal vein thrombosis shortly after completion of the infusion; a dose of 1.25×10^8 cfu was associated with 50% mortality.[15] Other investigators have targeted the liver in a similar fashion; but even when hepatocytes can be stimulated to undergo mitosis after partial hepatectomy and retroviral vectors are infused via the portal vein, only 5% of the cells are transduced.[16,17] For practical reasons, this approach has limited applicability for patients with HCC. Most of the neoplastic cells are not actively in the mitotic cycle at any given time; most tumors derive much of their vascular supply from the hepatic artery and not the portal vein; and many patients would not tolerate the surgery. A percutaneously placed catheter in the hepatic artery would be an answer for the latter two issues, but successful manipulation of the growth of the tumor is uncharted territory and potentially deleterious.

Retroviruses are unable to carry nucleic acids, which are much larger than approximately 8 kb, which may restrict the ability to carry larger genes along with their appropriate control elements (cis-acting sequences).

Adenoviruses have also been evaluated as a vector for genetic therapy. These viruses are capable of DNA transduction into both resting and divided cells, which is advantageous for malignancies with longer cell cycles, such as most solid tumors.[18,19] Unlike retroviruses, adenoviruses do not stably integrate the vector DNA into the host genome, so it is usually lost after several cell divisions. Furthermore, this vector can usually generate much higher titers than retroviruses, which is potentially useful in the setting of greater tumor bulk. As the virus requires intact immediate early E1a and E1b proteins to propagate and be infectious, and these proteins are lacking in host cells, vectors are designed with deleted E1 genes. These recombinant vectors are often produced in the embryonic kidney 293 cell lines, which contans the E1 gene products in trans, and allow assembly of the vector[20] However, as adenoviruses are ubiquitous, vector recipients have usually been exposed to some adenovirus strains (or may require multiple treatments with the same vector) and may mount an immune response that inactivates the vector prior to its reaching the intended target.[21,22] Cytotoxic T cells may be generated with the expression of some viral proteins; this reaction has been observed when E1-deficient vectors are transduced into murine liver or lungs, leading to the destruction of vector-infected cells.[21,23] This particular problem may be circumvented by iatrogenic immunosuppression, though an ideal regimen has not been determined.[24,25]

Adenoviruses have also been delivered via portal vein infusion. Li and coworkers determined that if 100 cfu/hepatocyte were infused, nearly 95% of murine hepatocytes could be transduced.[26] However, as expected, the transduction was not stable, and by 4 months fewer than 10% of the hepatocytes were expressing the exogenous gene (β galactosidase).

Other viruses have been evaluated as potential vectors. Some mammalian viruses, such as the herpes simplex viruses (HSV), already exhibit nonhepatic tissue tropism (neurotropism in the case of HSV), though they may be useful for targeting tumors derived from other tissues of interest. The adeno-associated virus has also been evaluated as a vector. This parvovirus is without known pathologic consequences, and it is capable of expressing the genes of interest without regard to the state of the mitotic cycle. The wild-type virus is capable of integration into a specific site on chromosome 19, though recombinant viruses appear unable to do so.[27] The size of the insert is relatively small, on the order of 5 kb; and the viral titers produced are usually several-fold lower than with other viruses. Moreover, this virus requires a helper virus (e.g., adenovirus) to provide the necessary genetic machinery for propagation, and the helper virus is a potentially problematic contaminant. Others, such as the insect-derived baculoviruses, are attractive because no viral genes seem to be expressed in mammalian cells; nucleotide segments in excess of 200 kb can be inserted into the vector[28,29]; high viral titers can be generated in insect packaging cells[30]; and baculoviruses do not seem to integrate the DNA into the host genome.[31] Although expression of the transduced gene is transient, potentially necessitating multiple injections, expression in normal hepatocytes has been achieved.[31]

Liposomes

Liposomes are essentially nontoxic vectors; and because of the similarity of the lipids in the cell membrane and within the liposomes themselves, in most instances fusion to the cell membrane occurs spontaneously. The first report of liposomal nucleic acid incorporation and the subsequent transfection of eukaryotic cells (a process now known as lipofection) dates from 1978 when a fragment of the human X chromosome was successfully transferred into murine cells.[32]

In contrast to viral vectors, there is no possibility of the liposome spontaneously mutating or recombining with another virus to become a more virulent or infectious form. Additionally, liposomes can hold much larger segments of DNA than can most viruses, and liposomally packaged genes can be prepared rapidly in large quantities, which is usually not the case for viral vectors. The constituents and physical characteristics of the liposome may be altered, which may allow organ targeting. Furthermore, liposomes are relatively easy to prepare in bulk, and incorporation of the nucleic acid may occur with no loss of integrity of the nucleic acid sequence of interest. Finally, liposomes may be constructed that contain constituents other than DNA; viral vectors are limited to DNA or RNA and must be separately devised, as a certain species of virus contains only DNA or RNA, depending on its parental nucleotide composition.

As may be expected, there are difficulties associated with the use of liposomes to introduce exogenous nucleic acid sequences. First, the efficiency of nucleic acid incorporation is usually low, with less than half of the liposomes containing the sequence of interest[33]; the percentage of incorporation is highly dependent on the methods used to prepare the liposomes. Additionally, the percentage of cellular uptake of the liposomal nucleic acid complex is often low; although chemical and physical methods exist that can be utilized to enhance uptake *in vitro,* they are not readily applicable *in vivo.* Finally, although incorporation of nucleic acids into liposomes may protect them from degradation by nucleases which are present within the serum, most liposomes are taken up by the cells of the monocyte/macrophage lineage, not the parenchymal cells of the target organ(s).

Multiple methods to incorporate molecules into liposomes have been reported. Some have already been brought to clinical practice, such as the investigation of encapsulated antibiotics and antineoplastic agents.[34-37] In general, this strategy is employed in an effort to reduce patient toxicity or to reverse drug resistance. However, not all methods are equally well suited for use with nucleic acids. In general, polynucleotides are easily damaged and may not tolerate certain solvents or vigorous encapsulation procedures. The application of certain methods has been successful in incorporating intact DNA, though occasional damage has been noted, such as nicking with the subsequent linearization of circular DNA.[38]

The efficiency of encapsulation of DNA or RNA depends on several variables, perhaps the most significant of which is the method of preparation, followed by the size (length) of the polynucleotide molecule. Supercoiled circular DNA occupies a smaller volume than either open circular (relaxed) or linear DNA, and this smaller volume allows more efficient encapsulation by liposomes. However, open circular DNA is less efficient in transfecting cells than linear DNA.[39] Furthermore, DNA often exists in its linear form in solution, as does RNA, so the degree of incorporation depends on the length of the nucleic acid molecule used. To encapsulate large molecules as polynucleotides efficiently, the liposomes must fairly large, often more than 100 nm in diameter.

In a manner similar to retroviral vectors, the amount of liposomal DNA taken up by cells depends on the phase of the cell cycle. For example, G_1 phase HeLa cells took up nearly twice as much of the plasmid DNA encapsulated in phosphatidylcholine (a neutral lipid) than HeLa cells in active mitosis.[40] Although the makeup of the liposomes appears to have little or no bearing on the amount of DNA that eventually finds its way into the nucleus, the addition of anionic phospholipids (e.g., phosphatidylserine) leads to preferential liposomal uptake during mitosis, in contrast to that in the G_1 phase.

Virosomes represent a form of hybridization between viruses and liposomes. Here, a viral envelope protein is added to the mixture of nucleic acid and phospholipid prior to the formation of the liposomal vesicles; the resulting liposome contains the virus which may confer some degree of stability or targeting. A variety of fusion proteins have been utilized, such as the HA2 influenza virus protein and the Sendai virus F and HN proteins, though none appears to be superior.[41,42] The inclusion of the viral protein should increase the likelihood of liposomal fusion, but the encapsulation efficiency is still low, and large amounts of the viral fusion protein are required.[43-46] A separate, but closely related, approach is to use the formation of cationic lipid complexes with DNA or messenger RNA to facilitate transfection.[47] In this instance, the nucleic acid is not truly encapsulated but lies on the outer surface of the lipid; the DNA remains "transfection competent." The exact mechanism remains unknown, but it has been postulated that the positively charged lipid more than neutralizes the negative charge carried by the DNA, and as the lipid–DNA complex retains a net positive charge, it may more readily interact with the negatively charged cell surface. Lipofectin is an example of a cationic lipid; a commercially available reagent (Gibco BRL, Gaithersburg, MD), it contains equal amounts of dioleylphospha-tidylethanolamine (DOPE) and N-[1-(2,3-dioleyloxy)propyl]-N,N,N-trimethylammonium chloride (DOTMA).

In an aqueous medium, DOTMA forms liposomes alone or in combination with other phospholipids. DNA and DOTMA spontaneously form complexes after mixing, though the ratio of the amounts of DOTMA to DNA determines the optimal efficiency of transfection; a 5:1 ratio (by weight) of lipid/DNA leads to encapsulation of all of the DNA.[8] By comparison, only 10% of DNA is encapsulated by neutral lipids. The greater degree of complex formation is due to the presence of opposing electrical charges on DNA and DOTMA. Ideally, the positive charge of the DOTMA within the complex should slightly exceed the negative charge contributed by the nucleic acid; this net positive charge enhances the association of the complex with the negatively charged cell surface.

The DOTMA-containing liposomes are highly efficient in delivering polynucleotides to the cell. In labeling studies 80–100% of the cells took up the tracer.[8] After fusion the label was noted to diffuse throughout the cellular membrane; in contrast, when a different lipid, dioleylphosphatidylcholine, was labeled and used, a lower level of fusion was observed, and the label remained in discrete areas within the membrane. Despite high levels of fusion, approximately 0.06% of the exogenous DNA can be recovered intact from the nuclei of transfected murine cells. This amount is 30-fold more DNA than the amount of intact DNA that may be found in the nuclei when utilizing other methods of transfection. Depending on the choice of cell line and vector, up to 10% of cells may be stably transfected by lipofection.[47]

Other agents have been synthesized that can form cationic liposomes. A class of similar agents are the lipopolyamines, formed by the linkage of a polyamine to a lipid via a peptide bond. Examples are dioctadecylamidoglycylspermine (DOGS) and dipalmitoylphosphatidylethanolamylspermine (DPPES).[48] DOGS is equally efficient to DPPES in terms of mediating transfection, though the latter is degraded more rapidly. As with DOTMA, these substances spontaneously form cationic liposomes in aqueous media and, if mixed with nucleic acids, form complexes that resemble the nucleic acid coated by a lipid bilayer. These agents have been used successfully to transfect a variety of cell lines and primary cultures with a variety of polynucleotides.[48]

It is also possible to utilize liposomal encapsulation to transfect intact messenger RNA. These interactions are transient owing to the nature of the polynucleotide and its inability to integrate into the host genome. mRNA transfection is simpler on a cellular level, as the mRNA needs only to reach the cytoplasm to be transcribed, whereas DNA must first reach the nucleus and then undergo translation before transcription. The *in vitro* transfection of DOTMA–RNA complexes is highly efficient, as approximately 60% of radiolabeled RNA is associated with the cells within 1 hour, and half of that is resistant to exogenous RNAse.[49] The level of the gene-specific protein product is increased further by the addition of carrier RNA, which presumably acts by competing for cytoplasmic RNAses; the presence of a 5' cap (capped RNA is 40 times more efficient than noncapped RNA), the inclusion of a 5' untranslated region, and the presence and type of the 3' untranslated region.

In contrast to providing a newly functional gene, as in the case of DNA transfection, RNA transfection utilizes mRNA more as a drug, that is, as an agent that temporarily affects and alters the function of one or more organs. For example, it has been shown that double-stranded synthetic polyribonucleotides, such as Ampligen [poly(rI:rC12-rU) and poly(rI;rC)], are capable of *in vivo* stimulation of a variety of cytokines, such as interferons α and β and interleukin 6, as well as enhancing the production of antibodies.[50]

In addition to the study of synthetic ribonucleotides, more work has been carried out with antisense olignucleotides. These substances are sequences designed to interfere with specific genes, such as by formation of a local triple DNA helix, which subsequently inhibits gene transcription, or by homologous recombination with pre-mRNA or mRNA, which interferes with RNA processing or translation. Initially, standard DNA oligonucleotides were evaluated, but these compunds are relatively instable and sensitive to nuclease degradation. By comparison, phosphorothioate and methylphosphonate oligonucleotides are more stable and more resistant to nucleases than unmodified phosphodiester oligonucleotides.[51] Both methylphosphonate and to a lesser degree phosphorothioate oligonucleotides are capable of directly binding to lipid membranes.

Naked DNA

If DNA is injected intravenously or intraarterially, it is usually rapidly degraded by the presence of serum nucleases. An exception has been observed by Budker and associates. In a murine system, DNA in a hypertonic saline/mannitol solution was infused into the portal vein while the hepatic veins were temporarily clamped.[52] They noted that intraportal delivery was three orders of magnitude more efficient in terms of gene expression than direct parenchymal injection, but only 1% of the hepatocytes were transduced.

Targeting Strategies

Possibly the easiest method for delivering DNA to the intended site is to apply the naked DNA directly into the tumor bed. It may be accomplished by intratumoral injection of the DNA, coating the DNA onto an angioplasty ballon and transferring to the endothelium, or binding the DNA to metallic particles, such as tungsten or gold, and then bombarding the target area with these bound particles at high velocity.[53,54] Related to this technique is the jet injection method, where a DNA solution is delivered under high pressure to a target area.[55] Each of these methods has demonstrated an ability to express genes *in vivo*.[56,57] In each case the individual tumors must be accessed separately, sometimes requiring a surgical procedure, which may be impossible for deep-seated lesions and certainly misses lesions small enough to be below the level of clinical detection.

Intraarterial or intraportal injections of DNA or viral vectors may also be accomplished. Some of these protocols involve temporary occlusion of the hepatic vein to prevent the rapid egress of DNA from the liver. In one report of a rat model, the superior portal vein (which supplies the left and medial hepatic lobes in the rat) was ligated, and a retroviral construct was administered via intraportal infusion at various time points.[58] Expression of the construct gene was noted as the portal vein occlusion induced apoptosis and subsequent hepatocyte regeneration, though at lower levels than observed at partial hepatectomy. Although the liver itself is targeted with these approaches, uptake throughout the organ tends to be low.

Ideally, one would employ a virus that normally targets the liver selectively or exclusively. As noted previously, the hepatitis B virus is too small to be useful, and other hepatitis viruses cannot be readily utilized. Hepatocytes also have receptors for several of the adenovirus subtypes (2 and 5), though enterocytes share these receptors.[59] As normal hepatocytes express the V3 and V5 integrins, which are the adenovirus-binding sites, it is unlikely that by itself the use of an adenovirus vector (or surface proteins from hepatotropic viruses) can form a strategy to target HCC cells selectively. In fact, the difficulty of using adenoviruses to target HCC cells was reported by Arbuthnot and colleagues, who noted that the recombinant adenoviral vector transduced an HCC cell line *in vitro*, but that rat and mouse HCCs were poorly tranduced *in vivo* despite efficient peritumoral and hepatocyte transduction.[60]

Most intravenously administered liposomes are taken up first by the reticuloendothelial system within the liver and to a lesser extent by the spleen. This hepatic uptake occurs rapidly, and in some models the circulating half-life of radiolabeled liposomes may be as short as two minutes.[33] The half-life in the circulation depends on the lipid composition and size of the vesicles, the use of other targeting strategies (e.g., incorporation of monoclonal antibodies or other proteins), and the state of the reticuloendothelial system. After uptake, release of liposomes by the liver occurs slowly. Although nearly two-thirds of the injected liposomes are found within the Kupffer cells of the liver within 2 hours of the injection, some are also found in the endothelial cells and hepatocytes themselves.[33] In general, liposomes larger than 200 nm are taken up by the Kupffer cells, as this size is the limit for any material to pass through the gaps in the sinusoidal capillaries.

Hepatocytes have several unique cell-surface receptors that can be exploited for targeting by genetic therapy. Possibly one of the best characterized systems is the asialoglycoprotein receptor. Here the vector can be modified by adding lactose, which facilitates binding to hepatocytes.[61-63] The difficulty arises in that such modifications can reduce the efficiency of infection with viral vectors. A similar strategy was utilized by Kasahara et al., who engineered a chimeric envelope protein/erythropoietin protein to be expressed. Although this method was active in the intended cells (erythropoietin-receptor-positive hematopoietic progenitor cells), it has not be adequately evaluated for hepatocytes *in vivo*.[64]

A related mechanism is to utilize bound monoclonal antibodies directed to cell-surface moieties as a mechanism to target the vector. This method is being actively evaluated with other therapeutic agents, such as bound radionucleotides or standard antineoplastic agents, in an effort to concentrate the therapy to the site of the malignant cells. This modality is potentially promising, especially for therapy of nonmalignant diseases, although several features of the neoplasms often compromise the results: Tumor clones may lose the ability to express the moiety or may have never expressed the antigen; additionally, tumors may shed or secrete an excess of the moiety such that the antigen forms complexes with the antibody in the serum, and the antibody–vector complex never reaches its intended target.

Target Specificity

Vectors may be taken up by a broad spectrum of cell types, regardless of the route of administration, so this method is not associated with any inherent specificity to HCC. Specificity may be conferred by the use of certain liver-specific *cis*-acting sequences. These control elements are naturally found in all tissues but are functional only in cells that have the appropriate DNA-binding proteins (i.e., the *trans*-acting factors) to recognize them. A variety of gene promoters and enhancers have been evaluated alone in various combinations, including those associated with apolipoprotein E, α_1-antitrypsin, and hepatitis B viral core promoter and hepatitis B virus enhancer I.[65,66] Although these *cis*-acting sequences are active in hepatocytes, they are not selective for neoplastic cells. As most patients with HCC overexpress α-fetoprotein, a protein not normally expressed in any appreciable amount in the adult liver, the control elements of this gene are a logical choice for evaluation.

Perhaps the greatest difficulty when attempting to augment the genetic function of a malignant cell is to determine which gene to modulate. As presently conceived, cancer is not a monogenic defect but probably the outcome of a cascade of errors in the apparatus that controls cellular growth and division. Inserting and expressing genes that code for anti-oncogenes is an obvious choice, especially for those tumors in which a defective anti-oncogene has been identified. However, to eradicate the neoplasm, all of the tumor cells would need to be transduced, which is a practical impossibility with present techniques. Furthermore, all of the tumor cells would have to be genetically identical, which is unlikely as tumors grow and develop multiple clones. This difficulty was demonstrated by Bao and coworkers, who treated transgenic mice (bearing HCCs induced by either the SV40 T antigen or the hepatitis B virus envelope protein transgenes) with intraportal infusions of a recombinant adenovirus containing a *p53* gene construct.[67] Despite documented expression of the *p53* gene within the tumor, nodules were observed. Similar limitations exist if RNA, antisense oligonucleotides, ribozymes, and nuclease genes are incorporated into a vector.

It is not currently possible to transfect 100% of the tumor cells, so an alternative strategy is needed. One such plan is to transduce a suicide gene into some of the tumor cells; the protein product of this gene then activates a relatively innocuous agent or produg, thereby converting it into a cytotoxic agent within the tumor cell. However, a "bystander effect" is created, such that nearby cells that are not transduced are killed along with the cells that have taken up the vector. This phenomenon has been well documented utilizing HSV thymidine kinase to activate ganciclovir by phosphorylating it.[68] Subsequently, host kinases convert ganciclovir monophosphate to the triphosphate form, which subsequently inhibits DNA polymerase.[69] Cells surrounding the transduced cell also die, even though they themselves are not transduced, apparently because the phosphorylated ganciclovir metabolites are transferred to neighboring cells via gap junctions.[70]

Previous HSV thymidine kinase constructs utilized strong promoters, such as the human cytomegalovirus immediate early promoter, which is active in a broad spectrum of cell types and thus fails to confer specificity to HCC. Kaneko and colleagues placed the HSV thymidine kinase gene under the control of α-fetoprotein (AFP) *cis*-acting sequences and demonstrated cytotoxicity in AFP-producing cell lines (but not in an HCC line that failed to produce AFP), as well as inhibition of tumor growth.[71] Su et al. confirmed these observations when an adeno-associated virus vector was utilized to transfer the HSV thymidine kinase gene under the control of the AFP gene promoter and the albumin gene enhancer; ganciclovir therapy caused the death of only AFP- and albumin-positive HCC cells but not those negative for AFP and albumin, or normal hepatocytes.[72] As reviewed by Deonarain and colleagues, a variety of other enzyme–prodrug systems have also been evaluated, though it is unclear if a bystander effect would be observed in any or all of them.[73]

A related strategy being evaluated is transfer of a cytokine gene into HCC cells. Huang and coworkers inserted an interleukin-2 (IL-2) gene into a recombinant adenovirus vector and then injected the vector directly into implanted murine HCCs. Half of the animals experienced a complete response; among the animals that responded, all were resistant to an intraperitoneal rechallenge by the same HCC cell line.[74] Cao and associates noted that when a murine HCC cell line was tranfected with a retroviral vector containing the tumor necrosis factor-α (TNFα) gene (under control of the albumin gene promoter) and the cells were then injected into a syngeneic host, the cells lost their tumorigenicity and furthermore inhibited the growth of established HCCs.[75] Intratumoral injection of the TNFα–retrovirus was active against established HCCs and resulted in significantly superior survival compared to that of control animals.

Conclusions

Gene therapy for a variety of diseases has now become a possibility, as investigators are better understanding the genetic involvement of a wide variety of diseases. In a sense, malignancy is likewise a genetic disease, though clearly not one associated with a single gene mutation. At present, efforts to manipulate single gene expression in neoplastic cells are limited by an inability to transduce all of the cells with the currently available vectors and by the biology of malignant lesions, which accounts for the development of mutant clones that may not respond as desired to the vector construct. Utilizing the vectors to deliver prodrugs is a promising strategy being evaluated in a number of preclinical models. As activity is being reported from an increasing number of investigators, it is only a matter of time until clinical trials in patients with HCC are conducted (some are now beginning), bringing hope to a population of patients to whom little could be offered until now.

References

1. Carr BI, Flickinger JC, Lotze MT. Hepatobiliary cancers. In: DeVita VT, Hellman S, Rosenberg SA (eds) Cancer: Principles and Practice of Oncology, 5th ed. Philadelphia, Lippincott-Raven, 1997, pp. 1087–1114
2. Hug P, Sleight RG. Liposomes for the transformation of eukaryotic cells. Biochim Biophys Acta 1097:1, 1991
3. Sorrentino BP, Brandt SJ, Bodine D, et al. Selection of drug-resistant bone marrow cells in vivo after retroviral transfer of the human MDR1. Science 257:99, 1992
4. Mickisch GH, Aksentijevich I, Schoenlein PV, et al. Transplantation of bone marrow cells from transgenic mice expressing the human MDR1 gene results in long-term protection against the myelosuppressive effect of chemotherapy in mice. Blood 79:1087, 1992

5. May C, Gunther R, McIvor RS. Protection of mice from lethal doses of methotrexate by transplantation with transgenic marrow expressing drug-resistant dihydrofolate-reductase activity. Blood 86:2439, 1995

6. Moritz T, Mackay W, Glassner BJ, Williams DA, Samson L. Retrovirus-mediated expression of DNA repair protein protection in bone marrow protects hematopoietic cells from nitrosourea-induced toxicity in vitro and in vivo. Cancer Res 55:2608, 1995

7. Spencer HT, Sleep SE, Rehg JE, Blakely RL, Sorrentino BP. A gene transfer strategy for making bone marrow cells resistant to trimetrexate. Blood 87:2579, 1996

8. Felgner PL, Gadek TR, Holm M, et al. Lipofection: a highly efficient, lipid-mediated DNA-transfection procedure. Proc Natl Acad Sci USA 84:7413, 1987

9. Graham FL, van der Eb AJ. A new technique for the assay of human adenovirus 5 DNA. Virology 52:456, 1973

10. Diacumakos EG, Gershey EL. Uncoating and gene expression of simian virus 40 in CV-1 cell nuclei inoculated by microinjection. J Virol 24:903, 1977

11. Graessmann M, Graessmann A. In: Celis JE, Graessmann A, Loyter A (eds) Microinjection and Organelle Transplantation Techniques. London, Academic, 1986, pp. 3–13

12. Fountain JW, Lockwood WK, Collins FS. Transformation of primary human skin fibroblasts by electroporation. Gene 68:167, 1988

13. Hama-Inaba H, Nishimoto T, Ohtsubo M, Sato K, Kasai M. Simple and effective method of electroporation for introduction of plasmid and cosmid DNAs to mammalian cells. Nucleic Acids Symp Series 19:149, 1988

14. Strauss M. Liver-directed gene therapy: prospects and problems. Gene Ther 1:156, 1994

15. Bowles NE, Eisensmith RC, Mohuiddin R, Pyron M, Woo SLC. A simple and efficient method for the concentration and purification of recombinant retrovirus for increased hepatocyte transduction in vivo. Hum Gene Ther 7:1735, 1996

16. Ferry N, Duplessis O, Houssein D, Danos O, Heard J-L. Retroviral-mediated gene transfer into hepatocytes in vivo. Proc Natl Acad Sci USA 88:8377, 1991

17. Kay MA, Li Q, Liu TJ, et al. Hepatic gene therapy: persistent expression of human alpha 1-antitrypsin in mice after direct gene delivery in vivo. Hum Gene Ther 3:641, 1992

18. Stratford-Perricaudet LD, Levrero M, Chasse JF, Perricaudet M, Briaand P. Evaluation of the transfer and expression in mice of an enzyme-encoding gene using an adenovirus vector. Hum Gene Ther 1:241, 1990

19. Levrero M, Barbaann V, Manteca S, et al. Defective and nondefective adenovirus vectors for expressing foreign genes in vitro and in vivo. Gene 101:195, 1991

20. Graham FL, Smiley J, Russell WL, Nairn R. Characterization of a human ccell line transformed by DNA from adenovirus 5. J Gen Virol 36:59, 1977

21. Yang Y, Li Q, Ertl HCJ, Wilson JM. Cellular and humoral immune responses to viral antigens created barriers to lung-directed gene therapy with recombinant adenoviruses. J Virol 69:2004, 1995

22. Yang Y, Greenough K, Wilson JM. Transient immune blockade prevents formation of neutralizing antibody to recombinant adenovirus and allows repeated gene transfer to mouse liver. Gene Ther 3:412, 1996

23. Yang Y, Ertl HCJ, Wilson JM. MHC class I-restricted cytotoxic T lymphocytes

to viral antigens destroy hepatocytes in mice infected with E1-deleted recombinant adenoviruses. Immunity 1:433, 1994

24. Dai Y, Schwarz EM, Gu D, et al. Cellular aand humoral immune responses to adenoviral vectors containing factor IX gene: tolerization of both factor IX and vector antigens allows for long-term expression. Proc Natl Acad Sci USA 92:1401, 1995

25. Fang B, Eisensmith RC, Wang H, et al. Gene therapy for hemophilia B: host immunosuppresssion prolongs the therapeutic effect of adenovirus-mediated factor IX expression. Hum Gene Ther 6:1039, 1995

26. Li QT, Kay MA, Finegold M, Stratford-Perricaudet LD, Woo SLC. Assessment of recombinaent adenoviral vectors for hepatic gene therapy. Hum Gene Ther 4:403, 1993

27. Halbert CL, Alexander IE, Wolgamot GM, Miller AD. Adeno-associated virus vectors transduce primary cells much less efficiently than immortalized cells. J Virol 69:1473, 1995

28. O'Reilly OR, Miller LK, Luckow VA. Virus host interactions. In: Baculovirus Expression Vectors: A Laboratory Manual. Oxford, Oxford University Press, 1994

29. Roth JA, Cristiano RJ. Gene therapy for cancer: what have we done and where are we going? J Natl Cancer Inst 88:21, 1997

30. Gruenwald S, Heitz J. Baculovirus Expressor System: Procedures and Methods Manual. San Diego, PharMingen, 1993

31. Sandig V, Hofmann C, Steinert S, et al. Gene transfer into hepatocytes and human liver tissue by baculovirus vectors. Hum Gene Ther 7:1937, 1996

32. Mukherjee AB, Orloff S, Butler JD, et al. Entrapment of metaphase chromosomes into phospholipid vesicles (lipochromosomes): carrier potential in gene transfer. Proc Natl Acad Sci USA 75:1361, 1978

33. Nicolau C, Cudd A. Liposomes as carriers of DNA. Crit Rev Ther Drug Carrier Syst 6:239, 1989

34. Lopez-Berestein G. Treatment of systemic fungal infections with liposomal amphotericin B. In: Liposomes in the Treatment of Infectious Diseases and Cancer. New York, Liss, 1989, pp. 317–327

35. Forssen EA, Tokes ZA. Use of anionic liposomes for the reduction of chronic doxorubicin-induced cardiotoxicity. Proc Natl Acad Sci USA 78:1873, 1981

36. Gabizon A, Dagan A, Goren D, Barenholz Y, Fuks Z. Liposomes as in vivo carriers of adriamycin: reduced cardiac uptake and preserved antitumor activity in mice. Cancer Res 42:4734, 1982

37. Perez-Soler R, Lopez-Berestein G, Lautersztain J, et al. Phase I clinical and pharmacological study of liposome-entrapped cis-bis-neodecanoato-trans-R,R-1,2-diaminocyclohexane platinum (II). Cancer Res 50:4254, 1990

38. Lurquin PF. Entrapment of plasmid DNA by liposomes and their interactions with plant protoplasts. Nucleic Acids Res 6:3773, 1979

39. Fukunaga Y, Nagata T, Takebe I. Liposome-mediated infection of plant protoplasts with tobacco mosaic virus RNA. Virology 113:752, 1981

40. Nicolau C, Sene C. Liposome-mediated DNA transfer in eukaryotic cells: dependence of the transfer efficiency upon the type of liposomes used and the host cell cycle stage. Biochim Biophys Acta 721:185, 1982

41. Kaneda Y, Uchida T, Sugawa H, Ishiura M, Okada Y. The improved efficient method for introducing macromolecules into cells using HVJ (Sendai virus) liposomes with gangliosides. Exp Cell Res 173:56, 1987

42. Lapidot M, Loyter A. Fusion-mediated microinjection of liposome-enclosed DNA into cultured cells with the aid of influenza virus glycoproteins. Exp Cell Res 189:241, 1990
43. Vainstein A, Razin A, Graessman A, Loyter A. Methods Enzymol 101:492, 1983
44. Jay DG, Gilbert W. Basic protein enhances the incorporation of DNA into lipid vesicles: model for the formation of primordial cells. Proc Natl Acad Sci USA 84:1978, 1987
45. Fraley R, Straubinger RM, Rule G, Springer EL, Papahadjopoulos D. Liposome-mediated delivery of deoxyribonucleic acid to cells: enhanced efficiency of delivery related to lipid composition and incubation conditions. Biochemistry 20:6978, 1981
46. Straubinger RM, Hong K, Friend DS, Papahadjopoulos D. Endocytosis of liposomes and intracellular fate of encapsulated molecules: encounter with a low pH compartment after internalization in coated vesicles. Cell 32:1069, 1983
47. Felgner PL, Ringold GM. Cationic liposome-mediated transfection. Nature 337:387, 1989
48. Loeffler J-P, Behr J-P. Gene transfer into primary and established mammalian cell lines with lipopolyamine-coated DNA. Methods Enzymol 217:599, 1993
49. Dwarki VJ, Malone RW, Verma IM. Cationic liposome-mediated RNA transfection. Methods Enzymol 217:644, 1993
50. Milhaud PG, Machy P, Colote S, Lebleu B, Leserman L. Free and liposome-encapsulated double-stranded RNAs as inducers of interferon, interleukin-6, and cellular toxicity. J Interferon Res 11:261, 1991
51. Akhtar S, Basu S, Wickstrom E, Juliano RL. Interactions of antisense DNA oligonucleotide analogs with phospholipid membranes (liposomes). Nucleic Acids Res 20:5551, 1991
52. Budker V, Zhang G, Knechtle S, Wolff JA. Naked DNA delivered intraportally expresses efficiently in hepatocytes. Gene Ther 3:593, 1996
53. Yang N, Burkholder J, Robert B. In vivo and in vitro gene transfer to mammalian somatic cells by particle bombardment. Proc Natl Acad Sci USA 87:9568, 1990
54. Zelenin AV, Alimov AA, Titomirov AV, et al. High-velocity mechanical DNA transfer of the chloramphenicol acetyltransferase gene into rodent liver, kidney and mammary gland cells in organ explants and in vivo. FEBS Lett 280:365, 1991
55. Furth PA, Shamay A, Wall RJ, Henninghausen L. Gene transfer into somatic tissues by jet injection. Anal Biochem 205;365, 1992
56. Cheng L, Ziegelhoffer PR, Yang NS. In vivo promoter activity and transgene expression in mammalian somatic tissues evaluated by using particle bombardment. Proc Natl Acad Sci USA 90:4455, 1993
57. Nicolet CM, Burkholder JK, Gan J, et al. Expression of a tumor-reactive antibody-interleukin 2 fusion protein after in vivo particle-mediated gene delivery. Cancer Gene Ther 2:161, 1995
58. Bowling WM, Kennedy SC, Cai S-R, et al. Portal branch occlusion safely facilitates in vivo retroviral vector transduction of rat liver. Hum Gene Ther 7:2113, 1996
59. Zern MA, Kresina TF. Hepatic drug delivery and gene therapy. Hepatology 25:484, 1997
60. Arbuthnot PB, Bralet M-P, Le Jossic C, et al. In vitro and in vivo hepatoma

cell-specific expression of a gene transferred with an adenoviral vector. Hum Gene Ther 7:1503, 1996

61. Wu G, Wu C. Receptor-mediated gene delivery and expression in vivo. J Biol Chem 263:14621, 1988
62. Wu G, Wu C. Receptor-mediated in vitro gene transfections by a soluble DNA carrier system. J Biol Chem 262:4429, 1987
63. Neda H, Wu CH, Wu GY. Chemical modification of an ectotropic virus results in redirection of its target cell specificity. J Biol Chem 266:14143, 1991
64. Kasahara N, Dozy AM, Kan YW. Tissue-specific targeting of retroviral vectors through ligand–receptor interactions. Science 266:1373, 1994
65. Okuyama T, Huber RM, Bowling W, et al. Liver-directed gene therapy: a retroviral vector with a complete LTR and the ApoE enhancer-α_1-antitrypsin promoter dramatically increases expression of human α_1-antitrypsin in vivo. Hum Gene Ther 7:637, 1996
66. Sandig V, Löser P, Lieber A, Kay MA, Strauss M. HBV-derived promoters direct liver-specific expression of an adenovirally transduced LDL receptor gene. Gene Ther 3:1002, 1996
67. Bao J-J, Zhang W-W, Kuo MT. Adenoviral delivery of recombinant DNA into transgenic mice bearing hepatocellular carcinomas. Hum Gene Ther 7:355, 1996
68. Moolten FL, Wells M. Curability of tumors bearing herpes thymidine kinase genes transferred by retroviral vectors. J Natl Cancer Inst 82:297, 1990
69. Matthews T, Boehme R. Antiviral activity and mechanism of action of ganciclovir. Rev Infect Dis 10:S490, 1988
70. Elshami AA, Saavedra A, Zhang H, et al. Gap junctions play a role in the 'bystander effect' of the herpes simplex virus thymidine kinase/ganciclovir system in vitro. Gene Ther 3:85, 1996
71. Kaneko S, Hallenbeck P, Kotani T, et al. Adenovirus-mediated gene therapy of hepatocellular carcinoma using cancer-specific gene expression. Cancer Res 55:5283, 1995
72. Su H, Chang JC, Xu SM, Kan YW. Selective killing of AFP-positive hepatocellular carcinoma cells by adeno-associated virus transfer of the herpes simplex virus thymidine kinase gene. Hum Gene Ther 7:463, 1996
73. Deonarain MP, Spooner RA, Epenetos AA. Genetic delivery of enzymes for cancer therapy. Gene Ther 2:235, 1995
74. Huang H, Chen SH, Kosai K, Finegold MJ, Woo SLC. Gene therapy for hepatocellular carcinoma: long-term remission of primary and metastatic tumors in mice by interleukin-2 gene therapy in vivo. Gene Ther 3:980, 1996
75. Cao G, Kuriyama S, Du P, et al. Complete regression of established murine hepatocellular carcinoma by in vivo tumor necrosis factor α gene transfer. Gastroenterology 112:501, 1997

Index

Lightning Source UK Ltd.
Milton Keynes UK
UKOW05f0131200913

217523UK00001B/9/P